Multiple Sclerosis

The Questions You Have, The Answers You Need

Multiple Sclerosis

The Questions You Have, The Answers You Need

Fifth Edition

Rosalind C. Kalb, PhD

Editor

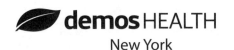

demos HEALTH

New York

ISBN: 978-1-936303-16-8
E-ISBN: 978-1-617050-76-3
Visit our web site at www.demoshealth.com

Acquisitions Editor: Noreen Henson
Compositor: Newgen Imaging
Printer: Bradford & Bigelow

Library of Congress Cataloging-in-Publication Data

Multiple sclerosis : the questions you have, the answers you need / Rosalind
C. Kalb, editor. — 5th ed.
    p. cm.
  Includes index.
    ISBN 978-1-936303-16-8 (pbk.)
  1. Multiple sclerosis—Popular works. 2. Multiple sclerosis—Miscellanea.
I. Kalb, Rosalind.
  RC377.M8685 2012
  616.8'34—dc23   2011032540

A

Special discounts on bulk quantities of Demos Health books are available to corporations, professional associations, pharmaceutical companies, health care organizations, and other qualifying groups. For details, please contact:

Special Sales Department
Demos Medical Publishing
11 W. 42nd Street
New York, NY 10036
Phone: 800-532-8663 or 212-683-0072
Fax: 212-941-7842
E-mail: rsantana@demosmedpub.com

Made in the United States of America
11 12 13 14 15   5 4 3 2 1

To the memory of Kathryn Dailey—a dear friend and respected colleague who worked tirelessly to improve the quality of life for people living with chronic illness and disability. In her 20 years at the National Multiple Sclerosis Society, Kathryn led numerous initiatives on behalf of people with MS, including creating the Society's standards for accessibility, developing programs for people newly diagnosed, and building the Society's national call center (800-344-4867), an invaluable resource referenced in every chapter of this book. As a result of her vision, the call center today fields 200,000 inquiries a year. Kathryn's wisdom, integrity, commitment, and humor enhanced the lives of all who knew her, and we hope that her motto—"People do not care how much we know, until they know how much we care"—echoes through these pages.

Contents

Note to the Reader

We first met on October 29, 2009, on the platform of the Princeton Junction, NJ, train station. Enroute to a business meeting in Princeton from Boston, her hometown, Lisa's ancient scooter—purchased in 1988 and veteran of hundreds of airplane flights—misbehaved badly as she headed from her arrival gate to the train station at Newark Airport, grinding to its final halt as she reached the train platform. The conductor pushed her onto the train and then pushed her off once she reached her destination. Michael, a Princeton Junction resident who uses a power wheelchair, got off the same train, heading home after a concert in Newark. He noticed Lisa, stranded and immobilized, recognized her obvious distress, and rolled over to offer his support. He waited with her for 45 minutes as the sun set and a chill settled in until the car, organized by Lisa's business hosts, arrived to cart her away. Michael's vigil was a show of solidarity with a fellow wheelchair traveler: he knew from similar misadventures over the years what trouble she was in. He would not leave until he knew she was safe.

Within perhaps 3 weeks, we knew much about each other—our familiarity accelerated by our common diagnosis of MS. We learned we are the same age; we are both scientists (Lisa has a medical degree from Harvard Medical School and Michael a Doctor of Philosophy in physics from Oxford University); we share a passion for classical music, art, and word play; and between us, with our combined 48 years of living with MS, we cover almost the full range of signs and symptoms the disease offers. With notable exceptions (neither of us has yet had noticeable visual or cognitive disturbances), one or both of us have exhibited, at some point, most of the diverse, sometimes overwhelming, and often confusing MS manifestations addressed in this extensive book.

We also have important differences—again, highlighting the bewildering diversity of MS chronicled in these pages. Lisa's first symptoms arrived when she was 22. She started with the most common initial form of MS—the relapsing-remitting pattern—and like many with that type of MS, she transitioned to secondary progressive MS. She began using a scooter at age 34. Lisa was diagnosed before MRI scans were available, and today's disease-modifying drugs were far in the future. With limited therapeutic options, she knew that there was little medically that could help her; she focused instead on healthy behaviors, maintaining her weight, exercising as possible, and striving for the sometimes elusive psychological resilience to keep on going. She continues working her customary 60 hours a week as a health policy expert.

Michael, in contrast, had been an insatiable athlete—a long-distance cyclist, speed skater, and cross-country skier. His MS came when he was age 42, in the primary progressive form, which affects only 10 percent of MS patients. He tried the new MS medications but to no avail. His disability progressed rapidly, and within 7 years, he no longer could move either leg, his left arm was coiled in a tight contracture (he is left handed), and he had only minimal use of his right arm and hand. He retired from work at age 50. Nonetheless, determined to live as independently and actively as possible, he purchased and renovated a small home, installing accessibility features throughout. Personal care assistants get him up in the morning, put him to bed at night, and feed him during the day. He audits classes at Princeton University, does disability advocacy work, and, most importantly, spends time with his two young daughters. Although no treatments yet touch PPMS, Michael has extensive interactions with diverse health care professionals described in this book: physiatrists, urologists, physical and occupational therapists, primary care physicians, and, most importantly, neurologists.

We find in this extensive and thoughtful book the many questions we have asked ourselves—and now sometimes ask each other—over the years we have lived with MS. We see reflected here our interest in science: being driven by evidence rather than by anecdote about what works. We also see an acknowledgment that MS touches not only myriad aspects of our bodies but also the ways we live our daily lives, interact with families and friends, and live within our communities. We encourage you to use this book to answer your questions about MS, help you manage your daily symptoms, inform conversations with your trusted clinicians, and live your lives as fully as you would wish.

Our friendship and mutual support ease those inevitable difficult moments, like the day Lisa's scooter died. With this emotional support bolstered by solid information about our options such as that ably offered here, we intend to continue living as fully as possible. We are both positive about what we have. While we welcome medical advances and understanding about MS, we do not put our lives on hold waiting for that "silver bullet," a cure for our disease. MS shapes our lives, but it does not define who we are.

Lisa I. Iezzoni, MD, MSc, and Michael Ogg, DPhil

Foreword

WHO IS THIS BOOK FOR?

This book is not just for people with MS and their families, friends, and colleagues. It is a "must read" for everyone. With one in 750 people living with MS, each of us knows, knows of, or will know someone with MS. We all have questions about MS that we need answered.

Nor is this book just for "lay" people. Although written in everyday language, it is "required reading" for all whose work affects people with MS: health care professionals, researchers, policymakers, and those in the pharmaceutical, medical equipment and supplies, and health and disability insurance industries.

I am a psychiatrist. For the past 30 years, I have worked with people with MS and their families as they faced the challenges and adapted to the demands of the illness. I also have conferred with neurologists, primary care physicians, and other mental health professionals, conducted research, and advised policymakers and pharmaceutical companies. This book has been my companion in these endeavors since its first edition. It helps me as a clinician hear more clearly and listen more empathically. It keeps me mindful as a researcher of the people my studies are intended to benefit. It is a resource I share with those who need to learn more about MS and experience what it is like to live with this illness.

WHAT DOES THIS BOOK DO?

This book asks Questions and gives Answers. The simplicity of the "Q and A" approach is deceptive because it serves many purposes. The Questions are my "Users' Guide" to the book. Set out from the rest of the text in their own font and bolded typeface, they make it easy for me to flip through a chapter to find exactly what I am looking for. The Questions are my "Teacher's Guide" to what is important to know about MS. These are *real* Questions from *real* people *really* living with MS. They teach me what my patients want to know and may not yet have asked, perhaps because the issue has not yet come up, they do not know how to ask, or are too uncomfortable to do so. With these Questions in mind, I am better able to help my patients think about the future, formulate their questions, and feel more at ease. I am also better able to teach others about the immediate and ongoing concerns of people with MS and their families. Reading the Questions, I hear the voices of people I know: not only their worries and fears, but also their determination to manage their illness and live full and meaningful lives.

It can be overwhelming to hear "you have MS," bewildering to make decisions about treatment, and anxiety-provoking to call the doctor. The Questions help put thoughts into words that are clear, succinct, and direct so people can get the best possible Answers. It is not easy for anyone to talk about bladder, bowel, and sexual function, memory problems, or anger and disappointment. The Questions give us a way to talk about issues like these that are so essential to good MS care and solid relationships. For me, the Questions are reminders of what my patients may be reluctant to share and what I must ask about: complementary therapies and alternative medicines; care partner abuse; marital discord; nursing home options. They also show me what people may not know and what I must address: the ins-and-outs of health insurance and the value of disability and long-term care insurance. Human resources and benefits managers, employers, and payers need to understand this knowledge gap too as they counsel, accommodate, and serve people with MS.

What I find especially intriguing are the comments that lead into the questions. Try this yourself. Go to a chapter. Read just the statements in sequence (skip the Questions for now). What emerges is an accurate, compelling picture of what it is like to live with MS. "I'm experiencing increasing weakness in my hands and fingers.... It seems to take so much effort just to get up in the morning.... I enjoy my work, but.... I feel so helpless when fatigue takes over.... Dressing is becoming tiring and a time-consuming task.... Being able to drive my care is very important to me.... I want to remain in my current home, but...." I use comments like these when I teach medical students, interns, and residents about MS: they "get it" in a way they never do from textbooks and scientific articles.

WHAT DOES THIS BOOK SAY?

The way the authors answer the Questions makes this book special. Of course there is solid factual information. See, for example, the chapters on the disease and its epidemiology and on the ADA, FMLA, SSDI, and PASS. Hear the sound advice on communication, planning for the future, and sexuality. Notice the wisdom on parenting, family dynamics, and how to "bank and budget energy."

I admire the authors for being frank, honest, and straightforward—they are good role models for us clinicians. I understand the challenge of answering tough Questions well. Consider, for example, "Should I start taking a disease-modifying medication right away?" Although the author says that patients and physicians should make this decision together, he does not stop there. Rather, he encourages careful consideration and explains why some people hesitate; he presents and documents the experts' opinion and lays out the scientific reasoning behind it. When there are no clear answers to questions—"Is my fatigue due to MS or depression?" "How does stress affect my MS?"—the authors tell us so. As they explain why, giving the available information on all sides of an issue, we are encouraged to think it through ourselves and make our own decisions.

I appreciate the authors debunking the myths that for years have troubled people with MS, their families, and some clinicians. Take, for example, depression. The many contributing factors—including genetics and biology—are thoroughly explained and discussed, effectively dispelling the notions that "anyone would be depressed" or that "trying harder" would make the difference. Consider also the old adage about pregnancy. The authors reject it—"a woman should not be discouraged from becoming pregnant simply because she has been diagnosed with MS"—but not without providing the evidence or discussing the challenges. Finally, put to rest is the notion that using a wheelchair *causes* difficulty walking.

To me, the tone of the Answers is as important as their content. Forthright and candid, the Answers manifest respect. Sensitive and compassionate, they model empathy. There is no "talking down" in this book: authors use medical terminology and educate through a glossary and anatomical drawings. The message this book sends to patients, families, and clinicians is loud and clear: nothing is too sensitive, too difficult, too complicated, or seemingly too simple to talk about. I would like to send a message as well. For those in the MS community who do not live with the illness or whose work does not bring them into direct contact with people who do, getting to know the patients, families, clinicians, and other experts who speak to us through this book can help you keep your work relevant and meaningful. For us all, this book can open our minds and give rise to new understanding.

Sarah Minden, MD

Acknowledgments

While working on the fifth edition of this book, I reflected on how much has changed since the first edition came out in 1996, and how much has stayed the same. People living with MS have more treatment options, new and better technologies to assist them, and a research horizon filled with more answers and greater promise than ever before. What has not changed at all is the commitment of the individuals engaged in this project. These authors, all recognized experts in their field, share a belief in the value of information and communication in today's complex health care environment—and each has worked to ensure that readers have the information they need to communicate most effectively with their health care team. Their shared belief in the importance of comprehensive and coordinated care for people with MS is what makes this book possible—and I deeply appreciate their efforts. I also want to thank Nancy Reitman, RN, MA, MSCN, for her invaluable assistance throughout the process, and Noreen Henson and the team at Demos Health for continuing to believe in the importance of this book—and, as always, I thank Nicholas LaRocca, PhD, my husband, friend, colleague, and go-to person for all the things that matter most.

About the Authors

Kristan J. Aronson, BSc, MSc, PhD
Professor in the Department of Community Health and Epidemiology and in the School of Environmental Studies, and a member of the Cancer Research Institute at Queen's University, Kingston, Ontario, Canada. Her research on multiple sclerosis began with a survey of health service utilization and quality of life among those with MS and their caregivers in Ontario, and continues with a focus on the potential interaction of environmental and genetic causes of MS. Dr. Aronson has received several awards for her research, and her volunteer service in MS was recognized in the awarding of the Golden Jubilee Medallion of Queen Elizabeth II.

Maria Teresa Benedetto-Anzai, MD
Assistant Professor at the New York University School of Medicine, Department of Gynecology, specializing in reproductive endocrinology and infertility, general comprehensive OB/GYN, and high-risk obstetrics. She is also the consulting gynecologist to the Initiative for Women with Disabilities Elly and Steve Hammerman Health and Wellness Center at New York University Hospital for Joint Diseases in New York City. Dr. Benedetto-Anzai was the center's gynecologist from 2000 to 2005, during which time she was instrumental in developing and expanding the gynecology practice and ensuring that women with multiple sclerosis and other physical disabilities received high-quality gynecologic care.

Francois Bethoux, MD
Director of Rehabilitation Services at the Mellen Center for MS Treatment and Research at the Cleveland Clinic Foundation in Cleveland, Ohio. Dr. Bethoux is a principal or coinvestigator in a number of research studies in the area of multiple sclerosis rehabilitation, ambulation, and spasticity management. He currently chairs the Research Interest Group on symptom management of the Consortium of Multiple Sclerosis Centers.

Allen Bowling, MD, PhD
Director of the Complementary and Alternative Medicine (CAM) Service at the Colorado Neurological Institute (CNI). He is also Medical Director of the Multiple Sclerosis (MS) Service at CNI and Clinical Associate Professor of Neurology at the University of Colorado. Dr. Bowling has more than 100 lay and professional publications. He is the author or coauthor of four books, including *Complementary and Alternative Medicine and Multiple Sclerosis*.

Kimberly Calder, MPS

Director, Federal Health Affairs and Insurance Policy at the National Multiple Sclerosis Society. As a specialist in access to care, health and disability insurance for high-risk and disabled individuals, she leads the Society's health care reform implementation team and advocacy efforts on public and private insurance at the federal level. Ms. Calder was a founding member of New Yorkers for Accessible Health Coverage, the Cancer Leadership Council, and the National Breast Cancer Coalition. In 2010, she became a Consumer Representative to the National Association of Insurance Commissioners.

Laura Cooper, Esq

Practicing attorney for the past 26 years, 2 years as counsel to the Chairman of the Interstate Commerce Commission in Washington, DC, 8 years focusing on disability rights and consumer-based health law on behalf of the National Multiple Sclerosis Society, and the past 11 years in private practice in Eugene, Oregon. She has also served the National MS Society as a consultant on life planning, legal, and employment issues, and as a member of the Services Subcommittee on Independent Living. Ms. Cooper made the decision to attend law school after developing MS. After receiving her degree, she was named one of the 20 outstanding young American lawyers "who make a difference" by the American Bar Association.

Frederick W. Foley, PhD

Professor of Psychology at Ferkauf Graduate School of Psychology of Yeshiva University, in Bronx, NY, and Director of Neuropsychology and Psychosocial Research at the MS Comprehensive Care Center at Holy Name Medical Center in Teaneck, NJ. He has served as a volunteer on a variety of projects for the National Multiple Sclerosis Society and is a past president of the Consortium of MS Centers, an organization of MS professionals dedicated to education, treatment, and research in MS.

Debra Frankel, MS, OTR

Associate Vice President of Chapter Programs and Services at the National Multiple Sclerosis Society. After working as an occupational therapist in rehabilitation settings for several years, Ms. Frankel joined the Central New England Chapter of the Society as Director of Chapter Programs. She also served as a consultant to the Society's home office, working with other chapters to strengthen their local programming. Ms. Frankel is author of numerous publications and articles about MS, long-term care, and other health promotion issues.

Cindy Gackle, OTR/L, MSCS

Staff occupational therapist in adult outpatient rehabilitation at the University of Minnesota Medical Center, Fairview, in Minneapolis, MN. Since 1997, her work has focused on treatment for people with multiple sclerosis. She is also a programs consultant with Can Do Multiple Sclerosis lifestyle empowerment programs, and participates in the National MS Society–Minnesota Chapter's Clinical Advisory Committee. Ms. Gackle also serves as the OT project leader for the Consortium of MS Centers' Web site. She has provided educational seminars for professionals and patients nationwide on rehabilitation for individuals with multiple sclerosis.

Barbara Giesser, MD

Clinical Professor of Neurology at the David Geffen School of Medicine at the University of California at Los Angeles (UCLA). Dr. Giesser has specialized in the care of persons with MS since 1982. She has served as Medical Director of the Gimbel MS Center at Holy Name Hospital in Teaneck, NJ, and Medical Director of the Rehab Institute of Tucson, AZ. Dr. Giesser is currently Clinical Director of the MS Program at UCLA and Medical Director of the Marilyn Hilton MS Achievement Center at UCLA. Her research interests include gender issues in MS and the role of exercise as a treatment. Dr. Giesser is coauthor with Dr. Kalb and Dr. Holland of *Multiple Sclerosis for Dummies.*

June Halper, MSN, ANP-C, FAAN, MSCN

A certified adult nurse practitioner, she has specialized in multiple sclerosis since 1978. Ms. Halper was a founder of the Gimbel MS Center in Teaneck, NJ, and Executive Director from 1985 to 2002. She is currently the Executive Director of the Consortium of Multiple Sclerosis Centers and the International Organization of Multiple Sclerosis Nurses. Her numerous publications include *Comprehensive Nursing Care in Multiple Sclerosis* (3rd ed.), *Advanced Concepts in Nursing Care in Multiple Sclerosis* (2nd ed.), and *Nursing Practice in Multiple Sclerosis: A Core Curriculum.*

Robert Herndon, MD

Professor of Neurology at the University of Mississippi Medical Center. He has directed MS clinics at Johns Hopkins University, the University of Rochester, and Good Samaritan Hospital in Portland, OR. Dr. Herndon is past president of the Consortium of MS Centers (CMSC) and serves on the National Clinical Advisory Board of the National Multiple Sclerosis Society and the Multiple Sclerosis International Federation. He has participated in numerous clinical trials of new treatments for MS and has published more than 100 papers and five professional books.

Nancy J. Holland, EdD, RN

Now retired, she has led clinical programs at the National Multiple Sclerosis Society for more than 25 years. Prior to joining the Society, Dr. Holland worked as a nurse and program director at the Medical Rehabilitation Research and Training Center in MS at the Albert Einstein College of Medicine in New York. She is a recognized expert on bladder and bowel management in MS and the author or editor of more than 60 MS-related articles, chapters, and books, including *Multiple Sclerosis: A Guide for Patients and Their Families, Multiple Sclerosis: A Guide for the Newly Diagnosed* (3rd ed.), *Comprehensive Nursing Care in Multiple Sclerosis,* and *Multiple Sclerosis: A Self-Care Guide to Wellness.* Dr. Holland is coauthor with Dr. Kalb and Dr. Giesser of *Multiple Sclerosis for Dummies.* She is a founding member of the Board of Directors of the International Organization of MS Nurses.

Rosalind C. Kalb, PhD

Vice President of the Professional Resource Center at the National Multiple Sclerosis Society in New York City, developing and providing educational materials and consultation services for health care professionals. As a clinical psychologist in private practice, Dr. Kalb has provided individual and family therapy for people living with MS for more than 25 years. She is the author of the National MS Society's *Knowledge is Power* series for individuals newly diagnosed with MS, senior author of *Multiple*

Sclerosis for Dummies (Wiley Publishing), and coauthor with Nicholas LaRocca, PhD, of *Multiple Sclerosis: Understanding the Cognitive Challenges* (Demos Health). Dr. Kalb is also the editor of two books—*Multiple Sclerosis: The Questions You Have, The Answers You Need*, now in its 5th edition, and *Multiple Sclerosis: A Guide for Families* (3rd ed.), also from Demos Medical Publishing.

Nicholas G. LaRocca, PhD

A clinical psychologist who has worked in the field of MS for more than 30 years. He was an Associate Professor at Albert Einstein College of Medicine and New York Medical College before joining the Society in 1997. He currently serves as Vice President of Health Care Delivery and Policy Research in the Research Programs Department at the Society's New York City home office. In this role, he has responsibility for Society funding of research to address the symptoms of MS, rehabilitation, epidemiology, and psychosocial aspects of MS, as well as health policy studies. He has a long-standing interest in cognition and rehabilitation and coauthored a book on cognitive changes in MS that was published in 2006.

Jeri A. Logemann, PhD

The Ralph and Jean Sundin Professor of Communication Sciences and Disorders at Northwestern University, and Professor of Otolaryngology, Head and Neck Surgery, and Neurology at Northwestern University's Feinberg School of Medicine, Evanston and Chicago, IL. She has published and lectured widely both nationally and internationally on normal swallowing and on the evaluation and treatment of swallowing disorders in specific populations, including multiple sclerosis.

Aaron Miller, MD

Medical Director of the Corinne Goldsmith Dickinson Center for Multiple Sclerosis at the Mount Sinai School of Medicine. Prior to assuming that position, he headed the Division of Neurology at Maimonides Medical Center in Brooklyn, NY, where he continues to serve as codirector of the MS Care Center. He is also a Professor of Neurology at the Mt. Sinai School of Medicine in New York City. Dr. Miller serves as the National MS Society's Chief Medical Officer and is past chairman of the Society's National Clinical Advisory Board. He is also a past president of the Consortium of MS Centers and served as the first chairman of the multiple sclerosis section of the American Academy of Neurology.

Deborah M. Miller, PhD, LISW

Director of Comprehensive Care at the Mellen Center for Multiple Sclerosis Treatment and Research and Associate Professor of Medicine of the Cleveland Clinic, with responsibility for program development, outcomes research, and clinical care for families. Dr. Miller's practice interests focus on marital and family adjustment to MS, and her research interests include quality-of-life assessment and the impact of clinical interventions on patients' assessment of health status. Dr. Miller has developed and facilitated group treatment programs for school-age children and teenagers whose parents have MS, and for adults who have parenting concerns because of MS.

Pamela H. Miller, MA, CCC-SLP

Has provided evaluation and treatment for the speech, swallowing, and cognitive-language problems of neurologically impaired adults since 1976. She has been the speech-language pathologist on the MS Clinical Team at the Denver Veterans Administration Hospital since 2007, and has been a consulting speech-language pathologist for Can Do Multiple Sclerosis since 1992. Ms. Miller served as Director of Speech-Language Pathology at the Rocky Mountain Multiple Sclerosis Center from 1988 to 1996. A past president of the Consortium of MS Centers, Ms. Miller has also served on the Employment Committee for the National Multiple Sclerosis Society and on the Editorial Advisory Board for the monthly publication *Real Living with MS* since 1996.

Steven W. Nissen, MS, CRC

Senior Director of Employment and Community Programs at the National Capital Chapter of the National Multiple Sclerosis Society in Washington, DC. Before coming to the National MS Society, Steve worked extensively in the vocational rehabilitation field. He worked for the Virginia Department of Rehabilitative Services and the state vocational rehabilitation agency, as well as for a private vocational rehabilitation and case management company where he provided job development and placement assistance to individuals with physical disabilities. He coauthored *Employment Issues and Multiple Sclerosis* (2nd ed., Demos Health) with Phillip Rumrill, Jr., PhD, and Mary Hennessey, PhD.

Phillip D. Rumrill, Jr., PhD, CRC

A Professor and Coordinator of the rehabilitation counseling program at Kent State University in Ohio. He is also the Founding Director of the Kent State University Center for Disability Studies. Dr. Rumrill has published numerous professional publications and books and research investigations regarding the employment of people with MS, and he has consulted with many chapters of the National MS Society in developing employment programs.

Randall Schapiro, MD

The founder of the Schapiro Center for Multiple Sclerosis at the Minneapolis Clinic of Neurology and current President of The Schapiro Multiple Sclerosis Advisory Group. He is a clinical professor of neurology at the University of Minnesota. Dr. Schapiro is the author of numerous books, book chapters, and articles, including *Managing the Symptoms of Multiple Sclerosis*, now in its fifth edition (Demos Health). As an invited speaker and visiting professor, he has lectured extensively throughout the country and around the world. He is currently a member of the Colorado/Wyoming Chapter of the National MS Society's Board of Directors and a former member of the National Board of Directors.

Charles Smith, MD

Specializing in both multiple sclerosis (MS) and neurorehabilitation, Dr. Smith is a practicing neurologist at the Scripps Clinic in La Jolla, California. Prior to joining Scripps Clinic, Dr. Smith was director of the Multiple Sclerosis Comprehensive Care Centers at White Plains and Bronx Lebanon Hospital Centers in New York. He also served as director of the federally funded Medical Rehabilitation Research and Training Center for Multiple Sclerosis at both Albert Einstein College of Medicine and New York Medical College. His scientific articles about MS and other neurological conditions have been published in more than 40 medical journals.

Matthew Sutliff, PT, MSCS

A physical therapist, Matthew Sutliff is Rehabilitation Manager at the Mellen Center for Multiple Sclerosis Treatment and Research, part of the Cleveland Clinic Neurological Institute in Cleveland, Ohio. He has published articles on MS and ALS rehabilitation. Mr. Sutliff has conducted research trials on new treatment options, and his development of the Hip Flexion Assist Device (HFAD), which is used to enhance walking ability in MS patients, earned him the Cleveland Clinic's 2005 Innovator Award. Mr. Sutliff is also a staff physical therapist with the Can Do MS Center in Edwards, CO, a wellness and educational program for people with MS. He is an active member within the Consortium of Multiple Sclerosis Centers.

Michael A. Werner, MD

A urologist who specializes exclusively in male infertility and male and female sexual dysfunction and lectures and writes extensively on these topics in medical journals and books. He has private practice offices in Purchase, NY, Manhattan, and Norwalk, CT. Dr. Werner is the medical director of MAZE Fertility Laboratories in Purchase, NY, Manhattan, and Clifton, NJ, and The Medical Center for Female Sexuality in Purchase, NY, and Manhattan.

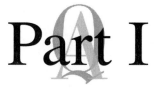

Part I

MS: What's It All About?

Multiple sclerosis (MS) is a complex disease for which the cause and cure are still unknown. In other words, there are still a lot of unanswered questions for anyone living with MS. In this part of the book, we provide an overview of the disease—describing what we know and do not know about MS. Experts in the field provide up-to-date answers to the most commonly asked questions about what happens in MS, who gets the disease and why, how it is diagnosed, and what kinds of symptoms can occur. We start with a chapter designed to help you figure out how to make the best use of a book that is filled with more information than you may ever need to know about MS.

What Should I Know About This Book?

Nancy J. Holland, EdD, RN

IS THIS BOOK FOR ME?

Multiple Sclerosis: The Questions You Have, The Answers You Need was written primarily for people with multiple sclerosis (MS). However, if you love someone with MS, work with a person who has MS, or are just curious about the disease, you will find this book helpful and informative. It covers a wide range of topics in a format that is familiar, accessible, and easily understood. The question-and-answer format was selected for several reasons. First, it reflects the collaborative relationship between individuals with MS and their health care professionals. The authors of each chapter answer the questions that they have been asked repeatedly in the course of their work with people with MS. Second, the questions included here provide a model and a vocabulary for those who are not certain what questions to ask or how to ask them. Third, the question-and-answer format makes it possible for readers to zero in on particular topics, and even particular questions, without having to wade through material that may be irrelevant to their individual needs.

The importance and value of this book to people with MS is underscored by this being its fifth edition. For many years, the MS community has looked to *Multiple Sclerosis: The Questions You Have, The Answers You Need* for information and clarification on perplexing and confusing issues related to MS. Having passed this test of time, the "MS Q&A book" should feel like an old and valued friend—one to approach again and again, as needs arise.

WHAT IS THE PURPOSE OF THIS BOOK?

It is important for someone with a *chronic* illness to understand its potentially far-reaching impact and to know what positive actions can be taken to manage this unexpected intrusion into daily life. An open dialogue with the physician and other professionals on the health care team is an important part of the adjustment process. This book answers specific questions about living with MS and can help prepare you to interact with health professionals as an informed and active participant in your health promotion plan. Factors such as the symptoms you are experiencing, the course of your MS, and career and family plans all must be considered in a thoughtful manner. This book provides one tool to help in that process. Concerned professionals will also assist and support you through the difficult aspects of adjusting to MS.

HOW WERE PEOPLE SELECTED TO ANSWER THE QUESTIONS IN THIS BOOK?
Beginning with the first edition, recognized experts in the field of MS were invited to participate. Over the years, the book's content has grown as these MS specialists have continued to share their expertise and experience, and new authors have joined along the way. Most of the authors are affiliated with an MS care center and/or the National MS Society; others work in related fields that target the medical, psychosocial, and economic challenges faced by those with chronic illness. All have extensive experience in assisting people to deal with MS-related problems.

HOW WERE THE QUESTIONS SELECTED FOR INCLUSION?
For the first edition of the book, each of the contributing authors was asked to provide a list of questions, related to his or her area of expertise, commonly asked by individuals with MS and their family members. Authors were also asked to include questions that they felt people should be encouraged to ask even if they were not routinely doing so. In addition, the Information Resource Center at the National MS Society provided a computerized listing of topics most frequently asked about on the telephone information line or by e-mail. The proposed questions for each chapter were then reviewed by a number of people with MS, family members, caregivers, and health professionals to ensure that the list of questions was both comprehensive and meaningful. The questions and topics that have been added to subsequent editions of the book were suggested by people with MS and their family members, professionals in the field, and other interested readers. The information has grown as knowledge about MS has grown.

HOW SHOULD I USE THIS BOOK?
There are a few factors to consider before deciding how to use this book. First, the symptoms and course of MS can vary significantly from one individual to the next, as can the individual's response to treatment. People also vary in the individual characteristics they bring to the situation—their age, gender, family composition, social support network, and occupation, to name a few. Personality characteristics can also influence how a person will deal with MS and how he or she will choose to use this book. For example, some people want to know everything about MS, regardless of immediate or long-term relevance to their own medical situation. For most people, however, this is not the case. They want to know answers to specific questions pertinent to decisions they need to make now and in the immediate future. You can use this book in any way that best suits your needs and your style of dealing with information.

The book attempts to answer questions for everyone living with MS—those who have the disease and those who share life with someone who has it. Although many people with MS do not have serious or debilitating symptoms, others face significant physical, cognitive, social, and/or emotional challenges. Since all of the information in this book will not pertain to everyone, some material may be upsetting to those not experiencing the more disabling problems. We recommend that you be selective in your reading; don't see this as a book you must read from cover to cover. No one person will face all the problems addressed here, and the full range of circumstances can be overwhelming if not dealt with selectively. Each chapter has a short introduction to the particular topic, a series of questions and answers relating to the topic, and a listing of recommended readings for people who wish to pursue the topic in greater depth. Where applicable, the authors have also provided a list of available resources, including organizations, agencies, product manufacturers, and other potential sources of relevant information or goods and services.

The best strategy is probably to use this book for reference purposes, reading it now for background information and answers to your immediate questions, and consulting it in the future as other problems or questions arise. The remaining chapters in Part I provide a useful overview of MS—including answers to questions about who gets the disease and why, and a quick look at the symptoms it can cause. Part II covers the complete range of treatments and strategies available to manage the disease. Part III addresses how people with MS and their family members react to the intrusion of MS in their lives and learn to cope with its challenges. Part IV will alert you to important issues that you should think about now to safeguard yourself and your family down the road.

- *Glossary.* Medical words and phrases appearing in bold type in the text are explained in the alphabetized glossary. Also included in the glossary are terms that you might encounter in other MS-related reading materials or in discussions with your health care providers. MS is surrounded by a new and unfamiliar vocabulary of neurologic terms, anatomic parts, and rehabilitation language. Learning the meaning of these terms will increase your understanding of this complex information and facilitate your efforts to communicate with your health care providers.
- *List of commonly used medications.* Many medications are used to deal with the MS disease course and the various symptoms that can occur. A particular medication will likely be of interest only if your physician has recommended it, or if you read or hear about it as a suggested therapy for a symptom you are experiencing. A table at the end of the book includes the commonly used medications and their usage in MS.
- *Recommended reading list.* Included in Appendix C are books and other publications relating specifically to MS or to chronic illness.
- *Resource list.* Your particular needs at any given time will direct your use of the Resource section at the back of the book. Included in this list are government and private agencies and organizations that provide information and/or services to deal with MS-related problems. Because many resources vary according to the state or community in which you live, the Resource List can also guide your efforts to identify local sources of information and assistance. Resources specifically relevant to the area covered in a particular chapter are listed at the end of that chapter.

WHAT IF I HAVE ONLY RECENTLY BEEN DIAGNOSED WITH MS?

In general, it will not be helpful for someone with a recent diagnosis to read the entire book. If you were only recently diagnosed, you probably have a relatively short history of MS symptoms to look back on and limited experience with the impact of these symptoms on your daily life. People differ in their responses to both the diagnosis and the challenges it poses. In addition, considerable variation can occur in disease course and symptoms in MS. Therefore, much of the material in this book will not be pertinent for you now, and may or may not be pertinent for you in the future. If your MS follows a mild or moderate course, some of this information will never be relevant to your situation.

MS is an unwelcome and distressing intruder for everyone involved. One way to reduce the discomfort is to have accurate information about what to expect and what can be done. Some people with MS have an easier time than others, but this book attempts to deal with the full range of possible problems, even the very difficult ones. Remember to focus on those topics that relate to your particular and unique situation and try not to become preoccupied with questions and problems unrelated to your own. If you continue to have questions or concerns about the information provided here, be sure to contact a member of your health care team for further discussion.

HOW CAN I GET ADDITIONAL INFORMATION ABOUT TOPICS ADDRESSED IN THIS BOOK?

Each chapter includes a list of recommended readings for people who wish to pursue more detailed information about a particular topic. Most of the recommended readings are for lay audiences. Articles from professional journals have been included in some lists, particularly in those areas in which little has been written for nonprofessionals (e.g., speech and swallowing disorders, *cognition*). Information about articles pertaining directly to MS may be available at your public library, through the library's interlibrary loan service, or from an online computer service. More general readings are listed in the Recommended Reading List. You can also contact a member of your health care team for additional recommendations.

The National MS Society is an excellent source of up-to-date information about MS. You can obtain information and print materials by calling 800-344-3867 or online at *www.nationalmssociety.org*. Obviously, no single book can include every possible question. Each individual is different and will experience MS in his or her own way. You will probably have questions of your own that do not appear in these pages. The goal of this book is to help you ask important questions—and find accurate, meaningful answers—so that you can manage life with MS in a way that best meets your needs.

Multiple Sclerosis:
An Introduction to the Disease

Charles Smith, MD

Multiple sclerosis (MS) is a ***chronic, immune-mediated disease*** that affects the ***central nervous system*** (CNS), which includes the brain, spinal cord, and optic *nerves* (see Figure 2-1). Although it appears most commonly in young adulthood, MS has been known to make its first appearance in early childhood or after the age of 60.

Fortunately, although MS is a chronic illness, it is not always a disabling one. Many people with MS lead fully active and productive lives. For them, the symptoms of MS are more of a nuisance than a hindrance to life's ambitions. For those whose MS is more severe and debilitating, there are management strategies that may help to keep the ***symptoms*** from compromising their daily activities or interfering with their active participation in society.

As you read this chapter, you will find that many unanswered questions about this disease still persist. For example, we still do not know what causes MS or why one person gets the disease and another does not (see Chapter 3 for more information about who gets MS and why), and we do not know why the disease is so variable from one person to the next or from one day or week to another for a given individual. This uncertainty has contributed to the frustrations faced by scientists as they search for a cure. The good news is that the search for answers and more effective treatments is moving at a faster pace than ever before and, in the meantime, physicians, nurses, ***rehabilitation*** specialists, and other health professionals are helping individuals with MS to feel and function at their best.

The following questions and answers highlight the primary concerns of people who are trying to understand this puzzling and unpredictable disease.

THE DISEASE PROCESS

WHAT HAPPENS WHEN A PERSON HAS MS?

MS is believed by most experts to be an ***autoimmune disease***, which means that the body's immune system mistakenly attacks an apparently normal tissue or organ of the body. In MS, the autoimmune attack involves ***inflammation*** directed against

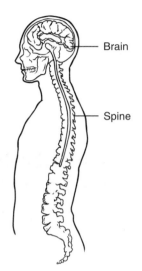

FIGURE 2-1. The central nervous system.

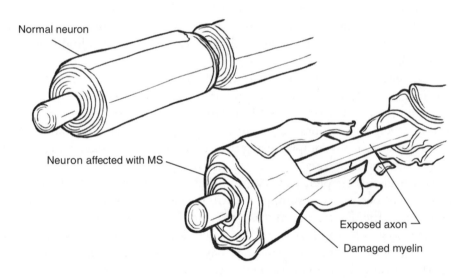

FIGURE 2-2. The healthy neuron and the neuron damaged by MS.

the *myelin* and the cells that make myelin, the *oligodendrocytes* of the CNS in a process called *demyelination*. *Neurons*, or nerve cells, in the CNS are made up of the cell body, dendrites (the processes of the cell body that receive nervous impulses from other nerve cells), and *axons* (the processes of nerve cells that conduct nervous impulses away from the cell body to allow communication with other nerve cells). Myelin is the insulation or coating that surrounds the axons and speeds nerve conduction. Demyelination results in *plaques* (also called *lesions* or *scars*) along the myelin sheath that interfere with nerve conduction (see Figure 2-2). The symptoms that occur in MS result from this inflammatory process, as well as from damage to the axons themselves. These symptoms can include loss of vision, double vision, stiffness, weakness, imbalance, numbness, pain, problems with bladder and bowel control, fatigue, sexual changes, speech and swallowing difficulties, emotional changes, and intellectual impairment. The type and number of symptoms vary from one individual to the next, depending on where in the CNS the damage to the myelin and axons occurs. At this time, we do not know exactly why the damage occurs or why some people get more or different symptoms than others.

The reasons for *axonal damage* in MS are not fully known. Although the inflammatory activity directed against myelin might damage axons via an "innocent bystander" effect, additional causes are likely to be discovered in the future. It is now believed that axonal damage, which begins in the earliest phases of the disease, is the likely cause of symptoms that do not improve (i.e., fixed disability). Progressive axonal damage and loss may also be the explanation for the brain *atrophy* seen later in the course of the illness, also known as the progressive phase of MS.

WHAT MAKES A DISEASE "AUTOIMMUNE?"
Most doctors believe that MS is an autoimmune disease because the plaques or scars in the myelin caused by MS appear to be the result of the person's immune system mistakenly attacking tissue in his or her own body. For example, immune cells such as *lymphocytes*, plasma cells (white blood cells that make *antibodies*), and *macrophages* (cells that destroy myelin) can be found around sites of active inflammation and scarring. Many plaques start around a small vein, suggesting that these immune cells escape from the blood, pass through the *blood-brain barrier*, and enter the brain and spinal cord to do damage. *Experimental allergic encephalomyelitis (EAE)*, an animal model for MS, is known to be an autoimmune disease. Scientists can cause EAE in laboratory animals, making it a valuable tool in the research efforts to find the cause and treatment of MS (see Chapter 5).

WHAT CAUSES A PERSON TO GET MS?
The cause of MS remains one of the big unanswered questions. The current thinking is that the disease occurs in people who have a genetic predisposition to respond to some environmental trigger(s), setting in motion the autoimmune process. However, we still have not identified what the specific trigger or triggers might be, or what other factors might be involved. Chapter 3 describes in detail what we know—and do not know—about the *epidemiology* of MS, including information about gender, ethnicity, and genetics, as well as environmental and lifestyle factors that may play a role.

WHAT CAUSES THE SYMPTOMS OF MS?
The body's actions and reactions to outside stimuli involve a lightning-quick and complicated process in which the body receives those stimuli through the various senses (vision or touch, for example), sends a report to the brain, and then responds to instructions from the brain about what to do next. This ongoing process depends on the coordinated transmission of nerve impulses from one nerve cell to the next. Nerve impulses pass along nerve fibers that connect at synapses. A fatty substance called myelin, which forms a sheath around the nerve fibers in the CNS (which is made up of the brain, optic nerves, and spinal cord), helps to speed this conduction of nerve impulses. The myelin, which is made and maintained by cells called

oligodendrocytes, has a whitish appearance, leading to the identification of MS as a disease that primarily affects the white matter of the CNS (although we now know that the gray matter in the CNS is affected as well).

Any damage to the myelin sheath results in some disruption of the impulse or message being transmitted, much as would occur in a damaged telephone wire. In MS, overactive, misguided cells of the immune system enter the CNS, causing inflammation in the brain and spinal cord. This inflammation causes damage to the myelin and the axons. Wherever myelin is destroyed, a plaque (lesion) forms, with a gradual buildup of hardened scar tissue (*sclerosis*) at the site. These sclerotic sites occur in varied locations throughout the CNS, giving rise to the name *multiple sclerosis*. Although many of these scars may be "silent," causing no apparent symptoms, others can interfere with sensation or function. In addition, demyelination may disrupt communication between different parts of the brain, even if the parts themselves remain intact.

Although the name of the disease comes from the multiple scarring sites (sclerosis) caused by demyelination, the disease also causes irreversible damage to the nerve fibers (axons) themselves. Recent studies of brain tissue (on biopsy or autopsy specimens) have clearly shown the presence of damaged axons in people with MS, even in the very earliest stages of the illness. It is now believed that damage to the axons is responsible for those symptoms that do not improve. Whereas myelin has the ability to regenerate, at least early in the course of MS, axonal damage is permanent.

THE DIAGNOSTIC PROCESS

WHY IS IT SOMETIMES SO DIFFICULT TO DIAGNOSE MS?

At present, no specific blood tests, imaging techniques (e.g., *magnetic resonance imaging* [MRI] or computed tomography [CT] scan), tests of immune function, or genetic tests can, by themselves, determine if a person has MS or is likely to have it in the future. The diagnosis is a clinical one, made on the basis of a person's medical history, an assessment of the *symptoms* experienced and reported by the person, and the existence of *signs* detected by the physician (but not necessarily noticed by the person) during the neurologic examination. Both symptoms and signs are necessary, because symptoms are subjective complaints that can vary tremendously from one individual to another, whereas signs are measurable, objective observations. Examples of the symptoms commonly reported by people with MS include problems with vision, walking, bladder control, fatigue, and uncomfortable sensations such as numbness or "pins and needles." Common signs that can be detected by the doctor during a physical examination—even if the person has never noticed or been troubled by these changes—include altered eye movements and abnormal responses of the pupils, altered *reflex* responses, *sensory* disturbances, and *spasticity* of the limbs.

To make a definite diagnosis of MS, the physician must:

● Find evidence of plaques (lesions) in at least two distinct areas of the CNS white matter

● Determine that the plaques have occurred at different points in time

● Be sure that these plaques in the white matter have no other reasonable explanation

In other words, MS is a diagnosis that should be made only after every other possible explanation of the signs and symptoms has been ruled out because there is no test, other than microscopic examination of the CNS lesions, that can unequivocally prove the diagnosis.

In 2001, the International Panel on the Diagnosis of Multiple Sclerosis, led by W. Ian McDonald, FRPC, published revised criteria for the diagnosis of MS. The "McDonald criteria," which were further revised in 2005 and again in 2010, specify the ways in which MRI findings (including the number, location, and quality of observed abnormalities) can be combined with other laboratory findings to diagnose MS more quickly and accurately.

HOW WILL THE DOCTOR DETERMINE IF I HAVE MS?

The physician will first take a very careful history, including any past and present complaints that you have, any pertinent family history of disease, the places you have lived and visited, substance use (alcohol, drug, and smoking habits), and any medications that you are taking. Through detailed questioning, the doctor can determine whether you have ever experienced other symptoms—no matter how slight or transient—that might be indicative of MS-related disease activity.

The physician will do a neurologic examination to check for signs that can explain the symptoms you are experiencing or point to disease activity of which you may have been totally unaware.

- An eye examination with an ophthalmoscope may reveal the presence of damage to the *optic nerve*. A pale optic nerve in MS is often indicative of earlier damage, even if the person reports no past or current visual symptoms. The doctor will also test visual acuity and look for evidence of double vision (***diplopia***) or incoordination of eye movements.

- The physician will test for evidence of weakness by asking you to resist efforts to pull or push your arms and legs. You may also be asked to squeeze the doctor's hand as hard as you can.

- Your coordination will be tested in a variety of ways, including the ***finger-to-nose test***, in which you are asked to bring the tip of your index finger to your nose rapidly, with your eyes open and then closed, and the ***heel-knee-shin test*** in which you are asked to move one heel up and down the shin of the other leg. The physician will evaluate your balance by asking you to perform a variety of tasks, including walking on your heels and then on your toes, performing a ***tandem gait*** (placing the heel of one foot directly against the toe of the other foot in an alternating fashion), and standing still with your eyes closed.

- Sensory changes will also be tested in a variety of ways. Your physician will determine if you can tell, with your eyes closed, where your body parts (e.g., fingers and toes) are in space (position sense). ***Vibration sense*** will be tested with a vibrating tuning fork placed against various points on your body. The physician may also use a (gentle) pinprick to test for changes in skin sensitivity. Unfortunately, many of the sensory changes experienced by people with MS, such as numbness, pain, or tingling, cannot be seen or objectively measured on examination, with the result that some physicians have tended to ignore or dismiss these uncomfortable symptoms as unimportant.

- The physician will test the reflexes in various parts of your body. Inequality of reflexes on the two sides of your body is indicative of an abnormal reflex. Absent reflexes, particularly in the abdomen, are also common in MS, although they can have other explanations such as obesity or multiple pregnancies. The **Babinski reflex**, a frequent *sign* found in MS, is clearly indicative of disturbances in major nervous pathways. This neurologic sign is elicited when the physician draws a bluntly pointed object along the outer edge of the sole of the foot from the heel to the little toe. Instead of the normal downward flexion of the toes, it results in an abnormal response in which the big toe extends upward and the other toes fan outward.
- **Lhermitte's sign**, a problem frequently described by persons with MS, can also be used to help confirm the diagnosis of MS. This neurologic phenomenon, which is elicited by flexing the head forward, results in an abnormal "electrical" sensation down the back or limbs. Even though the symptom is a subjective one, Lhermitte's sign can be used to confirm another site of MS involvement in the CNS, and it is routinely sought when evaluating patients for MS.

For some people, no tests beyond this history and neurologic examination are necessary to make the diagnosis. If the doctor is able to find evidence of multiple lesions in the CNS that have occurred at different points in time and have no other reasonable explanation, the diagnosis can be made without any other testing. However, most physicians will not rely entirely on this type of evaluation and will do at least one other test to confirm the diagnosis. This is especially true if the history and examination have not provided conclusive evidence of more than one lesion in the brain or spinal cord.

- The most commonly done test is the MRI of the brain, which is abnormal in about 90 to 95 percent of people with definite MS. MRI of the spinal cord can also be useful, but is not as frequently positive as MRI of the brain. Prior to the development of MRI, a specialized x-ray technique known as the CT scan was used to demonstrate the presence of lesions. However, MRI, which is safer and more accurate than any x-ray technique, provides better evidence of white matter lesions in the CNS.
- Another test often used to help confirm a diagnosis of MS is the **visual evoked potential (VEP)**. This test, which looks at the speed and efficiency of myelin conduction in the visual system, is abnormal in about 90 percent of people with MS. VEPs are particularly useful in confirming the diagnosis because they can demonstrate an asymptomatic lesion in the optic nerves that would otherwise go unnoticed. Like MRI, this test is noninvasive and painless.
- In some instances, a person will be advised to have a **lumbar puncture** (spinal tap). In this test, **cerebrospinal fluid** (fluid that bathes the spinal cord and brain) is collected for chemical analysis. In performing this test, the physician is looking for (1) elevations in IgG (**immunoglobulin** G, a protein fraction of gammaglobulin) and other proteins that are indicative of some abnormality in the immune system, and (2) the presence of a specific IgG that appears in the spinal fluid as **oligoclonal bands**. Neither of these is specific to MS, making a lumbar puncture primarily useful for confirming the diagnosis of MS when other suggestive evidence is present. Because a lumbar puncture is somewhat uncomfortable,

it is not done as frequently as MRI or evoked potentials. However, one of the most important reasons for doing diagnostic tests is to make sure that some other disease is not masquerading as MS, and a lumbar puncture is an effective means of ruling out other diagnoses.

Thus, a variety of diagnostic procedures may be used to help confirm the diagnosis of MS when inadequate evidence is present in the history and clinical examination. For example, if a person develops **optic neuritis** and, three months later, has a new lesion on a brain MRI, the diagnosis can be made because the physician now has evidence of two lesions that have occurred at different times in different places in the CNS. Keep in mind that the diagnosis cannot be made solely on the basis of these tests because MS is only one of several conditions that can cause them to be positive. Your medical history and the symptoms and signs of CNS demyelination that you and the doctor are able to piece together are the clearest evidence for the diagnosis of MS.

CAN THE DOCTOR DIAGNOSE MS AFTER ONLY ONE EPISODE OF NEUROLOGIC SYMPTOMS?
The diagnosis of MS always requires evidence of *dissemination in time and space*—which means evidence of at least two episodes of demyelination that have occurred in different parts of the CNS at different points in time. When a person experiences a single neurologic episode that lasts at least 24 hours, and which is caused by inflammation/demyelination in one or more sites in the CNS, it is called a **clinically isolated syndrome (CIS)**. When this occurs, the challenge for the doctor is to determine the likelihood that the person will go on to have a second episode of demyelination and, therefore, a confirmed diagnosis of MS. The best way for the doctor to make this determination is to look for MS-like lesions on the person's brain MRI. When a person with a CIS has lesions on the MRI that are not causing any symptoms but are consistent with MS, the likelihood that he or she will go on to develop MS at some time in the future is high. When the MRI is free of MS-like lesions, the chances are much smaller.

All four **interferon-beta** medications (Avonex, Betaseron, Extavia, and Rebif) and glatiramer acetate (Copaxone) have been shown to delay the second demyelinating event—and therefore the diagnosis of clinically definite MS—in people with a CIS. Avonex, Betaseron, Copaxone, and Extavia have been approved by the U.S. **Food and Drug Administration** for this use (see Chapter 6 for more information).

WHAT DOES MRI TELL THE DOCTOR?
MRI, or magnetic resonance imaging, is a powerful tool that can be used to directly see at least some of the effects of MS on the brain, optic nerves, and spinal cord.

- The plaques of MS can be directly seen and the number and volume of the plaques can be estimated. In other words, the doctor can estimate the "burden of the disease."
- MRI can also show the effects of atrophy ("shrinkage") of the brain and whether there are permanent "black holes," areas of severe damage to the brain. Both atrophy and "black holes" are worrisome signs that the disease may be entering the progressive stage.

- Doctors use MRI as an extension of the physical examination. In fact, the physical examination is an attempt to locate the sites of the plaques that cause the symptoms and signs. Because individual plaques in the brain may be in areas where damage does not result in any obvious symptoms, MRI may be a more sensitive test of the extent of the disease than relying on the symptoms and findings on physical examination. Experience has confirmed this sensitivity of MRI by demonstrating that for every plaque that causes a symptom, an average of nine are "silent."
- MRI also provides information about the degree of MS activity by allowing the doctor to count the plaques that have occurred since the previous MRI. Very recent plaques will enhance (show up as brighter) on an MRI scan that is done with *gadolinium*, a contrast agent that is injected into the person's body prior to the scan. To cause a new MS attack, immune cells must cross into the brain (or spinal cord) from the blood. This occurs because the immune cells make tiny holes in the walls of small blood vessels. When gadolinium is injected into the body, it also passes through these small holes into the attack site. The enhancement that results lasts until the blood vessels heal, typically 4 to 6 weeks after the immune attack stops. Thus, contrast enhancement gives the doctor an idea of how active MS is at a given point in time.
- In persons with a first episode that suggests MS *(CIS)*, research has shown that the presence or absence of plaques in the nervous system, other than the plaque causing the current symptom, can predict the likelihood that the patient will eventually develop definite MS.
- Further, the number of plaques and the rate of accumulation of new plaques, at least in the first years of the illness, can give some idea of the likelihood of disability later in the course of the disease.

Thus, MRI can provide important information to help the doctor decide when to start treatment and which disease-modifying drug to use at different stages of the disease.

HOW OFTEN DO I NEED TO GET AN MRI DONE?

If your history and physical examination confirm the diagnosis of MS, no additional testing is needed. However, most physicians recommend MRI of the brain at the time of diagnosis to help confirm that the problem is indeed MS rather than some other condition. Although MRI does not reliably predict the course of the disease, there is a growing body of evidence that suggests that changes on repeat MRIs, at least in the early years of the disease, may predict long-term outcome.

Many neurologists now recommend MRI as one means of assessing the effect of a disease-modifying therapy, such as interferon-beta or glatiramer acetate. In other words, the MRI can be done to ensure that a medication is successfully preventing new lesions from accumulating. Even though a person may feel stable or symptom-free, only a minority of plaques (about one out of 5–10), actually cause a symptom—which means that plaques may be forming without the person being aware of it. A chemical contrast agent called *gadolinium* can be administered during the MRI to help distinguish between new or active lesions and old ones, giving the physician information—like "a snapshot"—about the activity of the disease at the time of the

MRI. The MRI is best repeated with the same MRI machine used in the first study so that reasonable comparisons can be made.

THE DISEASE COURSE AND PROGNOSIS

ARE THERE DIFFERENT COURSES OF MS?

The different types of MS are now defined in the following way:

- *Relapsing-remitting MS* is characterized by clearly defined *acute attacks* (exacerbations) that last from days to weeks, with either full recovery or residual deficit(s) (remissions). Whether or not deficits remain after the attacks, the periods between attacks are characterized by stability and absence of disease progression.
- *Primary-progressive MS* is characterized by gradual progression of disability from onset, typically without any *attacks* or *remissions*. However, many patients experience variable periods of apparent stability.
- *Secondary-progressive MS* begins initially with a relapsing-remitting course, which later becomes a more consistently progressive course. A physician cannot reliably predict who will remain relapsing-remitting and who will eventually transition to a secondary-progressive disease course. Thus, it is difficult to give any person a firm *prognosis*.
- *Progressive-relapsing MS* shows clear progression in disability level from the onset of the disease, but with clear, acute relapses that may or may not have some recovery following the acute episode.

These definitions clearly convey that MS is an unpredictable disease that can change course along the way. Research indicates that the vast majority of people (approximately 85 percent) have relapsing-remitting disease at the time of diagnosis, whereas only 15 percent initially have progressive disease. From natural history studies in MS, we know that, in the absence of any disease-modifying treatment, more than half of those initially diagnosed with a relapsing-remitting course will develop secondary-progressive disease after 10 years or so; within a period of 25 years, approximately 90 percent will have changed from relapsing-remitting to progressive disease. The disease-modifying therapies now used in MS (see Chapter 6) have not yet been in use long enough for us to know their long-term impact on the disease course, but the hope is that they will significantly slow disease progression.

I HAVE A NEIGHBOR WITH MS, AND HER SYMPTOMS ARE COMPLETELY DIFFERENT FROM MINE. HOW CAN THE SAME ILLNESS CAUSE SUCH DIFFERENT SYMPTOMS IN PEOPLE?

Just as there are different courses of MS, there are different kinds of symptoms, even among people of the same gender and age who have had the illness for the same length of time. This results from the fact that the plaques of MS are scattered throughout the white matter of the brain and spinal cord. Although the plaques are more likely to occur in some areas than others, the distribution is fairly random. Therefore, one person might experience loss of vision and another might have problems controlling urination. All MS symptoms are caused by damage to the myelin sheath (demyelination) or axons in the CNS; however, the particular areas that become damaged vary from person to person.

HOW IS AN EXACERBATION (RELAPSE) DIFFERENT FROM A PSEUDOEXACERBATION, AND WHAT CAUSES EACH TO HAPPEN?

An *exacerbation* or "attack" of MS (also called a relapse) is caused by a new plaque of demyelination or the reactivation of an old plaque. For a symptom to qualify as an exacerbation it must, by definition, last for at least 24 hours and be separated from the previous attack by 1 month. Although these limits are somewhat arbitrary, it is important that they be considered, so that symptoms will not be misinterpreted.

A *pseudoexacerbation* is unrelated to new disease activity. It results from some other problem—such as an elevated body temperature from overexertion, an infection, or pain—which aggravates the neurologic effects of the preexisting plaques but does not create new or increased damage. For example, people with MS who develop a fever often feel—and appear—much worse as long as their temperature remains elevated. Once their temperature drops to normal, they return to their baseline neurologic function. Similarly, people with *spasticity* in their lower limbs notice more spasms and stiffness when they have a bladder infection. Once the bladder infection is cured with antibiotics, the spasms and stiffness return to their previous level.

Although many identifiable causes exist for pseudoexacerbations, nobody knows the cause of true MS exacerbations. Conflicting evidence exists concerning the role of stress or trauma in exacerbations (see Chapter 16). Some studies have indicated that viral infections such as the common cold or flu can trigger a true exacerbation. This may happen because viral infections trigger the body's immune response.

IS THERE ANYTHING I CAN DO TO PREVENT AN EXACERBATION?

There is no proven way to completely prevent MS attacks. There is no medical treatment that always works to prevent an exacerbation, or every person with MS would be taking it. No convincing evidence exists that a person can prevent an exacerbation by avoiding or controlling life stresses. However, we now have eight medications— the injectable drugs Avonex (interferon beta-1a), Betaseron (interferon beta-1b), Copaxone (glatiramer acetate), Extavia (identical formulation to Betaseron), Rebif (interferon beta-1a); the oral medication Gilenya (fingolimod); and the infused medications, Novantrone (mitoxantrone) and Tysabri (natalizumab)—that have been approved in the United States for the treatment of relapsing forms of MS (see Chapter 6 for more information about each of these medications). All of these medications have been shown to reduce the frequency of exacerbations and the number of new or active lesions visible on MRI, and some have been proven to reduce the progression of disability.

Because many scientists believe that some infectious agents (viral or bacterial) might trigger an exacerbation, it also makes sense to employ good personal hygiene to reduce the possibility of getting such an infection. For example, washing your hands is known to reduce the chance of getting many contagious viral illnesses, such as the common cold.

IS THERE ANYTHING I CAN DO TO PROLONG A REMISSION?

Medical treatments may help to prolong remission for some people. For example, the eight disease-modifying medications (Avonex, Betaseron, Copaxone, Extavia, Gilenya, Rebif, Novantrone, and Tysabri) have all been shown to reduce the frequency of exacerbations in some individuals with relapsing forms of MS. Although physicians differ somewhat in their use of these medications, Gilenya, Novantrone, and Tysabri are more often reserved for persons with continuing attacks or disease progression despite use of the interferon medications (Avonex, Betaseron, Extavia, and Rebif) or Copaxone.

Although doctors frequently use ***corticosteroids*** to treat MS attacks, there is insufficient proof that these medications prolong remission or prevent attacks from occurring. Once an exacerbation has begun, however, these treatments seem to make it resolve more quickly than if no treatment were given (see Chapter 6 for more information about the management of exacerbations).

HOW WILL MY MS AFFECT ME IN THE FUTURE? WILL I END UP IN A WHEELCHAIR OR BEDRIDDEN?

It is not possible for the physician to predict with sufficient accuracy what the future holds for any particular person with MS because it is such an unpredictable disease. However, many physicians will hazard a guess based on such factors as the frequency of attacks and the types of symptoms that the person has experienced.

Individuals who have frequent attacks, especially during the first few years of illness, seem to do less well than those who have infrequent attacks. People whose attacks last for a long time, especially if these attacks are characterized by weakness or incoordination, tend to do less well than those who have brief attacks consisting primarily of numbness or visual loss. Those individuals who have prominent weakness and/or incoordination that does not go away with time tend to have a worse prognosis, as do males and those people who are diagnosed at a later age. There is also evidence that continued MRI activity, especially in the early years following diagnosis, predicts a less favorable outcome in the long term.

Studies involving large populations of people have shown that about 50 percent of persons with the relapsing-remitting form of MS tend to convert to the secondary-progressive form about 15 years after the diagnosis of MS is made. As these studies were done before approved treatment was generally available, most MS experts believe that the progressive phase of MS can be delayed, or even prevented, by the early treatment with approved disease-modifying therapies.

WHAT IS THE EDSS?

Neurologists who see many people with MS need some basis of comparison so that they can communicate findings and conclusions about them in an effective and consistent way. Although the neurologic examination gives a great deal of useful information, it takes a long time to describe the different parts of the examination.

The ***Expanded Disability Status Scale (EDSS)***, which is part of the ***Minimal Record of Disability***, summarizes the neurologic examination and provides a measure of overall disability—at least as it relates to the ability to walk. It is a 20-point scale, ranging from 0 ("normal examination") to 10 ("death due to MS"). A person with a score of 4.5 can walk three blocks without stopping; a score of 6.0 means that a cane is needed to walk one block; a score over 7.5 indicates that a person cannot take more than a few steps, even with crutches or help from another person. The EDSS is used for many reasons, including deciding future medical treatment, establishing rehabilitation goals, and choosing subjects for participation in *clinical trials*. The major drawback of the scale is that its emphasis on gait impairment ignores disability that results from other impairments such as upper limb problems or memory problems. However, no other scale for MS is as widely used in clinical trials as this one.

FINDING THE RIGHT DOCTOR

WHAT TYPE OF PHYSICIAN SHOULD I SEE FOR HELP WITH MY MS?
WHAT ARE THE DIFFERENCES BETWEEN GOING TO AN MS CENTER AND SEEING A PRIVATE PRACTICE NEUROLOGIST?

You should get treatment from a doctor with whom you feel comfortable and who gives you sound advice. Of course, it is not always possible for someone to know when advice is sound or not. Look for a physician who listens carefully to your problems and concerns and offers suggestions on how to remedy them. A good physician will explain what is known about your disease and its symptoms and what treatment options are available. A physician who merely answers all your questions with "That's caused by MS and there's nothing that can be done…go home and learn to live with it" is not giving you the best possible service.

Generally, *neurologists* are best equipped to answer your questions and give you the guidance you need. Obviously, physicians who see many people with MS, and work at an MS center, are more likely to have a broad base of experience. They also tend to work within a multidisciplinary team of professionals (including, for example, nurses, *physical therapists*, *occupational therapists*, psychologists, and social workers) who are knowledgeable about specialized aspects of MS care. The variable and complex symptoms of MS have the potential to affect many different aspects of a person's physical, emotional, and social functioning. The members of a multidisciplinary MS team have the expertise to diagnose and treat the varied problems potentially associated with the disease. In addition, the team approach ensures that a person's care is coordinated rather than spread out among several specialists who are working independently without communicating with one another.

WHAT IS A PHYSIATRIST?

A *physiatrist* is a physician whose specialty is *rehabilitation* medicine. Although these physicians prescribe medication, their primary emphasis is on physical treatments (e.g., *orthotics*, mobility aids, and exercise) designed to ease or improve important functions such as walking. While some physiatrists treat MS patients and manage the full range of symptoms, others see MS patients who are referred to them specifically for rehabilitation purposes.

THE NEUROLOGIST IN MY MANAGED CARE PROGRAM DOES NOT SPECIALIZE IN MS. HOW WILL I KNOW IF I AM GETTING APPROPRIATE OR UP-TO-DATE MEDICAL CARE?

Although it is not always easy to tell if you are getting the most up-to-date treatment and advice, there are several ways that you can educate yourself about current treatment strategies in MS. The National MS Society publishes pamphlets and brochures describing the symptoms of MS and their management, as well as information about what can be done to control the disease. The Society also makes this information available on its web site (www.nationalmssociety.org/Treatments). Most Society chapters sponsor open lecture and discussion meetings throughout the year, as well as support groups. Support groups may be particularly helpful because you can listen to what other people with MS have to say about their experiences. If you have a computer and modem, you can access several Internet forums to raise questions and discuss topics of interest with other individuals who have MS (http://www.nationalmssociety.org/onlinecommunity).

If you learn about a treatment, medication, or management strategy that you think might be beneficial for you, ask your doctor about it and see what kind of response you get. If you always seem to know more than your doctor about what is available, it may be time to consider a change.

RECOMMENDED RESOURCES
....

Holland N, Murray TJ, Reingold S. *Multiple Sclerosis: A Guide for the Newly Diagnosed* (3rd ed.). New York: Demos Medical Publishing, 2007.
Kalb R, Holland N, Giesser B. *Multiple Sclerosis for Dummies*. Hoboken, NJ: Wiley, 2007.

Resources from the National MS Society
Brochures available by calling 800-Fight-MS or online at www.nationalmssociety.org/brochures
- *What is multiple sclerosis?*
- *Choosing the right health care provider*
- *What everyone should know about multiple sclerosis* (suitable for the whole family; available only in a print version)?
- *The history of multiple sclerosis*

General information about MS at www.nationalmssociety.org/aboutms
MS Learn Online programming about all aspects of MS at www.nationalmssociety.org/mslearnonline

The Epidemiology of Multiple Sclerosis—Who Gets MS and Why?

Kristan J. Aronson, BSc, MSc, PhD

The answers to questions about who gets multiple sclerosis (MS) and why are important to many different people for many different reasons. First, any person who is diagnosed with this disease wants to know why it happened and how many other people are dealing with the same diagnosis. And, those who are diagnosed with MS are also worried about what it may mean for their family members—particularly, their children. Scientists look at the geographic, gender, and ethnic distribution of the disease for clues to the causes of MS. Policy makers look to the numbers of people with MS and other diseases to make important decisions about research funding, insurance regulations, and legal protections for individuals with disabilities. In this chapter, we provide answers—or observations and estimates, to be more precise—to some of the most commonly asked questions about the *epidemiology* of MS.

HOW MANY PEOPLE HAVE MS?

Although this question might seem easy to answer, it is actually quite difficult to come up with a precise estimate. MS is not a disease that must be reported to health authorities. As a result, no central registry or database of cases exists for the United States. Thus, in order to determine how many people have MS, it is necessary to perform complex and expensive studies throughout the country. Such studies have not been conducted in more than 30 years. It is, however, possible to estimate the number of people who have MS by examining evidence from smaller studies focused on specific geographic areas.

We talk about the number of people who have MS in two different ways: *Prevalence* is the number of all new and existing cases diagnosed with a disease in a defined population at a defined point in time. *Incidence* is the number of new cases diagnosed in a specified population over a defined period of time. Both prevalence and incidence can be expressed in two different ways: either as total number of cases (400,000 in the United States), or as the number of cases per segment of the population (e.g., 135 per 100,000).

Currently, the National MS Society estimates that approximately 400,000 people in the United States have been diagnosed with MS (prevalence), and that approximately 10,000 new cases are diagnosed each year (incidence). Because of the uncertainty in estimating incidence and prevalence, different authors may come up with different numbers—either lower or higher.

To put these numbers in perspective, it is estimated that approximately 3 million Americans alive today have suffered a stroke, 2.5 million have Alzheimer's disease, 2.1 million have rheumatoid arthritis, 1.5 million have Parkinson's disease, and 250,000 have experienced a spinal cord injury.

I'VE HEARD THAT THERE IS MORE MS NOW THAN THERE USED TO BE. IS IT TRUE THAT THE NUMBER OF PEOPLE WITH MS IS INCREASING?

More people are identified as having MS today than at any time in the past. However, what this means is not entirely clear. Does it mean that more people are *getting* MS? Does it mean that more people with **symptoms** are seeking medical help? Does it mean that doctors have better tools to help them make the diagnosis—for example, magnetic resonance imaging—or are more willing to communicate the diagnosis to their patients? Or, does the increase in the number of people with MS simply reflect the growth of the population and the fact that more people are living longer?

Scientists are not entirely sure what might account for the increase. In all likelihood, the answer is a combination of some or all of these factors.

It is certainly true that the tools available to aid in the diagnosis of MS have improved over the past 20 years or so. If, in addition, the disease is actually occurring in more people than it used to, the possible causes might be environmental factors such as exposure to one or more viruses or bacteria or to one or more toxic substances, or changes in people's lifestyles. Or, some unknown factor may be present that has not yet been considered (see "What causes MS?").

The National MS Society, Parkinson's Action Network, and Centers for Disease Control and Prevention have been looking into the development of a shared national registry for MS, Parkinson's disease, and other chronic neurologic conditions to get a clear picture of the numbers of people living with these conditions.

WHO GETS MS?

The majority of people with MS are diagnosed between the ages of 20 and 50, although MS has been known to make its first appearance in early childhood or after age 60. The average age of disease onset (the appearance of first symptoms) is between 30 and 35. MS is two to three times more common in women than in men. It is most common among people of northern European ancestry, appearing more frequently among Caucasians than among Hispanics or African Americans. It is relatively rare among Asians and some other groups. MS appears to be more common in areas farther from the equator. Although MS is not an inherited disease like Huntington's or cystic fibrosis, we know that there is a genetic component to a person's risk of developing it, and that approximately 20 percent of people who are diagnosed with MS have a family member with the disease.

IS MS MORE COMMON IN SOME PARTS OF THE WORLD THAN IN OTHERS?

The risk of developing MS has long been thought to be greater in areas farther from the equator—for example, in the northern United States and Canada and in southern Australia. This is known as a "latitude gradient." The reason for this difference is not understood. One theory is that individuals growing up closer to the equator have greater exposure to sunlight that stimulates the body to produce higher levels of vitamin D, which may have a protective effect. However, genetic, ethnic, and lifestyle differences associated with distance from the equator may also play a role in the risk for developing MS. One example of the complex interplay between geographic and other factors is seen among Inuits of the polar regions; although they live in an area that is far from the equator, their risk of developing MS is virtually nil.

Some recent studies have suggested that the latitude gradient may be less significant than originally thought. It is clear that additional research is needed to clarify the significance of this issue.

CAN I LOWER MY CHILDREN'S RISK OF GETTING MS BY MOVING TO AN AREA WHERE MS IS LESS COMMON?

Where you lived as a child (before puberty) may have some influence on MS risk. Studies have shown that people who move from a high-risk to a low-risk area after puberty retain the risk associated with their place of origin. On the other hand, people who move very early in life from a high-risk to a low-risk area seem to acquire a level of risk similar to the area to which they move. In both cases, the opposite—moving from a low-risk to a high-risk area—would have similar effects. These simple conclusions, however, have been shown by researchers to be complicated by a variety of other factors, including lifestyle and genetics, so it remains unclear whether moving to a low-risk area is a reasonable strategy if you are worried about your children's risk of MS. The bottom line is that moving to a part of the world where risk may be lower is probably not justified by the current scientific evidence.

WHAT CAUSES MS?

The causes of MS are unknown, but most experts agree that the causes are likely a combination of a person's genetic predisposition, a malfunction in the *immune system*, and one or more environmental factors. In other words, the disease seems to occur when a person, whose genetic makeup predisposes him or her to MS, comes into contact with some environmental factor(s) that sets in motion an attack by the person's immune system on the *central nervous system* (CNS) (see Chapter 2). Although a number of environmental factors have been studied, none has been confirmed as a definitive cause of MS onset or worsening:

- *Epstein-Barr virus* (EBV): Some research has suggested that increased levels of immune *antibodies* that fight EBV—the very common herpes virus that causes infectious mononucleosis and other disorders—may be associated with an increased risk of developing MS. However, while the evidence supporting this is increasing, the role of EBV as a causative or triggering agent of MS has not yet been established.

- *Smoking:* Several studies have shown an association between smoking and an increased risk of developing MS; smoking may also increase the risk of disease progression.
- *Low levels of vitamin D early in life:* Studies suggest that low levels of vitamin D in a person's blood are associated with a higher risk of developing MS. This finding may explain why people who live closer to the equator during their early years—and therefore experience greater exposure to vitamin D from the sun—are at lower risk for developing MS. Recent research—which is still in need of confirmation—has suggested that high levels of maternal vitamin D during the third trimester of pregnancy may protect offspring from MS.
- *Factors with contradictory research findings:*
  - *Early childhood infections:* Although some studies have found an increased risk of MS in individuals who acquired certain childhood infections later in life, a large-scale study in Denmark found no association between childhood infections (either the total number of infections or the age at which they occurred) and increased risk of MS. The infections studied were measles, rubella, varicella (chicken pox), mumps, pertussis (whooping cough), and scarlet fever.
  - *Chlamydia pneumoniae:* Although some research has suggested that this bacterial agent may be a trigger for MS, the connection has not been proven.
  - *Vaccinations:* Although many people are concerned that vaccinations may cause MS or trigger acute **relapses**, most scientists have concluded that the vaccinations for hepatitis B, influenza, measles, and rubella (German measles) do not play a role in MS onset and are safe for people already diagnosed with the disease. A recent small study suggested an increased risk of relapse in people receiving the yellow fever vaccine. For more information about vaccinations and MS, go to www.nationalmssociety.org/Vaccinations.
  - *Stress:* Researchers continue to explore possible relationships between stress and the onset of MS or MS exacerbations. These studies are complicated by the fact that different types of life stress (e.g., ongoing vs. acute) affect people in very different ways. Although acknowledging that stress affects the functioning of the immune system, the question remains how—and to what degree—varying kinds of stress might influence a person's risk of developing MS or of having relapses. And research on stress is complicated by the difficulty in measuring it accurately.
  - *Cerebrospinal venous flow obstruction* (chronic cerebrospinal venous insufficiency—CCSVI): Recent studies suggest venous flow obstruction is not a primary cause of MS, but may be a consequence of the disease (see Chapter 6). Studies are ongoing to determine the precise relationship, if any, that CCSVI has with MS.
- *Factors found to have no link to the onset of MS:*
  - *Physical trauma:* Although the possible role of physical trauma in MS has been a long-standing subject of controversy, research has demonstrated no link between physical trauma and the onset of MS or MS exacerbations.
  - *Heavy metals:* Studies have shown no link between heavy metal poisoning—from mercury amalgams (dental fillings) or any other source—and the onset of MS.

DO GENETICS PLAY A ROLE IN DETERMINING WHO GETS MS?

We pass on to our children the genes that determine many of their characteristics, including the ways their immune systems behave. In MS, some people may inherit a genetic pattern that makes them more susceptible or reactive to whatever agents are the true causes of MS. And, in response to this environmental trigger, the person's immune system initiates the attack on the *myelin* in the CNS. So, MS is not directly inherited, like blue eyes or brown hair, but the susceptibility to develop the disease is likely determined at least in part by heredity.

The general conclusion is that people of northern and central European ancestry, as well as those whose ancestry has become mingled with this group, seem to have some genetic predisposition to the disease. Current research is trying to identify additional factors that may make people more susceptible to MS, such as specific genetic variants that could be affected by environmental exposures. Although we do not know as yet what factors within the environment cause MS to make its appearance in some of these individuals and not others, most researchers continue to believe that some unidentified infectious agent (e.g., viral or bacterial) is the likely culprit.

IS THERE AN MS GENE, AND CAN PEOPLE BE TESTED FOR IT?

In the 1990s, three large "whole genome" screens focusing on the MS markers were performed in the United States, the United Kingdom, and Canada. The studies were completed and published in 1996. The investigators reported that as many as 20 locations in the human genome may contain genes that contribute to MS susceptibility. Moreover, no single gene was shown to be the major influence on MS susceptibility. Since then, other studies have identified even more possible locations. Larger and more advanced genetic studies are under way using new technology, and results are expected soon. The bottom line, though, is that to date, no test can determine if a child or adult is at increased risk for developing MS.

ARE MY CHILDREN MORE LIKELY TO GET MS BECAUSE I HAVE IT?

The risk of developing MS for anyone in the general population is 1 in 750 or 0.13 percent: That's thirteen-hundredths of a percent. When a person has a close relative with MS—a parent, child, or sibling—the risk rises to 2 to 5 in 100 or approximately 3 percent. Thus, although your children have a higher risk of developing MS than someone in the general population, their risk is still relatively low. These risk estimates are complicated by certain other factors: If there are other people in your family who have MS, then your children's risk would be somewhat higher, because the more people with MS in a family, the greater the risk for other family members. It is unclear whether the sex of the parent with MS affects the child's risk.

WHY DID I GET MS, AND MY IDENTICAL TWIN SISTER DID NOT?

We know that MS is not directly inherited like eye color or hair color. This means that factors other than a person's genetic makeup help to determine if he or she is going to develop MS. Scientists believe that the disease occurs in a genetically susceptible individual only if that person comes into contact with some kind of environmental trigger or triggers. If the disease was directly inherited, then **monozygotic***, or identical twins who come from a single egg and share all the same genes, would both develop MS. Studies of identical twins have demonstrated, however, that when one twin develops MS, the risk for the other twin is only about 25 to 30 percent. The risk for a nonidentical or **dizygotic** twin, who comes from a different egg, is about 3 percent—the same as any close relative.

MY SISTER AND I BOTH HAVE MS, AND WE ALSO HAVE AN AUNT AND A GRANDMOTHER WITH THE DISEASE. WHY DOES OUR FAMILY HAVE SO MANY PEOPLE WITH MS IN IT?
It is important to keep in mind that, if other members of a person's family have virtually any disease—for example, breast cancer, prostate cancer, heart disease, and so on—the person is at greater risk for developing that disease. And the situation is no different in MS; the risk of developing MS is higher for any person who comes from a family in which other family members have the disease. We know from genetic studies that there are some families in which several members have MS—and scientists are interested in studying these families to identify possible clues to the role of genetics in MS. At present, we don't know why some families seem to have several members with MS, while other families have none or only one.

FOUR PEOPLE IN MY HIGH SCHOOL GRADUATING CLASS HAVE MS. WAS THERE SOMETHING ABOUT MY SCHOOL OR MY TOWN THAT MADE THAT HAPPEN?
Whenever several people in close proximity to one another—in the same class, on the same block, in the same town—develop a disease, people begin to wonder if something about that particular environment has caused this apparent "cluster" of cases to occur. It turns out that very few of these suspected disease clusters turn out to be true clusters—and none has ever been proved in MS. Upon investigation, it often turns out that the number of cases does not actually exceed the number that would be expected, given the size of the population. In MS, the investigation of clusters is further complicated by the fact that a significant amount of time may pass between disease onset and diagnosis. So, for example, three or four people in the same town may be diagnosed with MS at the same time, but one or more of them may actually have developed the disease years earlier, and perhaps in a different place.

Possible MS "clusters" have been studied in the Faroe Islands; Galion, Ohio; DePue, Illinois; Rochester, New York; and El Paso, Texas, among others. To date, however, scientists have not been able to confirm any environmental factor that might account for them. In 2002, the federal Agency for Toxic Substances and Disease Registry awarded research grants to five investigators to evaluate possible environmental risk factors for MS and amyotrophic lateral sclerosis in several communities located near hazardous waste sites. These studies are ongoing in Illinois, Texas, Massachusetts, Eastern Washington, and Missouri, but nothing has been found to suggest that MS is linked to hazardous waste.

I WAS JUST DIAGNOSED WITH MS. IS IT GOING TO SHORTEN MY LIFE?
Most people with MS live very close to a normal life span—and most will die of cancer, heart disease, or stroke like everyone else (see Chapter 8 for information

about health and wellness). In rare instances, a person develops a form of MS that is very rapidly progressive, leading to an early death. This form of MS is so severe—and occurs so infrequently—that it is thought by many experts to be separate and distinct from the more typical disease courses (see Chapter 2 for a description of the four disease courses).

People with MS can also develop life-threatening complications, such as intractable urinary tract infections or pneumonia. Fortunately, more is known today about how to treat infections and prevent unnecessary complications so that the life span of a person with MS is significantly longer today than in years past.

Another important factor that contributes to the slightly lower life expectancy for people with MS is the high rate of suicide. Research indicates that the rate of suicide is approximately 7.5 times higher among people with MS than in the general population. Most people assume that this increased rate of suicide relates to the fact that MS is a *chronic*, potentially disabling disease—in other words, that people who become severely disabled over time are more likely to commit suicide. However, studies have shown that the greatest risk factor for suicide in MS is depression, which is a common but highly treatable symptom in people with MS. You can read more about depression—including how it is diagnosed and treated—in Chapter 16.

IS MS CONTAGIOUS? DO I NEED TO WORRY THAT MY FAMILY MEMBERS, FRIENDS, OR COLLEAGUES WILL CATCH THIS DISEASE FROM ME?

No evidence suggests that one person can "catch" MS from another person. You do not need to be concerned that close contact with other people will put them at risk for developing MS.

RECOMMENDED RESOURCES

Kantarci O, Wingerchuk D. Epidemiology and natural history of multiple sclerosis: New insights. *Current Opinion in Neurology.* 2006;19(3):248–254.

Information available from the National Multiple Sclerosis Society (800-344-3867) or online:
- *www.nationalmssociety.org/Brochures:*
  - *Genetics: The Basic Facts*
- *www.nationalmssociety.org/WhoGetsMS*
- *www.nationalmssociety.org/Vaccinations*

Symptom Management at a Glance

Randall Schapiro, MD

An important part of living comfortably with a ***chronic*** illness like multiple sclerosis (MS) is learning how to manage the various kinds of ***symptoms*** that can occur. While the chapters in Part II of this book answer very specific questions about treatment strategies and the health professionals who offer them, this chapter provides an overview of the kinds of symptoms that MS can cause and emphasizes the importance of ongoing management to ensure personal comfort, safety, and independence.

IF THERE IS NO CURE FOR MS, WHY DO I NEED TO BOTHER SEEING A DOCTOR AT ALL?
A close look at medical practice today reveals that relatively few chronic diseases can actually be cured. Most must be treated on an ongoing basis to allow individuals who are living with the disease to function at their best—comfortably and productively. This is particularly true of MS, which can be so varied and unpredictable in its symptoms and associated problems. Periodic medical follow-up will help you manage the symptoms you have to increase your mobility, enhance day-to-day functioning, improve your comfort and, most important, help you avoid needless complications. In addition, these visits with your physician will help to ensure that you have up-to-date, accurate information about available medications and treatments so that you can be an active participant in the management of your MS. You may also be able to learn about upcoming ***clinical trials*** in which you might be eligible to participate (see Chapter 5 for further discussion of clinical trials).

WHAT KIND OF SYMPTOMS CAN MS CAUSE?
Because MS can cause ***inflammation*** and ***demyelination*** throughout the central nervous system (CNS), the list of *possible* symptoms is very long. Fortunately, however, most people never experience all these symptoms, and many experience only a few. Possible symptoms, which can range from mild to severe, include fatigue, visual problems, walking difficulties (due to problems with balance, weakness, stiffness, or numbness in the feet or legs), bowel and bladder changes, sexual problems, pain and other ***sensory*** changes, tremor, problems with speech and swallowing, depression

and other mood changes, and problems with thinking and memory. Any one of these symptoms could be a first sign of MS, and the challenge for people is that there is no way to predict which symptoms will occur, how long they will last, or how severe they will be.

HOW OFTEN DO I NEED TO BE SEEN BY THE DOCTOR?

How frequently you should be seen, and how long a visit should take, will be determined by the types of problems you are experiencing. A person with relatively stable MS who has very few symptoms can probably do well with just a thorough yearly examination. The person who has more complicated symptoms that require ongoing medical management and a *rehabilitation* regimen will need more frequent visits. Because the symptoms of MS can come and go over time, you may find that you need to see your physician more frequently at some times than at others. Of greatest importance is that your questions be answered and that a workable treatment and management strategy be understood and agreed upon by you and your physician.

WHY DO SOME SYMPTOMS COME AND GO, WHILE OTHERS SEEM TO STAY FOR A LONG TIME?

Symptoms of MS initially appear because of inflammation within the brain and spinal cord. The inflammation results in swelling (edema), which can cause symptoms. The symptoms start to go away as the swelling gradually subsides. Sometimes the inflammation in a particular area is severe enough to cause demyelination and *axonal damage*. Once the *axons* have been severely damaged, the symptoms are likely to remain. Symptoms of MS can also worsen temporarily for reasons unrelated to the disease process itself. Temporary elevations in body temperature, such as those caused by infection or overexertion, can cause a person's symptoms to flare until the body temperature returns to normal. Similarly, symptoms may temporarily worsen during periods of intense fatigue and subside following a period of rest. These episodes are called *pseudoexacerbations* because they do not reflect an actual change or progression in the disease.

TO ME, EVERY NEW SYMPTOM FEELS LIKE AN EMERGENCY. HOW DO I KNOW WHEN IT'S IMPORTANT TO CALL THE DOCTOR?

A disease such as MS, with its varied symptom picture and unpredictability, tends to make a person very aware of day-to-day changes in the way he or she feels. Each new symptom or sensation feels strange and perhaps somewhat frightening. In general, if you are experiencing a symptom that is puzzling or bothersome, a telephone call to your doctor is appropriate. As you become more familiar with your MS and the patterns your symptoms tend to follow, you may find that you are comfortable waiting a few days to see if the problem goes away before making the call. Keep track of the changes so that, when you do call your physician, you are able to describe how and when the problem started. Keep in mind that very few MS-related symptoms are medical emergencies and most can be handled safely and effectively during normal working hours.

MY SYMPTOMS ARE SO VARIED AND UNPREDICTABLE THAT IT'S HARD FOR ME TO KNOW WHICH ARE CAUSED BY MS AND WHICH MIGHT BE DUE TO SOME OTHER MEDICAL PROBLEM. HOW DO I KNOW WHICH DOCTOR TO CALL FOR A NEW PROBLEM OR SYMPTOM?

The symptoms of MS can be quite varied, appearing in many different parts of your body. It is important for you to be educated about MS and the types of symptoms it tends to cause so that you can make reasonable judgments about what is MS related and what is not. In general, any symptom that seems to be neurologic, and is not otherwise easily explained by some other common illness, should be reported to the doctor who is treating your MS. Symptoms that are not common in MS, such as chest pain, shortness of breath, stomach pain, and so on, should be discussed with your family physician. Because the ***neurologist*** functions as the principal physician for many people with MS, he or she will make an appropriate referral if the problem you are having is unrelated to your MS.

FATIGUE HAS BECOME MY MOST TROUBLESOME SYMPTOM. SOMETIMES I EVEN FEEL IT RIGHT AFTER I WAKE UP IN THE MORNING. IS THERE ANY TREATMENT FOR THIS PROBLEM?

Fatigue is the most common symptom of MS, with many people reporting it as their most disabling problem. It is, in fact, one of the primary reasons for people with MS leaving the workforce. Several distinct types of fatigue can occur in MS, each with its own management strategy:

- The fatigue that seems to be unique to this disease is also referred to as "lassitude." It is described as an overwhelming tiredness that seems unrelated to activity level or even time of day. While most people report this type of fatigue in the late afternoon or early evening, it can also occur in the morning. And, even though some people find that a brief rest alleviates this fatigue to some degree, others report that it is unaffected by sleep or relaxation. Lassitude of this type often responds to neurochemical medications (see Appendix B) such as Symmetrel (amantadine) and Provigil (modafinil), as well as to a personalized regimen of aerobic exercise. Your physician will try to identify and address all other factors that might be contributing to your fatigue before prescribing one of these medications. Other contributing factors might include:
  - *Temporary muscle fatigue* can occur in an arm or leg following repetitive movements. After walking some distance, for example, you might find that one leg begins to drag and feel very weak. This type of fatigue is caused by a temporary blocking in the ***nerve*** and is best managed by stopping the walk long enough to allow nerve conduction to restart. Cooling strategies may also be beneficial. A new medication called Ampyra (dalfampridine) has been approved by the U.S. Food and Drug Administration (FDA) to improve walking in people with MS. This medication is a potassium channel blocker that helps demyelinated nerve fibers conduct impulses more efficiently. Ampyra has the potential to help over one-third of people (known as "responders") who have walking problems due to weakness, so if you are having difficulty walking, with or without a mobility aid, you may want to ask your physician whether Ampyra might be appropriate for you.

- *Deconditioning fatigue* results when muscles are underutilized. People with MS who experience weakness, heat sensitivity, and fatigue tend to become less active. This inactivity, in turn, leads to greater fatigue and weakness. Therefore, it is important to engage in some form of regular exercise to increase your stamina. Your doctor or ***physical therapist*** can help you design an exercise regimen that is suited to your needs and abilities (see Chapter 9 for more information about physical therapy).
- *Neuromuscular fatigue* results from the impact of MS on muscle control, ***coordination***, strength, and the increased effort and energy needed to accomplish routine tasks. This kind of fatigue is best managed with ***assistive technology*** (e.g., tools and devices to simplify everyday activities and mobility aids to ease ambulation problems).
- *Depression-related fatigue* is very common in anyone experiencing significant depression. This type of fatigue is best managed by addressing the depression itself with a regimen of psychotherapy and, if needed, antidepressant medication.
- *Medication-induced fatigue* can be an unfortunate side effect of some of the medications used in MS. Clearly, the best strategy is to identify the medication that provides the greatest amount of symptom relief with the least amount of associated fatigue. When it is necessary to use a medication that causes significant fatigue, it can be helpful to start with a very low dose, building up gradually to allow your body to become adjusted to it.
- *Fatigue from sleep disturbances* is usually managed by addressing the symptoms or problems that interfere with sound sleep.

WHAT CAUSES THE STIFFNESS IN MY ARMS AND LEGS, AND WHAT IS THE BEST TREATMENT FOR THIS PROBLEM?

Muscle stiffness associated with MS is called ***spasticity***, an increase in muscle tone that can interfere with normal movement of the affected limb even though the strength of that limb might be normal. This increased muscle tone is caused by a dysregulation of nerve impulses in the spinal cord, resulting in too much stimulation to some muscles and too little to others. One of the interesting features of spasticity is that it is "velocity dependent"—which means that the faster you move the arm or leg the stiffer it feels. Therefore, to move efficiently with spasticity the movement must be slow and steady rather than fast and jerky. Spasticity tends to occur most frequently in postural muscles (those that enable us to stand upright), including muscles in the calf, thigh, groin, buttock and, occasionally, the back, but it can also occur in the arms. Spasticity does not need to be treated unless it is uncomfortable or otherwise problematic, and appropriate stretching and range of motion exercises may be enough to relieve very mild stiffness (see Chapter 9).

If exercises alone are too uncomfortable or do not provide adequate relief and mobility, antispasticity medications may be used. A variety of medications are available for this purpose, including Lioresal (baclofen), Zanaflex (tizanidine), Klonopin (clonazepam), Valium (diazepam), Dantrium (dantrolene), and Neurontin (gabapentin). Your physician will select the particular medication best suited for your needs; Lioresal is the drug most commonly used (see Appendix B). The correct dosage of

Lioresal will differ from one individual to another. The goal of treatment is to find the dosage level that provides adequate muscle relaxation without producing excessive fatigue or weakness. Zanaflex has been shown to relieve spasticity without causing muscle weakness, but it tends to be very sedating.

Occasionally, people with MS-related spasticity develop **flexor spasms** or **extensor spasms**. These spasms, which typically last two or three seconds, are disinhibited (hyperactive) spinal *reflexes* that can occur in response to the slightest of noxious stimuli (e.g., the rubbing of bed sheets against the foot during sleep). Flexor spasms cause both legs to pull upward into a clenched position, while extensor spasms cause the legs to straighten into the stiff, extended position. These uncontrolled spasms can be sufficiently intense and sudden to propel the person out of his or her chair. Requip (ropinirole hydrochloride), Mirapex (pramipexole dihydrochloride), Lioresal (baclofen), Neurontin (gabapentin), Valium (diazepam), Klonopin (clonazepam), and Zanaflex (tizanidine) are the medications of choice for the management of this problem (see Appendix B).

In the case of severe spasticity that cannot be managed comfortably or effectively with Lioresal tablets, a pump can be surgically implanted in the abdomen to automatically administer low doses of intrathecal baclofen (baclofen in liquid form) directly into the spinal canal (the **intrathecal space**). The pump's usefulness stems from its ability to reduce spasticity using a much lower dose of medication, thus eliminating the side effects (e.g., severe drowsiness, dizziness, weakness, or nausea) that can occur with higher oral doses.

In some instances of spasticity, Botox (made from botulinum toxin) may be used to block a nerve's function. When Botox is injected into the affected muscle at the point where the nerve enters the muscle, it prevents the nerve from exciting the muscle to contract. Botox, which can be administered by the neurologist, may require repetitive injections to achieve sustained blockage of the nerve. It is best used for focal spasticity in small muscles like those at the ankle or in the upper limbs.

In the past, severe spasticity that did not respond to oral medications, or for which Botox was not suitable, might have required **nerve blocks (motor point blocks)** or even cutting of nerve roots. Fortunately, because of the baclofen pump and other advances in spasticity management, such drastic, irreversible treatment is rarely required.

MY DOCTOR HAS TOLD ME THAT I MAY BE A SUITABLE CANDIDATE FOR A BACLOFEN PUMP. HOW DOES THE PUMP WORK, AND HOW WILL I KNOW IF IT IS THE RIGHT TREATMENT FOR ME?
Your physician may recommend the baclofen pump (SynchroMed Infusion System) if your spasticity is not adequately controlled by oral spasticity medication, or if you are experiencing intolerable side effects such as drowsiness, dizziness, weakness, or nausea. The pump is a surgically implanted device programmed to deliver the prescribed dose of intrathecal baclofen (liquid baclofen) on a continuous basis, directly into the area surrounding your spinal cord (intrathecal space). Because the drug is administered in this way, it is possible to obtain positive results using a lower dose with fewer side effects.

Before implanting the baclofen pump, your doctor will inject a test dose of liquid baclofen into the intrathecal space of your lower back to see how you respond to the medication. The test dose is given in the hospital, so that you can be observed for changes in rigidity and spasms and for any side effects you might experience. If the test dose proves effective, you and your physician will decide whether to proceed with the baclofen pump.

To receive liquid baclofen on a regular, long-term basis, it is necessary to implant a pump and catheter into your body. The pump (a round metal disk weighing about 6 ounces) is placed under the skin of the abdomen during a surgical procedure. A catheter connects the pump to the intrathecal space in your back. The pump is refilled at periodic intervals by injecting the baclofen through your skin into the pump's drug reservoir.

The pump has been shown to be a safe and effective treatment for the management of severe spasticity. Its potential to reduce the discomforts and possible complications associated with spasticity makes it a valuable treatment option for you and your physician to consider. The, pump is, however, an invasive and expensive intervention and should be reserved for those who have not responded to other treatments or have experienced unacceptable side effects.

WHAT ARE CONTRACTURES, AND HOW ARE THEY TREATED?
Contractures are an abnormal, sometimes permanent flexion (bending) of a joint that can occur if significant spasticity goes untreated. When spasticity prevents a limb from moving freely about the joint, some of the muscles and tendons around the joint become shortened. This shortening further constricts movement of the joint. Without treatment, the joint may freeze and become immobilized. Contractures can usually be prevented with a careful regimen of antispasticity medication (e.g., Lioresal [baclofen] or Zanaflex [tizanidine]) and physical therapy techniques designed to maintain joint flexibility, mobility, and full range of motion. Severe contractures may require more drastic treatment measures to reduce the intractable pain, positioning problems, and possible skin complications that can result. For example, surgery may be performed to sever the affected tendon, thus allowing the contracted limb to be straightened. This irreversible procedure is used only in individuals whose prolonged spasticity has resulted in permanent ***paralysis*** of the contracted limbs. By far the best treatment of contractures is to prevent them from occurring in the first place. With the availability of the baclofen pump, this type of unmanageable spasticity should be seen less frequently.

AT NIGHT I EXPERIENCE PAINFUL SPASMS IN MY LEGS THAT MAKE IT VERY HARD FOR ME TO SLEEP. IS THERE ANYTHING I CAN DO ABOUT THIS PROBLEM?
These painful flexor spasms are involuntary muscle contractions that result from spasticity or increased muscle tone. They seem to occur in response to such stimuli as sheets being rubbed over the skin of the lower limbs. Stretching exercises before bedtime may be helpful, but medication is often necessary. Requip (ropinirole hydrochloride), Mirapex (pramipexole dihydrochloride), Lioresal (baclofen), Valium (diazepam), Klonopin (clonazepam), Neurontin (gabapentin), Sinemet (L-dopa/carbidopa), and Zanaflex (tizanidine) are the medications most commonly used to treat these spasms. Valium and Klonopin are somewhat sedating and slowly

metabolized, making them particularly useful for the management of nighttime spasticity. Both these drugs can be habit forming, however, and must therefore be prescribed and used with some caution (see Appendix B).

MY HANDS AND FEET OFTEN GET NUMB OR FEEL LIKE "PINS AND NEEDLES."
ARE THERE ANY MEDICATIONS FOR THIS PROBLEM?
"Pins and needles" are one example of sensory symptoms in MS. Sensory symptoms are those that a person can feel, but for which the physician cannot see objective evidence during the neurologic exam. Other examples include numbness, tingling, decreased or blurred vision, dizziness, or pain. These symptoms occur because of demyelination in the sensory pathways of the spinal cord or brain. Although they can be quite uncomfortable, sensory symptoms are generally considered relatively benign because they tend to come and go without severely restricting a person's ability to function. Although there is no specific medication for most sensory symptoms, anti-seizure medications such as Neurontin (gabapentin), Lyrica (pregabalin), Topamax (topiramate), Trileptal (oxcarbazepine), Tegretol (carbamazepine), and Depakote (valproic acid) may decrease their intensity. A tricyclic antidepressant medication such as Elavil (amitriptyline) can provide some relief, particularly if the symptoms are painful (see Appendix B). In the meantime, remember that these symptoms tend to go away on their own and seldom signal significant *impairment*.

WHAT CAUSES TREMOR IN MS, AND ARE THERE ANY TREATMENTS AVAILABLE FOR IT?
Tremor is an involuntary, relatively rhythmic movement of the arms, legs, or head. While several types of tremor can occur in MS, the most common one results from demyelination in the pathways leading to or from the balance center of the brain (***cerebellum***). Damage in this area of the brain causes an ***intention tremor***, a relatively slow, oscillating (back and forth) movement of a limb engaged in purposeful movement. For example, a person with an intention tremor finds it difficult to perform the ***finger-to-nose test*** on the neurologic exam because the intentional movement of the finger toward the nose triggers a tremor in that arm.

   Tremor is one of the most difficult symptoms to treat and can be among the most disabling. Balance and coordination exercises (see Chapter 9) can help a person to develop compensatory techniques, but the results are far from satisfying. Weights can be placed on the affected limbs to lessen the oscillations somewhat, or weighted utensils can be used for such activities as eating, dressing, and writing (see Chapter 10).

   No medication has been developed specifically for tremor. However, some medications designed to treat other conditions have secondary antitremor properties. These include the beta-blocker Inderal (propranolol), Klonopin (clonazepam), Mysoline (primidone), and BuSpar (buspirone). A medication used for nausea resulting from cancer treatment, Zofran (ondansetron), may be helpful, but is prohibitively expensive on a long-term basis. Although these medications are not usually effective with MS-related tremor, it is impossible to predict who will respond to one or another of the medications and who will not. Therefore, it is worthwhile to try them singly or in combination in an effort to control the tremor.

I TAKE A LOT OF DIFFERENT MEDICATIONS NOW—SOME PRESCRIBED BY MY NEUROLOGIST AND OTHERS BY MY FAMILY DOCTOR. DO I NEED TO BE CONCERNED ABOUT THE INTERACTIONS OF ALL THESE DRUGS?

Everyone must be concerned about the actions and interactions of the drugs they take. Each physician involved in your care must know all the prescription and non-prescription medications that you are taking. Keep a list of all your medications and ask that a copy of that list be included in your medical chart. When the doctor prescribes a new medication for you, feel free to ask about its possible interactions with others you are taking. Many pharmacy computer systems have the capacity to track an individual's prescription medications and automatically detect potential drug interactions. Interaction problems are rare, but it makes good sense to raise the question with your physician and pharmacist. You can refer to the Medication Information Sheets on the National MS Society Web site (www.nationalmssociety.org/meds) for information about the drugs commonly used in MS. It is also recommended that you pay close attention to the pharmacy instruction sheet or "package insert" that comes with each medication or read about your medication(s) in one of the standard drug references.

IS THERE ANY TREATMENT FOR MY BALANCE PROBLEMS? PEOPLE WHO SEE ME ON THE STREET THINK I'M DRUNK.

Balance problems in MS, like tremor, are usually caused by damage in the cerebellum. Balance and coordination exercises may offer some compensatory strategies, but there is no effective treatment at this time for damage to the cerebellum. Assistive devices such as a cane, crutches, or a walker will offer you varying degrees of stability and, just as importantly, tell the world that you are not drunk (see Chapter 9). Many people initially take the emotional plunge of using an assistive device for this reason; they would rather be identified as having a physical impairment than as having had too much to drink.

I HAVE ALWAYS GOTTEN A LOT OF EXERCISE AND BEEN IN PRETTY GOOD SHAPE. NOW I FEEL WEAKNESS IN MY LEGS DESPITE THE EXERCISE. WHAT IS CAUSING THIS WEAKNESS, AND IS THERE ANYTHING I CAN DO ABOUT IT?

Weakness in MS is caused by faulty transmission of impulses from the brain through the spinal cord to the muscle. The problem is not due to a bad or weak muscle. Weakness from poor nerve transmission will not be altered by exercise and, in fact, may seem temporarily aggravated by aggressive exercise that produces fatigue. At the same time, however, inadequate use of the muscle will produce its own kind of weakness, which is really a result of deconditioning. Therefore, an effective exercise program for weakness must include exercises to strengthen the muscles that have adequate nerve conduction, as well as useful movements for those weakened muscles that lack adequate nerve conduction (see Chapter 9).

A new medication called Ampyra (dalfampridine) is used to improve walking in MS. It is a potassium channel blocker that helps demyelinated nerve fibers conduct impulses more efficiently. In the clinical trials leading to its approval by the FDA, in 2010, the medication was found to increase walking speed in a little more than a third of those tested (called "responders").

Weakness in the muscles that lift the foot may lead to "foot drop," which is particularly obvious and bothersome during ambulation. The toes tend to drag, causing the person to trip or fall. Bracing the foot may improve ambulation. Electrical stimulation (e.g., with a Walk-Aide or Bioness) to the nerve going to the foot can provide a similar result if foot drop is the principal reason for the ambulation difficulty (see Chapter 9 for more information about bracing and functional electrical stimulation).

I DON'T SEEM TO SLEEP AS WELL AS I USED TO.
COULD THIS HAVE ANYTHING TO DO WITH MY MS?
Many people with MS report problems with their sleep. For most, "not sleeping well" means that the time spent in bed trying to sleep is substantially greater than the total time they actually sleep. This kind of reduced sleep efficiency often results from an increase in the number of awakenings during the night.

There are many reasons why a person's sleep might be interrupted. We know that periodic limb movements (PLMs) are more common in people with MS than in the general population. Although PLMs are often very slight movements (a flexion of the big toe, for example), they alter the quality of the person's sleep. Therefore, people with MS can have PLMs that interrupt or disturb sleep without even being aware of them. In addition, people with MS are often awakened by spasms in their limbs or the need to urinate. Finally, stress and depression, both of which are quite common in MS, can result in insomnia. There are several kinds of insomnia, including trouble falling asleep, trouble staying asleep, and early morning awakening.

A variety of medications and behavioral strategies are available to manage sleep disturbances. To determine which interventions would be most helpful for you, it is necessary to identify the source(s) of your sleep problems. Talk to your doctor, being as specific as possible about your sleep schedule and habits. Your sleep partner may also be able to provide valuable information about limb movements or spasms that occur during the night. The doctor may refer you to a sleep specialist (usually a physician or psychologist with specific training in this area) if the specific causes of your sleep disturbance are not readily apparent. The sleep specialist will use a variety of techniques to identify the source(s) of your problems and recommend a treatment regimen. It is important to address any sleep problems you are having because they can contribute significantly to your daytime fatigue.

MY MS SEEMS TO GET WORSE EVERY SUMMER. I FEEL SO WEAK AND TIRED
WHEN IT'S HOT THAT I CAN HARDLY MOVE. WHY DOES THIS HAPPEN,
AND IS THERE ANY SOLUTION TO THIS PROBLEM?
For many people, heat temporarily worsens MS symptoms. This can occur with as little as a one-degree elevation in body temperature. There is no evidence that heat actually makes the disease worse. Instead, heat alters nerve conduction (the passage of nerve impulses) and causes a feeling of weakness in the limbs. This same phenomenon often occurs when a person becomes overheated following strenuous exercise or develops an elevated body temperature due to a viral or bacterial infection. In fact, the "hot bath test" for MS was used (before current imaging techniques made

it unnecessary) to capitalize on this heat sensitivity; a person suspected of having the disease was put in a bathtub of hot water to see if MS symptoms could be elicited.

Thus, it is not surprising that the heat and humidity of summer make your symptoms feel worse.

Keeping your body cool helps to alleviate this problem and is certainly the best management strategy for the heat of summer and of a fever. Avoid unnecessary heat—hot showers and sunbathing, for example, are not good activities for someone with MS—and make use of air conditioning, cold drinks, cooling hats or kerchiefs, or a body cooling system like those designed for laborers in heat-intensive occupations. Body cooling systems come in two basic types, and seem to be most helpful for those individuals who are sensitive to the heat rather than to the humidity of summer. The simplest cooling system is a vest designed to hold frozen gel packs in front and back compartments (e.g., Steele Vest). A person can wear this type of vest for driving in a warm car, engaging in outdoor activities, cooking over a hot stove, or just staying cool in a warm house. A somewhat more complex cooling system electronically pumps a cold liquid through a specially designed garment (e.g., the cooling suits made by Life Enhancement Technologies, LLC). The Multiple Sclerosis Association of America provides free cooling vests to individuals who qualify for the program (call 800-523-7667 or email clientservices@ msassociation.org).

WHAT TYPES OF PAIN CAN BE CAUSED BY MS? WHAT ARE THE BEST TREATMENTS FOR THE DIFFERENT TYPES OF PAIN?

Pain in MS falls into two basic categories: primary *(neurogenic)* pain that results directly from demyelination in the CNS, and secondary pain that results indirectly from other MS symptoms.

● Primary *(Neurogenic)* Pain: The demyelination causes distorted and unpleasant sensations—including burning, tingling, itching, and numbness—called *dysesthesias*. One particular type of dysesthesia, called *trigeminal neuralgia*, is caused by damage to the trigeminal nerve that runs down the side of the face. It is often described as a stabbing or shock-like pain along the cheek.

Neurogenic pain does not respond to ordinary pain medications. The preferred treatment is to try to alter the faulty nerve conduction with other types of medications, including antiepileptic drugs such as Neurontin (gabapentin), Lyrica (pregabalin), Tegretol (carbamazepine), Dilantin (phenytoin), and Depakote (valproic acid). Antidepressant medications such as Elavil (amitriptyline) and Cymbalta (duloxetine hydrochloride—which is approved for the treatment of neurogenic pain caused by diabetes) may also relieve the pain (see Appendix B). Some people find that acupuncture and meditation are effective for dysesthesias.

Unusually severe cases of trigeminal neuralgia that do not respond to any of these interventions can also be treated with an outpatient surgical procedure called a *percutaneous rhizotomy*. Under local anesthesia, the surgeon makes a tiny incision in the side of the face and blocks the function of the trigeminal nerve using one of several possible techniques, including laser surgery, cryosurgery (freezing), and cauterization.

● Secondary Pain: A relatively common type of secondary pain or discomfort in MS results from the symptom of spasticity—increased muscle tone and muscle spasms can be quite uncomfortable. Antispasticity medications are the most effective treatment for this type of discomfort.

Secondary orthopedic pain can result from changes in a person's posture or gait. If a person begins to walk or stand differently because of weakness or spasticity, for example, these changes can in turn cause pain in the knees, back, or hips. It is important to identify the causes of this type of secondary pain so that an appropriate treatment regimen of physical therapy, gait training, seating assessment (for someone in a wheelchair), exercise, and pain relief can be implemented.

MY EYE DOCTOR SAYS HE CAN'T GIVE ME GLASSES TO CORRECT THE VISION PROBLEMS CAUSED BY MS. WHAT IS CAUSING MY VISION PROBLEMS, AND WHY CAN'T THEY BE CORRECTED?

Visual symptoms are quite common in MS. They can result from damage to the optic nerve or from an incoordination in the eye muscles, neither of which is correctable with eyeglasses.

● *Damage to the Optic Nerve:* The optic nerve connects the eye to the brain. Inflammation or demyelination in the optic nerve causes *optic neuritis*, which is experienced as a temporary loss or disturbance in vision and possibly pain behind the affected eye. Typically, vision returns partially or fully within a few weeks. Although it is quite rare for a person with MS to become totally blind, it is not at all uncommon for an individual to have recurrent episodes of optic neuritis over the course of the disease, usually in one eye at a time. Damage to the optic nerve can result in a blurring of vision, which may or may not totally resolve. This blurring of vision is not correctable with eyeglasses because it is the result of nerve damage rather than changes in the shape of the eye. Color vision requires a great many nerve fibers from the eye for accurate transmission and is particularly susceptible to changes from demyelination.

Although episodes of optic neuritis typically resolve spontaneously, **acute** loss of vision used to be treated fairly routinely with low doses of oral cortisone to end the episode more quickly. Research has demonstrated that high-dose **corticosteroids** (commonly referred to as "steroids" even though they are different from the steroids talked about in the sports news) such as Solu-Medrol (methylprednisolone) or Decadron (dexamethasone) are more effective in the treatment of optic neuritis. If vision loss is relatively mild and manageable, the best alternative is probably to wait for the episode to remit on its own. However, a course of high-dose steroids may be prescribed if everyday functioning becomes too impaired.

Optic neuritis can cause a large, noticeable "blind spot" in the center of the visual field, and the person experiences a visual image with a dark, blank area in the middle. This is called a central **scotoma** and is not correctable with either eyeglasses or medication, although steroids may be helpful in the early, acute phase.

● *Incoordination of the Eye Muscles*: **Diplopia** (double vision), the experience of seeing two of everything, is caused by weakening or incoordination of eye muscles.

This symptom is typically treated with a short course of steroids. Patching one eye while trying to drive or read will stop the double image; however, permanent patching of the eye will slow the brain's remarkable ability to accommodate to the weakness and produce a single image despite the weakened muscles. Some physicians prescribe eyeglasses with special prisms that help to minimize double vision.

Upon examination, the physician may detect a rhythmic jerkiness or bounce in one or both eyes. This relatively common visual finding in MS is called *nystagmus*. Nystagmus does not always cause symptoms of which the person is aware. In the event that it does become troublesome, Klonopin (clonazepam) is sometimes effective in reducing this annoying but painless problem.

I HAVE DEVELOPED A LOT OF PROBLEMS WITH MY MEMORY AND THINKING IN THE LAST FEW YEARS. IS THERE ANY MEDICATION I CAN TAKE TO HELP WITH THESE PROBLEMS?

Some degree of measurable cognitive change occurs in 50 to 60 percent of people with MS. Fortunately, the majority of these changes progress quite slowly and are relatively mild. For a complete discussion of *cognition* in MS, please refer to Chapter 14.

The answer to your specific question is that no medication has been shown to resolve memory problems. Early and ongoing use of one of the approved disease-modifying therapies (see Chapter 6) may help slow the progression of cognitive problems. Although cognitive changes in MS are not related to time since diagnosis or level of physical disability, they have been found to correlate with *lesion* load—the total amount of lesion area in the brain. Because all the approved disease-modifying therapies have been shown to reduce the number of relapses a person experiences, as well as the number of new lesions on magnetic resonance imaging, it is reasonable to conclude that they might also slow the progression of cognitive changes.

You and your doctor should also be alert to any signs of depression, which can sometimes mimic changes in cognition and are far more amenable to treatment.

SOMETIMES THE TREATMENT I GET FOR ONE SYMPTOM MAKES ANOTHER PROBLEM WORSE (E.G., MY BLADDER MEDICATIONS CAUSE *CONSTIPATION* AND MAKE MY MOUTH UNCOMFORTABLY DRY, THE ANTIDEPRESSANT I TAKE INTERFERES WITH MY SEX LIFE, THE MEDICATION I TAKE FOR PAIN MAKES ME SLEEPY). HOW CAN I LEARN MORE ABOUT THESE SIDE EFFECTS SO THAT I CAN MAKE REASONABLE DECISIONS ABOUT WHAT IS BEST FOR ME?

Side effects are very common with certain medications and should be discussed with your physician. The MS health care team is quite knowledgeable about frequently used medications and has a great deal of experience with people's reactions to them. Using the information you give them about your symptoms, as well as feedback about the positive and not so positive responses you are having to the medications, your health care team can help you maximize the positive treatment effects while minimizing side effects. They will usually be able to reduce any unpleasant side effects to a manageable level with minor adjustments in level and timing of dosages. For additional information about medication side effects, you can refer to the Medication

Information Sheets at www.nationalmssociety.org/meds, read the "package insert" available at your pharmacy, or consult a drug reference book or online computer service for information about a particular medication that has been prescribed for you (e.g., www.medlineplus.gov).

I'VE READ THAT PEOPLE WHO AREN'T VERY MOBILE ARE AT GREATER RISK FOR OSTEOPOROSIS. I AM NOW IN A WHEELCHAIR MOST OF THE TIME. HOW CAN I PREVENT OSTEOPOROSIS, AND WHAT IS THE TREATMENT FOR IT?

Osteoporosis, defined as a gradual loss of calcium from the bones, which causes them to be fragile and easily broken, is caused by a combination of factors. Hormones, vitamins, genetic predisposition, and level of physical activity all play a role. Any person—female or male—who has decreased mobility, particularly a loss of weight-bearing activity (as would be true of a person using a wheelchair most of the time) must be concerned about osteoporosis. Postmenopausal women are also at increased risk of osteoporosis. In addition, excessive or prolonged use of steroids can lead to osteoporosis. Talk to your physician about your risk for osteoporosis and the advisability of a baseline evaluation to determine the health of your bones. You may be referred to a physical therapist for a regimen of weight-bearing exercises to enhance bone strength, given dietary recommendations, and possibly medications, to enhance bone strength. Do not begin any exercise program or medication regimen without first consulting your physician.

RECOMMENDED RESOURCES

BOOKS

Holland N, Halper J. (eds.). *Multiple Sclerosis: A Self-Care Guide to Wellness* (2nd ed.). New York: Demos Medical Publishing, 2005.

Kalb R, Holland N, Giesser B. *Multiple Sclerosis for Dummies.* Hoboken, NJ: Wiley Publishing, 2007.

LaRocca N, Kalb R. *Multiple Sclerosis: Understanding the Cognitive Challenges.* New York: Demos Medical Publishing, 2006.

Lowenstein N. *Fighting Fatigue in Multiple Sclerosis.* New York: Demos Medical Publishing, 2009.

Schapiro R. *Symptom Management in Multiple Sclerosis* (5th ed.). New York: Demos Medical Publishing, 2007.

NATIONAL MS SOCIETY RESOURCES

Brochures available by calling 800-344-3867 or online at *www.nationalmssociety.org/ Brochures:*

- *Bowel Problems: The Basic Facts*
- *Controlling Bladder Problems in MS*
- *Controlling Spasticity in MS*
- *Depression and MS*
- *Fatigue: What You Should Know*
- *Gait or Walking Problems: The Basic Facts*
- *MS and the Mind*

- *Pain: The Basic Facts*
- *Sleep Disorders and MS: The Basic Facts*
- *Solving Cognitive Problems*
- *Speech and Swallowing: The Basic Facts*
- *Tremor: The Basic Facts*
- *Vision Problems: The Basic Facts*

Information about MS symptoms and their management available at
www.nationalmssociety.org/Symptoms

MS Learn Online programming about symptom management and other issues available at
www.nationalmssociety.org/mslearnonline

Part II

How Is Multiple Sclerosis Treated?

To most people, being "treated" for an illness means that they report their symptoms to a physician, follow the doctor's orders, and get better. In another familiar scenario, the person gets a cold or the flu, goes to the pharmacy for some medications to relieve discomfort, and waits patiently for the virus to run its course. In the case of physical injury, the treatment may be even more direct and clear-cut. The person who temporarily cannot walk because of a broken leg is treated for the injury, and walking ability is restored. Of course, the best strategy of all is a vaccine to prevent the disease in the first place.

At present, none of these familiar notions of treatment apply in multiple sclerosis (MS): We are unable to prevent the illness from occurring, we do not know how to cure it, efforts to restore lost functions are still in their infancy, and the disease is a chronic one that does not just go away on its own. The good news is that exciting progress is being made on every front. While efforts continue in the scientific community to find the answers we are all waiting for, the day-to-day treatment of MS includes five important strategies:

- Management of MS relapses
- Management of the disease course
- Management of MS symptoms
- Rehabilitation
- Psychosocial support

In this part of the book, we answer the most frequently asked questions about each of these treatment strategies, beginning with a chapter that describes the lengthy steps involved in developing a new treatment.

How Multiple Sclerosis Treatments Are Developed

Robert Herndon, MD

Those with multiple sclerosis (MS), their caregivers, and the health care profession-als who treat them are impatient for treatments that are more effective than those we have today, and for a cure. To understand why efforts to find a cure or more effec-tive treatment for MS have been so frustrating, it is important to review some of the characteristics of the disease. Although we believe MS to be an ***autoimmune disease*** that is triggered in genetically susceptible individuals by some infectious agent in the environment (see Chapter 2), we do not yet have any definitive answers. There is good epidemiologic evidence that Epstein-Barr virus (the virus that causes infectious mononucleosis) is somehow involved in many instances but it does not appear to be, in and of itself, the cause of MS. Not knowing the cause of a disease makes looking for ways to prevent or cure it significantly more challenging. In addition, the disease tends to progress slowly in most individuals, with ***symptoms*** that are highly variable from one person to the next. These characteristics make it difficult for researchers to know how to evaluate the efficacy of any particular treatment. If the disease mani-fests itself differently from one person to the next, what symptom or other aspect of the disease should be evaluated to determine if a treatment is working?

Furthermore, although a review of treatments used in MS over the 15-year period from 1935 to 1950 indicated that 66 percent of the patients improved, none of these interventions have been shown over time to be any more effective than no treatment at all. Other studies have demonstrated that 70 percent of individuals treated for a recent worsening of their disease will improve, at least temporarily, with a ***placebo*** or inactive medication. Thus, treatment of a recent ***relapse*** (also called an ***exacer-bation*** or ***attack***) in MS can only be considered effective if it leads to long-lasting improvement in significantly more than 70 percent of people who are given it. This brings us back to the question of measuring the outcomes obtained when evaluating experimental treatments. Recent research efforts have targeted the number of exac-erbations, length of exacerbations, length of time between exacerbations, severity of exacerbations, progression of disability, and the total area or volume of ***plaques*** (also called *lesions* or *scars*) shown on magnetic resonance imaging (MRI) as reasonable indicators of an "effective" treatment in ***relapsing-remitting MS***.

In 1981, at the first international conference on therapeutic trials in MS, it was clear that only one successful treatment trial in MS met the scientific standards of its time. That trial of corticotropin hormone (ACTH) demonstrated that ACTH could shorten attacks even though it had no effect on the ultimate degree of recovery or long-term disability (see Chapter 6 for more information about ACTH). Since that time, there have been numerous high-quality drug trials in MS. More *clinical trials* are currently in progress in North America and Europe than at any time in the history of the disease. For an up-to-date list of ongoing trials, visit the Research section of the National MS Society Web site at www. nationalmssociety.org/ClinicalTrials. These include small-scale (fewer than 20 patients) and large-scale (many hundred patients) trials, targeting *acute attacks* as well as relapsing-remitting, *secondary-progressive*, and *primary-progressive MS*. They involve experimental therapies designed to affect immune function, fight infectious agents, restore *myelin*, and improve symptoms. The trials are evaluating new drugs, old drugs, drugs used primarily in other diseases, and drug combinations. In addition, treatments that have already been approved for use in MS are being compared to one another.

This is an exciting time for individuals with MS and their health care providers. Before 1993, no approved treatments for preventing attacks or slowing disability progression in MS existed. Since 1993, eight drugs have been approved by the *U.S. Food and Drug Administration (FDA)* for the treatment of MS following rigorous, high-quality clinical trials (see Chapter 6):

- Betaseron (*interferon* beta-1b) in 1993
- Avonex (interferon beta-1a) in 1996
- Rebif (interferon beta-1a) in 1998
- Copaxone (glatiramer acetate) in 1996
- Novantrone (mitoxantrone) in 2000
- Tysabri (natalizumab) in 2006
- Extavia (interferon beta-1b—identical formulation to Betaseron) in 2009
- Gilenya (fingolimod) in 2010

WHAT MAKES IT SO DIFFICULT FOR SCIENTISTS TO FIND A CURE FOR MS?
Physicians and researchers have found it difficult to find a cure for MS because the underlying cause of the illness is not known. Current thinking is that some "environmental" trigger (a viral infection, for example) initiates a process in which the individual's *immune system* inappropriately attacks the *myelin* in his or her own *central nervous system (CNS)*. This process is thought to occur more readily in people born with a genetic predisposition to the disease. Because we do not know the exact triggers for the initial and ongoing immunologic assault, it is difficult to devise specific treatments to prevent it.

The ultimate result of the immunologic process in MS is damage to the myelin and destruction of *nerve* fibers (*axons*). Whereas myelin has the potential to regenerate to some degree, and is known to do so early in the course of the disease, damaged axons do not regenerate. This explains why much of the function lost during acute attacks early in the disease tends to be recovered; the remaining nerve fibers compensate for those that are lost. As the disease progresses, however, cumulative damage to myelin and nerve fibers leads to increasing, persistent neurologic dysfunction.

TABLE 5-1. Summary Table of Steps Involved in the Development of a New Drug

• Preclinical phase	Animal studies
• Phase I	Preliminary human clinical trials—small, unblinded, open-label trials (for evaluating safety)
• Phase II	Small human clinical trials—often *double-blind*—for gathering efficacy data and additional safety data
• Phase III	Large, multicenter, randomized, double-blind, *placebo*-controlled trials needed for FDA approval
• Data analysis	
• Application for approval of drug by the FDA	
• Pharmaceutical company brings drug to market	

FDA, Food and Drug Administration.

Insufficient nerve fibers are left to carry out normal functions, and permanent weakness, numbness, visual loss, or other problems begin to occur.

Research has also demonstrated that some degree of brain *atrophy*, or shrinkage, occurs in MS, even in the early years of the illness. This results from loss of nerves and nerve fibers, scars that occur in the damaged areas that shrink over time, and probably other poorly understood processes. At present, we do not know how to repair or restore myelin or replace axons. We are, therefore, unable to reverse the neurologic symptoms—that is, cure the disease. Research has demonstrated, however, that mammals, including humans, have the capacity for spontaneous repair of CNS myelin. To take advantage of that natural repair process, some scientists are working to identify and reduce those mechanisms that have been shown to inhibit neural repair, while others are working simultaneously to identify and mimic the natural mechanisms that stimulate neural repair.

ONCE A PROMISING NEW TREATMENT HAS BEEN IDENTIFIED, WHY DOES IT TAKE SUCH A LONG TIME FOR IT TO BE AVAILABLE FOR PEOPLE WITH MS?

Unfortunately, the process of new drug development is very slow, particularly for a chronic disease like MS. The typical sequence begins with animal studies (see Table 5-1), often using an experimental, animal model of MS, *experimental allergic encephalomyelitis*, which exists in laboratory rodents (as well as other species). These studies allow a quick assessment of the possible benefits of a treatment, as well as the preliminary evaluation of its safety. A promising agent then moves into human *clinical trials*.

● Human clinical trials begin with very small open-label (unblinded) trials in which the physicians and subjects know what drug is being taken. These trials, which are usually done first in individuals without known disease in order to demonstrate the safety of a treatment, may then be followed by an open-label trial in a few patients with known disease. These trials are typically of much shorter duration than later studies, but still take many months to a year or longer because of the variable nature of MS.

- The open-label trials are then followed by relatively small, usually double-blind, Phase II pilot trials that are designed to give stronger evidence of a new treatment's effectiveness and safety. "Double-blind" means that neither the subject nor the investigators know which subjects are receiving the real medication and which are getting the placebo (an inactive substance). This procedure is followed to prevent hopes and expectations on the part of researchers or subjects from affecting the course or evaluation of the treatment.

- If the drug still appears promising, testing will move into Phase III, involving large, multicenter, randomized, placebo-controlled, double-blind trials. In this stage of drug development, typically hundreds of subjects are entered into a study in which some are randomly assigned to receive the medication and others to get placebo. Now that we have many approved treatments for MS, many of the large-scale controlled trials compare a new treatment to an existing treatment rather than—or in addition to—a placebo. Because MS is a chronic disease, in which changes occur relatively slowly in most people, these Phase III trials typically last for several years to obtain enough information on which to base fair and statistically valid conclusions. These trials are expensive, costing many millions of dollars that are essentially wasted if the drug does not work or proves to be more dangerous than is acceptable. The high cost of clinical trials accounts, in part, for the high cost of new drugs.

- Following the completion of the trial, another 6 months may be necessary to analyze the large quantity of data and prepare submission of documents to the FDA (or, in other countries, to their equivalent regulatory agency). The FDA, which is ultimately responsible for the approval of new drugs in the United States, carefully reviews both the data and the methodology of the trial. This agency must be convinced of both the effectiveness and safety of the treatment before giving its approval. The review process typically takes another 6 to 12 months. Finally, after approval of a drug, the pharmaceutical company typically needs a few more months to get the drug to market.

Thus, the process is extremely long and arduous, as well as very frustrating for people with MS and for their families. For example, beta-interferon trials began in 1981, yet the initial approval of Betaseron did not occur until 1993. However, it is a process designed to assure that everyone receives safe treatments and that no one misses out on the opportunity to take other, potentially useful treatments while taking something that is ineffective.

The problem with many of the publicly acclaimed "treatments" that receive so much attention in the press (e.g., snake venom, venous stenting to treat *chronic cerebrospinal venous insufficiency* [CCSVI; see Chapter 6], and the removal of tooth amalgams) is that they have not been through this process. In other words, they have not been proven to be safe or effective in a clinical trial and some of these unproven remedies can be dangerous or harmful. For example, venous stents have been known to come loose and wind up in the heart causing death or requiring open heart surgery for removal.

WHAT IS THE "PLACEBO EFFECT?"

A placebo is a nonactive substance designed to look just like the drug that is being evaluated in a research protocol. Investigators repeatedly find that a substantial proportion of people with a variety of diseases experience some benefit even when they are treated with a placebo. This phenomenon is known as the *placebo effect*. Although this effect may occur in part through unconscious psychological mechanisms, some studies have also demonstrated the production of certain chemicals in such individuals that may contribute to this improvement. Even though the benefits are not usually sustained, this short-lived effect confounds the study of new drugs. Randomized, placebo-controlled, double-blind trials are used to determine the advantage (if any) that the new drug shows over placebo effects. Thus, to demonstrate the value of a new treatment, it must be proven to have a benefit superior to that offered by a placebo.

It is important to remember that being treated with a placebo is not the same as receiving no treatment. Taking the placebo fosters certain expectations for improvement that are not present when no treatment is given. Thus, new drugs are either compared with a placebo or with an existing treatment, rather than with no treatment at all. The drug must demonstrate a specific benefit beyond the placebo effect or the improvement that might occur spontaneously with no treatment or with an existing treatment.

Now, with the availability of several approved treatments for relapsing forms of MS, it is likely that most future trials will compare a new drug with an existing drug rather than with placebo, to ensure that participants are either receiving the new, experimental treatment or an approved treatment known to be effective. Neither people with MS nor their physicians would want them to risk being on an inactive placebo over a prolonged period when effective treatments are available.

WHO DESIGNS CLINICAL TRIALS AND DECIDES WHEN AND WHERE THEY WILL TAKE PLACE, AND WHO CAN PARTICIPATE?

Clinical trials may originate from several different sources. Early trials are often initiated by investigators interested in MS, whereas more definitive trials of promising new treatments are generally undertaken by pharmaceutical companies interested in marketing a product. Although these companies often have physicians and basic scientists in their direct employment, they usually recruit outside investigators to help plan a clinical trial. Then, depending on the size of the study, additional investigators are invited to participate in the trial in order to enter the required number of subjects as quickly as possible. The lead investigators design the protocol or format for the trial, deciding how the trial will be carried out and who will be eligible to participate. The design of the trial is then submitted to the FDA for approval before the trial is begun.

HOW CAN I GET INTO A CLINICAL TRIAL?

Various sources of information about clinical trials are available (see Resources at the end of the chapter). The best place to start is with your own physician, who will often be able to direct you to a particular trial. Studies that are recruiting subjects are listed on the National Multiple Sclerosis Society Web site at www.nationalmssociety.

org/ClinicalTrials. Additional information is available at www.clinicaltrials.gov, a database produced and maintained by the U.S. National Institutes of Health. Some of the chapters of the National Multiple Sclerosis Society publish newsletters in which they announce trials in their area. NARCOMS (North American Research Consortium on MS) is a registry that people with MS can join if they are interested in participating in a clinical trial. It is important to remember that each trial has a very specific protocol that details the types of patients who are eligible to participate. For some trials, the eligibility criteria are quite restrictive; for others, the criteria are more liberal. Your willingness to participate in a clinical trial is greatly appreciated by investigators, because successful completion of such studies is the only way that we will definitively identify effective new treatments. Do not be discouraged if you do not meet the entrance criteria for a particular trial. Keep informed—the next one might be right for you.

WHY SHOULD I PARTICIPATE IN A CLINICAL TRIAL IF I HAVE A SIGNIFICANT CHANCE OF GETTING THE PLACEBO INSTEAD OF THE REAL DRUG?

There are several reasons to participate in clinical trials:

- It has been demonstrated repeatedly in MS trials that even those subjects who receive the placebo usually do better than they would have done without any intervention. The quality of medical care in trials tends to be very high, and it is provided without cost to the participants.
- Clinical trials are the best mechanism currently available to identify effective treatments; therefore, your participation ultimately helps investigators answer important questions.
- Standard, accepted treatments continue to be allowed under the research protocols of most placebo-controlled trials. For example, acute exacerbations could be treated with *corticosteroids* in the Betaseron (interferon beta-1b), Avonex (interferon beta-1a), Rebif (interferon beta-1a), Copaxone (glatiramer acetate), and Gilenya (fingolimod) trials.
- With eight drugs currently available in the United States and Canada, we are gradually shifting away from placebo-controlled trials in MS to drug-comparison trials in which a proposed new drug is compared with an effective drug that is already available. Thus, any proposed new drug would have to demonstrate its superiority over those that have already been approved for use. Participants in this type of drug-comparison trial would therefore be randomly assigned to either the proposed drug or one that has already been shown to be effective in treating MS.

WHY DO SO MANY CLINICAL TRIALS REQUIRE THAT PARTICIPANTS BE ABLE TO WALK?

The entrance criteria for particular trials are very specific. Many of the trials require that subjects be able to walk, sometimes without the use of walking aids. This requirement is made because it is often more difficult to detect changes in disease activity in individuals whose illness is more advanced, and the inclusion of people with more advanced disease might cause investigators to discard potentially useful treatments because they erroneously failed to detect a benefit.

TABLE 5-2. New Medications Currently in Clinical Trials

	Type(s) of MS
Oral agents	
Albuterol	Relapsing forms
Alemtuzumab	Relapsing forms
BG-12 (dimethyl fumarate)	Relapsing forms
Cladribine	Relapsing forms
Estriol	Relapsing forms
Gilenya (Fingolimod)	Primary progressive
Idebenone	Primary progressive
Lipitor (atorvastatin)	CIS
Minocin (minocycline)	CIS
Teriflunomide	Relapsing forms; CIS
Laquinomod	Relapsing forms
Rilutek (riluzole)	Early MS; CIS
Injected agents	
Pegylated interferon beta-1α	Relapsing forms
Monoclonal antibodies	
Alemtuzumab (Campath)	Relapsing forms
Ocrelizumab	Relapsing forms
Daclizumab (Zenapax)	Relapsing, SPMS

CIS, ***clinically isolated syndrome*** (first demyelinating event suggestive of MS); MS, multiple sclerosis; PPMS, primary-progressive MS; RRMS, relapsing-remitting MS; SPMS, secondary-progressive MS.

ARE ANY NEW MEDICATIONS BEING EVALUATED IN CLINICAL TRIALS?
A number of drugs are in clinical trials at the present time—probably more than at any time in history (see Table 5-2). Some of these drugs have been around for some time but are undergoing further study; others are new agents that have not yet been used to treat people with MS. In one way or another, all these drugs work to reduce ***inflammation*** in the brain and spinal cord. Many suppress the immune system in a general, nonspecific way. Others, such as ***monoclonal antibodies***, have highly specific effects on the immune system. All these agents are extremely potent, and all carry some risks. Only time will tell which are effective for people with MS and how safe they will prove to be.

For more information about ongoing clinical trials in MS, go to www.clinicaltrials. gov or www.nationalmssociety.org/ClinicalTrials.

RECOMMENDED READINGS

Quinn S. *Human Trials: Scientists, Investors, and Patients in the Quest for a Cure.* New York: Perseus Publishing, 2001.
Weiner HL. *Curing MS: How Science is Solving the Mysteries of Multiple Sclerosis.* New York: Crown Publishing, 2004.

RECOMMENDED RESOURCES

CenterWatch: A publishing and information services company that provides information on clinical trials, including a list of MS studies currently recruiting patients (www.centerwatch.com)

MS-CORE: A cooperative of investigators dedicated to fostering multicenter, investigator-led clinical research aimed at improving care for persons with MS. Established with funding from the National Multiple Sclerosis Society (www. ms-core.org)

Multiple Sclerosis International Federation (MFIS): Offers extensive information about clinical trials (www.msif.org/en/research/clinical_trials)

NARCOMS: The North American Research Consortium on MS is a database of individuals willing to participate in MS research, including clinical trials (narcoms@mscare.org)

National Multiple Sclerosis Society: Offers an overview of the clinical trial process and information about trials that are recruiting participants at www.nationalmssociety.org/ClinicalTrials

National Institutes of Health (NIH): Maintains a registry and results database of federally and privately supported clinical trials conducted in the United States and around the world (www. clinicaltrials.gov)

Considering Options for Managing Relapses and the Disease Course

Aaron Miller, MD

Although we do not yet have a way to cure multiple sclerosis (MS) or completely stop its progression, much can still be done to manage the disease. Two important components of MS treatment include reducing disease activity as much as possible with a disease-modifying medication and managing the **relapses** (also called exacerbations or attacks) that occur in spite of the best available disease-management strategies. In this chapter, we answer the questions most commonly asked about the options for managing the disease course and treating MS attacks.

MANAGEMENT OF RELAPSES

SOMETIMES, WHEN I HAVE A RELAPSE, MY DOCTOR PRESCRIBES INTRAVENOUS STEROIDS (E.G., SOLU-MEDROL). WHY ARE STEROIDS PRESCRIBED, AND HOW DOES MY DOCTOR DECIDE WHEN I NEED THEM AND WHEN I DON'T?

Corticosteroids (also referred to as "steroids") are a group of chemicals, some of which are naturally occurring hormones. They have many important hormonal functions, but they have various additional effects when administered as medications (usually in synthetic preparations). Their usefulness in MS stems from their ability to decrease **inflammation** in the central nervous system (CNS), at least in part by closing the damaged **blood–brain barrier**. The steroids used in MS should not be confused with the anabolic steroids used by athletes to build muscle; the corticosteroids used in MS suppress inflammation.

Under normal circumstances, many potentially damaging substances are prevented by the blood–brain barrier from passing out of the bloodstream into the brain and spinal cord. During attacks of MS, this barrier can break down and allow damaging chemicals and cells to leak into the CNS. This leakage produces inflammation that results in both **acute** neurologic injury—sometimes with accompanying **symptoms**—and **chronic** damage to **myelin** and **axons**. Steroids appear to decrease this inflammation.

Since most MS relapses eventually resolve on their own, MS specialists tend to prescribe corticosteroids only if the attack is severe enough to interfere with a person's functioning—for example, if you are having problems with seeing or walking that interfere with work or parenting activities. A mild attack of ***sensory*** changes (e.g., numbness and tingling) or weakness on one side might not require treatment unless you are very uncomfortable.

HOW DO STEROIDS TAKEN ORALLY DIFFER FROM STEROIDS TAKEN INTRAVENOUSLY?
Most ***neurologists*** caring for people with MS believe that a regimen of high-dose corticosteroids is the best treatment for those relapses that require treatment. However, there is some difference of opinion among MS specialists about whether the medication should be delivered *intravenously* (directly in the vein) or orally. They also differ in their opinions about the exact dosage used, the timing of the treatment, and whether or not to use a gradual tapering dose of oral steroids following the short, high-dose regimen.

The most common regimen used today is 500 to 1,000 mg of intravenous Solu-Medrol (methylprednisolone) for 3 to 5 days, with or without a tapering dose of oral steroids (most often prednisone) for 1 to 3 weeks. This high-dose treatment regimen is preferred because data from ***clinical trials*** indicate that it is more effective than a low-dose regimen. Although clinical studies have demonstrated the safety of high-dose steroids given orally, we still do not have studies that clearly demonstrate their effectiveness.

Some MS specialists opt to treat milder exacerbations with a 10- to 12-day course of low-dose oral steroids. However, the evidence to support the use of low-dose steroids is not clear.

I FEEL MUCH STRONGER WHILE I'M TAKING STEROIDS, BUT MY DOCTOR SAYS THEY SHOULD NOT BE USED FREQUENTLY OR FOR VERY LONG PERIODS. WHY NOT?
Continuous administration of steroids has never been shown to provide long-term benefits for people with MS. There is some suggestion that periodic short courses of high-dose steroids (referred to as "pulse steroids") may have a longer-term benefit in delaying further disease activity, but the research findings are not conclusive. Many people feel better while taking steroids, in part, because these drugs can have a mood-elevating effect. However, the chronic use of steroids is fraught with many potentially dangerous side effects and is currently thought to be unwise in the treatment of MS. Their long-term use can be associated with such side effects as hypertension, diabetes, bone loss (***osteoporosis***), cataracts, and ulcers. These potential detrimental effects outweigh the possible benefits when steroids are used on an extended basis.

WHEN I TAKE STEROIDS, I GET VERY EMOTIONAL AND HAVE INTENSE MOOD SWINGS. I ALSO FEEL VERY DOWN OR DEPRESSED TOWARD THE END OF THE TREATMENT. WHY DOES THIS HAPPEN, AND IS THERE ANYTHING TO DO ABOUT IT?
Short courses of steroids, even in very high doses, are usually well-tolerated. Many people, however, do have some minor mood changes, both highs and lows. Others may have difficulty sleeping. A much smaller group of individuals may have more severe disturbances in mood or behavior. Eskalith (lithium), a medication often prescribed for people with bipolar disorder (formerly called manic-depressive disorder), is sometimes used to prevent or manage these mood swings. Tegretol (carbamazepine)

and Depakote (divalproex) have also been shown to be very effective. On occasion, antidepressant medications may be prescribed, but they are seldom needed because the "blues" associated with a short course of steroids usually disappear spontaneously before the antidepressants would begin to take effect (usually a few weeks).

ARE OTHER TREATMENT STRATEGIES AVAILABLE IF A RELAPSE DOES NOT RESPOND TO INTRAVENOUS CORTICOSTEROIDS?

The vast majority of people experiencing acute attacks respond well to the standard high-dose corticosteroid treatment. Another treatment, called plasma exchange or *plasmapheresis*, may be used in the case of a severe exacerbation that has not responded to steroid treatment. Plasmapheresis involves the following steps:

- Whole blood—which is part liquid (plasma) and part solid (red and white blood cells)—is withdrawn from the person's body.
- The liquid portion of the blood—the plasma—is separated from the solid portion and replaced by an artificial plasma (made from albumin).
- The new plasma is combined with the person's red and white blood cells and transfused back into the person.

This process is a successful method for treating some autoimmune diseases such as myasthenia gravis and Guillain-Barré syndrome because it removes the circulating antibodies that are thought to be active in these diseases. Because MS is also thought to involve an autoimmune process, and because damaging factors have been found in plasma from people with MS, plasmapheresis has been studied as a treatment for MS.

In 2011, the American Academy of Neurology issued a revised set of guidelines concerning the use of plasmapheresis in autoimmune diseases, including MS. The guideline specifically states that plasmapheresis may be useful as a secondary therapy for people who experience a severe relapse that does not respond to treatment with corticosteroids.

The plasma exchange procedure can be performed at most major medical centers, sometimes without hospitalization. It usually involves seven treatments over a 14-day period and can be very costly. The procedure carries with it certain risks, including anemia and infection, so it will continue to be used primarily for those unusual exacerbations that do not respond to steroid treatment.

IF I HAVE A RELAPSE WHILE I'M TAKING A DISEASE-MODIFYING THERAPY TO MANAGE MY MS, CAN I STILL BE GIVEN INTRAVENOUS STEROIDS?

Individuals taking any of the medications approved by the U.S. Food and Drug Administration (FDA) to manage their MS can still be treated with intravenous steroids in the same manner as those not on any of these medications.

MANAGING THE DISEASE COURSE

WHAT MEDICATIONS HAVE BEEN APPROVED TO TREAT MS?

As of the printing of this book, eight medications have been approved by the FDA to treat MS. Of these, five are delivered by injection, one is taken orally, and two are delivered by intravenous (into the vein) infusion. Each group of medications will be described here, but you can obtain the most current information about disease-modifying therapies by calling the National MS Society at 800-344-4867 or online at www.nationalMSsociety.org/DMD.

While these medications differ in several ways, including route of delivery, dosing and schedule, short-term side effects, and longer-term risks, they have all been shown in *controlled clinical trials* to reduce the frequency of exacerbations and development of lesions in the brain as seen on MRI (magnetic resonance imaging) in relapsing forms of MS. They also appear to slow down the accumulation of disability. Unfortunately, none of these medications has been found to be of benefit in *primary-progressive MS* (PPMS), a disease course that is progressive from the beginning, without relapses.

These medications, which are generally taken on a long-term basis, are the best defense currently available to slow the natural course of MS. Even though the disease-modifying medications are not designed to treat symptoms and do not generally make a person feel better, they can be looked upon as an investment in the future.

Injectable Medications

The injectable medications were the first to become available for the management of the disease course in MS. Since the first of these medications—Betaseron (interferon beta-1b)—came to market in 1993, the injectables have been the mainstay of MS treatment. They have proven to be safe and effective medications and are considered by most MS experts to be the first-line option for most people with MS.

Of the five injectable medications, four are interferon-beta products:

Avonex (interferon beta-1a) is administered once a week by intramuscular (into the muscle) injection.

Rebif (a different formulation of interferon beta-1a) is administered three times a week by subcutaneous (under the skin) injection.

Betaseron and *Extavia* (identical formulations of interferon beta-1b) are administered every other day by subcutaneous injection. (Note: Because Extavia is identical to Betaseron, the FDA did not require it to be tested in clinical trials before approving it in 2009.)

All of these medications are approved for use in relapsing forms of MS—which includes *relapsing-remitting MS* (RRMS), as well as *secondary-progressive MS* (SPMS) and *progressive-relapsing MS* (PRMS) in those individuals who are experiencing relapses. Each has also been shown to be effective in delaying a second inflammatory, demyelinating episode, and, therefore, a confirmed diagnosis of MS in those individuals who have a clinically isolated syndrome (CIS—a first episode of neurologic symptoms) and have findings on MRI that are consistent with MS. Avonex, Betaseron, and Extavia have been approved by the FDA to treat CIS. The manufacturers of Rebif have applied to the FDA for this approval. See Chapter 2 for more information about CIS and the criteria for the diagnosis of MS.

The fifth injectable medication—Copaxone (glatiramer acetate)—is unrelated to the interferon products. It is administered daily by subcutaneous injection. Copaxone is approved to treat RRMS as well as CIS.

The interferon-beta medications and glatiramer acetate work in different ways to modify the disease course. The interferons are a group of natural proteins that are produced by human cells in response to viral infection and other stimuli. They work, at least in part, by inhibiting the entry of inflammatory cells into the CNS. Copaxone is a synthetic polypeptide (like a protein) that may act by stimulating the production of immune cells (T lymphocytes) that act to decrease inflammation in the brain and spinal cord rather than those that promote inflammation. This decrease in inflammation reduces the immune attack on myelin. (Table 6-1)

TABLE 6-1. Comparison of Injectable Medications

Brand Name and Generic Name

Betaseron® Extavia® interferon beta-1b	Avonex® interferon beta-1a	Rebif® interferon beta-1a	Copaxone® glatiramer acetate

Manufacturer/Distributor

Bayer HealthCare Pharmaceuticals Novartis Pharmaceuticals	Biogen Idec	EMD Serono/ Immunex	Teva Pharmaceuticals Industries

Approval

Betaseron—1993 US 1995 Can (RRMS) 1999 Can (SPMS) Extavia—2009 US, 2009 Can	1996 US 1998 Can	1998 Can 2002 US	1996 US 1997 Can

Frequency/Route of Delivery

Every other day; subcutaneous injection	Weekly; intramuscular injection	Three times per week; subcutaneous injection	Daily; subcutaneous injection

Common Side Effects

Flu-like symptoms following injection, which lessen over time for many people; injection site reactions. Less common: Depression, elevated liver enzymes, low white blood cell counts.	Flu-like symptoms following injection, which lessen over time for many people. Less common: Depression, mild anemia, elevated liver enzymes, liver toxicity.	Flu-like symptoms following injection, which lessen over time for many people; injection site reactions. Less common: Elevated liver enzymes, low white blood counts.	Injection site reactions. Less common: A reaction immediately after injection—lasting 5–10 minutes—which includes anxiety, chest tightness, shortness of breath, flushing. This reaction has no known long-term effects.

Patient Information and Financial Support Programs

BETAPLUS 1-800-788-1467 betaseron.com Extavia Patient Support Program 1-866-925-2333	MS Active Source 1-800-456-2255 avonex.com msactivesource.com	MS Lifelines 1-877-44-REBIF rebif.com mslifelines.com	Shared Solutions 1-800–887-8100 copaxone.com sharedsolutions.com

Oral Medication

The first oral medication to treat MS—*Gilenya* (fingolimod)—was approved by the FDA in 2010 to treat relapsing forms of MS (see Table 6-2). This medication is a capsule that is taken once daily. Gilenya is a new class of medication called a sphingosine-1-phosphate receptor modulator, which is thought to act by retaining certain white blood cells (lymphocytes) in the lymph nodes, thereby preventing those cells from crossing the blood–brain barrier into the CNS. Preventing the entry of these cells into the CNS reduces inflammatory damage to nerve cells.

Like the injectable medications, the FDA has indicated that this medication can be prescribed as a first treatment option, without requiring that any other disease-modifying medication be tried first. Because this medication is relatively new, however—with long-term benefits and risks yet to be confirmed—MS specialists vary in how they are prescribing Gilenya. Some are "saving" it as an option for those in whom the injectable medications provide insufficient benefit while others are opting to use it as the first treatment option. Coverage by insurers is also highly variable at this time.

Infused Medications

Two medications are delivered by intravenous infusion (see Table 6-2).

Tysabri (natalizumab) has a totally different mechanism of action from the interferon-beta products or Copaxone. It is a laboratory-produced ***monoclonal antibody*** that is designed to hamper the movement of potentially damaging immune cells from the bloodstream, across the blood–brain barrier, and into the brain and spinal cord. The drug inhibits this movement by attaching to alpha-4-integrin, a protein on the surface of immune ***T cells*** that normally enables them to adhere to and pass through the blood–brain barrier. Because of this mode of action, Tysabri is called a selective adhesion molecule inhibitor. Tysabri was approved by the FDA in 2006 as a monotherapy (not to be used in combination with another disease-modifying therapy) to treat relapsing forms of MS.

Tysabri has not been compared with any of the injectable medications in a head-to-head clinical trial, which is the only way to reliably compare their effectiveness. However, clinicians generally agree that each of the injectable drugs approved for use in MS reduces the rate of relapses by about one-third in comparison with ***placebo***. By contrast, after 2 years, Tysabri reduced the rate of relapses by about two-thirds as compared with placebo. Along with this apparent increase in efficacy, however, come more significant risks.

Because this medications increases a person's risk of developing a very serious brain infection known as progressive multifocal leukoencephalopathy (PML—see pp. 63–64), it is generally recommended for people who have had an inadequate response to, or cannot tolerate, other MS therapies. Some MS specialists, however, opt to use Tysabri as an early treatment option for individuals with particularly active disease. Recent preliminary data using a specific immunological assay suggest that PML may occur exclusively (or nearly so) in people who test positive for an antibody to JC virus, the agent that causes PML. This finding indicates that it may be safe to use Tysabri early in patients who test negative in that particular assay. So far, slightly more than half the patients tested have been antibody positive.

TABLE 6-2. Comparison of Other Treatment Options

Oral Medication	Infused Medications	
Brand and Generic Name		
Gilenya® fingolimod	Tysabri® natalizumab	Novantrone® mitoxantrone
Manufacturer/Distributor		
Novartis Pharmaceuticals	Biogen Idec/Elan Pharmaceuticals	EMD Serono/Immunex
Approval		
2010 US—to treat relapsing forms of MS; 2011 Can—to treat relapsing-remitting MS in those who did not respond or were unable to tolerate other MS medications	2006 US—to treat relapsing forms of MS; 2006 Can—to treat relapsing forms of MS	2000 US—to treat secondary-progressive MS with or without relapses, progressive-relapsing MS, and worsening relapsing-remitting MS
Frequency/Route of Delivery		
Every day: capsule taken orally	IV infusion every 4 weeks in a registered infusion center	Four times a year by IV infusion in a medical facility. Lifetime cumulative dose limit of approximately 8–12 doses over 2–3 years
Common Side Effects (see text for more information about potential risks)		
Headache, flu, diarrhea, back pain, liver enzyme elevations, cough. Less common: Slowed heart rate following first dose, infections, swelling in the eye.	Headache, fatigue, urinary tract infections, depression, lower respiratory tract infections, joint pain, chest discomfort. Less common: Allergic or hypersensitivity reactions within two hours of infusion (dizziness, fever, rash, itching, nausea, flushing, low blood pressure, difficulty breathing, chest pain).	Blue-green urine 24 hours after administration; infections, bone marrow suppression (fatigue, bruising, low blood cell counts), nausea, hair thinning, bladder infections, mouth sores. Patients must be monitored for serious liver and heart damage.
Patient Information and Financial Support Programs		
Patient Support Program 877-408-4974 gilenya.com	MS Active Source 800-456-2255 tysabri.com	Patient Information 877-447-3243 novantrone.com

Novantrone (mitoxantrone) is a chemotherapy that belongs to the general group of medicines called antineoplastics. Prior to its approval for use in MS, it was used only to treat certain forms of cancer. It acts in MS by suppressing the activity of T cells, B cells, and macrophages that are thought to lead the attack on the myelin sheath. Novantrone was approved by the FDA in 2000 for:

1. Patients with SPMS (disease that has changed from RRMS to a more consistently progressive course);
2. PRMS (disease characterized by gradual increase in disability from onset with clear, acute relapses along the way);
3. Worsening RRMS (disease characterized by clinical attacks without complete remission, resulting in a step-wise worsening of disability).

Novantrone is the only disease-modifying therapy approved specifically for SPMS. Because this medication can affect a person's cardiac function (see p. 64), it is delivered once every 3 months for approximately 2 to 3 years until a maximum life-time dose is reached. Like Tysabri, it is generally recommended for those who have not received adequate benefit from other MS medications.

WHY WERE THE INJECTABLE MEDICATIONS ORIGINALLY TESTED ONLY IN PEOPLE WITH RELAPSING-REMITTING DISEASE?

These agents were originally tested on people with RRMS because investigators thought those with early, milder disease would be more likely to show a benefit from the treatment. Also, previous studies had shown that it might be easier to demonstrate a treatment effect by measuring a reduction in relapse rate than by showing a reduction in disease progression, particularly since most trials only last two to three years. As investigators try to study potential disease-modifying therapies for PPMS, they will need to identify practical and effective ways to measure treatment outcomes in people whose disease course progresses at a slow but steady rate, without relapses.

WITH SO MANY TREATMENTS TO CHOOSE FROM, HOW WILL I KNOW WHICH ONE IS BEST FOR ME?

You and your doctor will consider a variety of factors when choosing which medication to use:

- The type of disease course and amount of disease activity you are experiencing
- Your lifestyle and personal preferences
- Your ability to give yourself injections or receive injections from someone else
- Your tolerance for possible short-term side effects and potential longer-term risks
- Your age, sex, and family-planning priorities
- Your insurance coverage

Clearly, there are many issues involved in this decision, and the option that you and your doctor choose may be the same or different from the option chosen by other people you know with MS. The goal is to find a treatment that works effectively for you and that you can tolerate well and use consistently until such time as you require a different treatment or something more appropriate for you is available.

WHAT KIND OF SIDE EFFECTS CAN I EXPECT FROM THE DISEASE-MODIFYING MEDICATIONS?

Side effects vary from one medication to another and from one individual to another (see Tables 6-1 and 6-2). So as you read this summary, keep in mind that your experience with a particular treatment may differ from that of someone else who is using the same one. One of the benefits of having several disease-modifying medications from which to choose is that you can switch medications if the side effects do not improve with time or you are unable to tolerate them.

Injectable Medications

Flu-like symptoms (e.g., fever, chills, muscle aches, fatigue) following injection are common with all of the interferon-beta medications (Avonex, Betaserson, Extavia, and Rebif). Taking ibuprofen or acetaminophen prior to each dose helps relieve these symptoms for most people, and many people find that this side effect improves or disappears after the first few months. Changes in liver functions and white blood cell counts can also occur with the interferon medications, but generally return to baseline as soon as the medication is stopped. The FDA recommends that anyone taking an interferon medication be monitored periodically (with a simple blood test) for these kinds of changes.

Copaxone does not cause any flu-like symptoms or changes in liver functions or white blood cell counts. However, people who are taking Copaxone should be aware of one peculiar reaction that, although infrequent, can be quite alarming. On rare occasions (perhaps once in 800 to 1,000 injections), a person taking Copaxone may experience an immediate postinjection reaction involving sensations of tightness in the chest and flushing of the face, perhaps accompanied by palpitations, shortness of breath, or anxiety. This reaction passes within 15 to 30 minutes and has never proved to be serious.

People who are taking medications that are delivered by subcutaneous injections (Betaseron, Copaxone, Extavia, and Rebif) also need to be aware of skin reactions, including lumps, bruises, pain, and infections, which can occur at the injection site. In rare situations, the skin around the injection site can die (necrosis). Good injection techniques can minimize these problems and autoinjection devices may be helpful. The pharmaceutical company patient support programs offer injection training and helpful tips for avoiding or limiting site reactions (see Recommended Resources).

Avonex, which is a deeper injection into the muscle, does not produce injection-site reactions.

Oral Medication

Immediately following the first dose, Gilenya may cause a person's heart rate to slow, with the drop being most significant at about 6 hours after the dose is taken (see Table 6-2). The FDA has recommended that people be monitored in a medical facility during this 6-hour period. The heart rate is likely to return to normal within 1 month of starting the medication. Other side effects that occurred in the clinical trials of Gilenya included headache, influenza, diarrhea, back pain, abnormal liver tests, and cough.

Infused Medications

The short-term side effects most commonly associated with Tysabri infusions include headache, pain in the arms or legs, fatigue, joint pain, diarrhea, and pain in the stomach area (see Table 6-2).

Novantrone infusions may be followed by nausea, temporary hair loss, and menstrual disorders in women (see Table 6-2). People taking Novantrone may also experience fever or chills, lower back or side pain, painful or difficult urination, swelling of feet and lower legs, black, tarry stools, cough or shortness of breath, sores in mouth and on lips, and stomach pain. Because the fluid for infusion is dark blue, it may cause a person's urine to become blue-green in color for a period of 24 hours after each infusion. For the same reason, the whites of a person's eyes may appear bluish.

WHAT KINDS OF LONGER-TERM RISKS ARE ASSOCIATED WITH THE DISEASE-MODIFYING MEDICATIONS?

Each of the disease-modifying medications has some associated long-term risks. The risks described for the injectable medications—which are all relatively mild and manageable—have become clearer as research data and clinical experience with these medications have accumulated over the past few decades. Some of the risks associated with the infused medications were apparent during the initial clinical trials, while other risks have become apparent with time. The clinical trials for Gilenya identified some of the risks associated with its use, but the relative newness of this medication means that we do not yet know what all of the long-term risks might be.

Injectable Medications

No severe, long-term safety issues have emerged with further experience with the interferon-beta medications or Copaxone. However, it is important to know about some problems that can occur.

Interferon-beta Medications

- Regular monitoring of blood counts and liver enzymes (with a simple blood test) is extremely important for any person taking one of the interferon-beta medications, particularly in the months following initiation of treatment. Occasional elevation of liver enzymes or reduction in blood counts may occur with any of the interferon-beta medications, and will correct with dose reduction or discontinuation of the medication. Cases of severe liver toxicity are extremely rare and are likely to be prevented by regular surveillance of liver enzymes. People with MS should also make sure that their physician knows of any prior history of liver disease (e.g., hepatitis) and has a complete list of all the other medications they are taking.
- Mood changes and acute depression, which are common in people with MS, may occur with greater frequency in people who are also taking an interferon-beta medication. While the research in this area has produced contradictory findings, people with MS, their families, and their physicians must be attentive to signs of depression, which will generally respond to treatment. In rare instances, the mood disturbances may require discontinuation of interferon therapy.

Oral Medication

The longer-term risks associated with Gilenya will become clearer as more people take the medication over longer periods of time.

- At the present time, we know that Gilenya reduces the number of white blood cells in the body, leading to an increased risk of infection. To address this risk, a blood test to measure white blood cell count is recommended prior to starting treatment. After starting treatment, a person who experiences fever, unusual tiredness, body aches, chills, nausea, or vomiting should report it to his or her physician. In addition, if a person has not had chicken pox (varicella) or prior varicella immunization, his or her doctor may recommend the varicella vaccine prior to starting this medication.

- Gilenya can cause a swelling of the macula in the eye, resulting in vision changes. For this reason, an examination by an ophthalmologist is recommended prior to starting treatment and 3 to 4 months later to look for evidence of macular swelling.

- Because Gilenya can cause liver problems, a blood test for liver function is recommended prior to starting treatment. Any signs of altered liver function (nausea, vomiting, stomach pain, loss of appetite, unusual tiredness, dark urine or a yellowish tint to the skin, or the whites of the eyes) should be reported to the physician.

Infused Medications

Tysabri

- Tysabri increases a person's risk of developing a rare, often fatal, disease called PML, which is caused by a common virus called the JC virus. As of mid-2011, there have been 150 confirmed cases of PML among the 88,100 people worldwide who have used Tysabri since it came on the market—which means that the overall risk of developing PML is about 1.70 per 1,000 patients. The accumulated data on people taking Tysabri suggest that the risk of developing PML gradually increases the longer a person takes the medication.

    Of the 150 people who developed PML, 29 have died (approximately 1 out of 5). The degree of disability in those who survived ranges from mild to severe. Some people have recovered enough to return to work, while others are confined to bed, requiring extensive assistance with activities of daily living. Still others are somewhere in between.

    In an effort to reduce the risk of PML as much as possible, the FDA has recommended that Tysabri be used only as a monotherapy (not in combination with any other MS medication), and that it not be taken by anyone whose immune system is suppressed—for example, by people with HIV/AIDS or leukemia or lymphoma, or those who are taking medications that partially or totally suppress the immune system (including chemotherapy agents, the MS injectable medications, or pulse steroids). People taking Tysabri can, however, receive a short course of steroids to treat an exacerbation.

    In conjunction with the FDA, the manufacturers of Tysabri have established the TOUCH (Tysabri Outreach: Unified Commitment to Health) Program to ensure the appropriate use of Tysabri and to monitor, on an ongoing basis, the incidence and risk factors for PML and other serious infections associated with Tysabri treatment. To receive Tysabri, the patient and the physician who has prescribed the medication must be enrolled in the TOUCH program. To enroll, the patient must discuss the potential benefits and risks of Tysabri with his or her doctor and sign a special consent form. The infusions can only be given by specially trained personnel at infusion centers enrolled in the TOUCH program. Prior to each infusion, the infusion nurse will review the patient's symptoms and check for any problems that may be indicative of PML.

If a person begins to show signs of new or worsening neurologic symptoms, the doctor will immediately test the blood and spinal fluid and obtain an MRI scan of the brain to help determine whether the JC virus that causes PML is present and active. If the virus is found to be active, Tysabri treatments are stopped immediately. There is no specific therapy to treat PML, but the best hope is to rebuild the person's immune system in an effort to avoid the fatal progression of the virus. In most of the cases of PML that have occurred, Tysabri was removed from the person's system as quickly as possible by plasmapheresis (see p. 55) or another blood-cleansing process called immunoadsorption.

- In addition to increasing the risk of PML, Tysabri increases a person's risk for other types of infections because it inhibits the recruitment of immune cells to sites of infection in various parts of the body. During the clinical trials, those taking Tysabri experienced infections, including pneumonia, urinary tract infections, gastroenteritis, vaginal infections, tooth infections, tonsillitis, and herpes infections, somewhat more often than those taking placebo.

Novantrone

- People taking Novantrone for MS or cancer are at risk of heart damage and secondary acute myelogenous leukemia (AML). The most recent report from the Academy of Neurology indicates that systolic dysfunction (an inability of the heart to pump enough blood to provide sufficient oxygen to the body) occurs in about 12 percent of MS patients treated with Novantrone, congestive heart failure occurs in about 0.4 percent, and leukemia occurs in about 0.8 percent.

- The FDA has recommended that Novantrone only be used by people with normal heart function. To ensure that someone is an appropriate candidate, the physician will carefully evaluate the person for signs and symptoms of heart disease prior to starting the medication. In addition, the doctor will ask if he or she is taking any other medications that are known to affect the heart. After starting the medication, the doctor will reevaluate the person's cardiac function prior to each dose, and limit the total cumulative dose to 140 mg/m^2, which comes to approximately 8 to 12 doses over 2 to 3 years.

- Because the immunosuppressant effects of Novantrone can increase a person's risk of various types of infections, the doctor will also do a blood test prior to each dose, to measure blood counts and liver functions. Between doses, patients are instructed to report problems such as chills and fever, pain on urination, or unusual bleeding to your doctor immediately.

- The doctor will also ask if a person has taken any chemotherapeutic agents in the past, because secondary AML is known to occur more often in people who have previously been treated with other types of chemotherapies called anthracyclines.

MY FAMILY IS WORRIED ABOUT MY USING AN INTERFERON MEDICATION BECAUSE OF THE WARNINGS IN THE PRESCRIBING INFORMATION ABOUT DEPRESSION AND SUICIDE. WHAT IS THE RISK OF DEPRESSION AND/OR SUICIDE WITH THE INTERFERON MEDICATIONS?

Depression is very common in people with MS. The good news is that it is usually not severe and typically responds well to a combination of psychotherapy and medication.

Nevertheless, suicide occurs more frequently among people with MS than among comparable groups of people without the disease. In the pivotal Betaseron trial, four suicide attempts and one completed suicide occurred. Because of the frequency of depression and suicide in the MS population (see Chapter 11) and the small number of events in the trial, one cannot conclude that these episodes of depression were caused by the drug. In the subsequent Avonex and Rebif trials, no differences in rates of severe depression or suicide attempts were found between those taking the interferon medication and those taking the placebo.

It is known, however, that very high doses of interferon, such as those used in cancer treatment, can cause depression. And, data collected since the MS pivotal trials of the interferon medications (referred to as "postmarketing data"—see Chapter 5) include reports of people experiencing depression while on treatment. As a result of concerns about the potential of interferon medications to cause or worsen depression, the FDA has required the manufacturers of these medications to include warnings about depression and suicide in their labeling information.

The safest strategy is probably for people with a previous history of severe affective disorder (depression or bipolar [manic-depressive] illness), or previous suicide attempts, to avoid the interferon medications. Individuals with milder forms of depression can probably safely take any of these medications under close supervision. Family members, other loved ones, and caregivers should be advised to be alert to any changes in mood and report them promptly to the physician. Sometimes the physician will wish to consult with a psychiatrist before starting a person on Avonex, Betaseron, Extavia, or Rebif.

MY DOCTOR HAS RECOMMENDED THAT I BEGIN TAKING ONE OF THE INTERFERON MEDICATIONS (AVONEX, BETASERON, EXTAVIA, OR REBIF). I'VE BEEN READING ABOUT THEM ON THE INTERNET AND HEARING ABOUT THE FLU-LIKE SIDE EFFECTS PEOPLE EXPERIENCE WITH THESE DRUGS. I'M RELUCTANT TO START AN INTERFERON BECAUSE I DON'T WANT TO FEEL WORSE THAN I ALREADY DO.

The Internet has been a useful forum for people to exchange views and information about MS. It is probably a fact of life, however, that people tend to report side effects and problems more commonly than they "go on record" with positive feelings. Certainly, side effects do occur with the interferon medications. Most common are flu-like symptoms that occur primarily in the first few months of treatment. For the majority of people, these are relatively mild and can be managed by starting the medication at a low dose and gradually building up to a full dose, and by taking the injections at night and using minor analgesics (pain relievers), such as ibuprofen or acetaminophen.

People taking Betaseron and Rebif (which are both delivered by subcutaneous injection) also experience local injection-site reactions. Most typically, these are confined to the appearance of red blotches and, perhaps, minor pain. Only infrequently do more severe reactions occur that may necessitate stopping the medication.

We now have experience with many thousands of people taking interferon medications. In general, with proper education and support from physicians and nurses, people tolerate the medications well and can readily continue taking them. Overall, perhaps about 15 percent of people must discontinue treatment for one reason or another and, certainly, not all of these are because of side effects.

MY DOCTOR WANTS ME TO START TREATMENT WITH ONE OF THE INJECTABLE MEDICATIONS. WITH SO MANY OPTIONS, HOW CAN I FIGURE OUT WHICH ONE IS THE BEST CHOICE FOR ME?

Although the modes of action of interferon beta-1b (Betaseron and Extavia) and interferon beta-1a (Avonex and Rebif) are probably identical, the fourth drug, Copaxone (glatiramer acetate), is completely unrelated to the interferons. All five medications appear to reduce disease activity by about 30 percent.

We now have some data comparing the relative effectiveness of the five drugs. Several studies have indicated that the beneficial effects of the interferon medications may be dose related. In the INCOMIN study comparing Avonex (interferon beta-1a) and Betaseron (interferon beta-1b), MRI, and *clinical findings* showed that Betaseron reduced *signs* of disease activity and progression more effectively than Avonex, and the difference between the two treatments increased during the second year of the study. In the EVIDENCE trial, Rebif (interferon beta-1a), administered three times a week, reduced the relapse rate, reduced active inflammation as seen on MRI, and extended the time to first relapse more so than Avonex, which was given once a week. Rebif and Betaseron both deliver a higher dose of interferon-β than Avonex. However, the implications of these differences are not clear since it has also been shown that *antibodies* that may neutralize the effect of interferon medications increase as the dosage of interferon increases.

Two studies have compared the effectiveness of Copaxone and a "high-dose" interferon in head-to-head trials. In the REGARD trial, Rebif was compared to Copaxone. Both drugs were equally effective on the primary endpoint of time to first relapse. In the second trial, known as BEYOND, Betaseron was compared to Copaxone and both drugs performed equally well on the primary endpoint of relapse risk. Thus, Copaxone and those interferons that are given several times per week appear to be comparably effective.

It is important for you to discuss with your physician the benefits and risks of the respective medications in order to reach a comfortable decision. The discussion should include the different routes of injection (subcutaneous vs. intramuscular), schedule of injection (ranging from once a week to every day), and possible side effects. Your physician will recommend the medication that he or she feels is best suited to your MS and to your lifestyle.

WHAT ARE NEUTRALIZING ANTIBODIES, AND WHAT IMPACT DO THEY HAVE ON THE EFFECTIVENESS OF THE INJECTABLE THERAPIES?

Antibodies are proteins of the immune system that arise in response to foreign substances, including viruses and bacteria. Some people who receive interferon-beta develop a form of antibody to the injected protein; it is called a "neutralizing antibody" (NAb) because some biologic property of the interferon is inactivated by it. Those who do develop NAbs when taking interferon-beta medications (Avonex, Betaseron, Extavia, and Rebif) typically do so about 12 to 18 months after the start of treatment. However, the frequency of the occurrence of such antibodies differs among the various interferon products, with an *incidence* of about 5 percent with Avonex, 15 to 20 percent with Rebif, and 30 to 40 percent with Betaseron. People who develop persistently high levels of NAbs appear to lose the benefit of treatment. The situation is complex, however, because some people also seem to lose their NAbs as time goes by. This is an area of continuing research and evolving understanding. Neutralizing antibodies do not appear to develop to Copaxone.

DO ANY OTHER MS MEDICATIONS PRODUCE NEUTRALIZING ANTIBODIES?
Approximately 6 percent of people taking Tysabri develop neutralizing antibodies that persist over time. When this occurs, there is evidence that the medication becomes less effective, so antibody testing may be considered for any person taking Tysabri who continues to have a higher than expected level of disease activity.

ONCE I START TAKING ONE OF THE INJECTABLE DRUGS (AVONEX, BETASERON, COPAXONE, EXTAVIA, OR REBIF), HOW LONG WILL I NEED TO STAY ON THE MEDICATION?
Follow-up data for each of these medications indicate that they continue to be safe and effective over time. In general, a person taking one of these medications should remain on it unless clear indications arise—such as frequent attacks, new lesions on MRI, or significant disease progression—that the treatment is not providing sufficient benefit, or the person is experiencing intolerable side effects. If any of these problems should occur, the physician would likely recommend switching to one of the other injectable medications or to Gilenya or Tysabri. Of course, the availability of newer, more effective treatments would require reassessment of an individual's situation.

Because none of these medications completely prevent disease activity, the occurrence of an occasional attack in someone taking one of these medications does not necessarily mean that the drug is not working. Each of the five injectable drugs has been shown in clinical trials to reduce the annual rate of exacerbations by about 30 percent—which means that a person will continue to have occasional relapses with these medications.

I HAVE BEEN TAKING ONE OF THE INJECTABLE AGENTS FOR MORE THAN 2 YEARS, AND I STILL DON'T FEEL BETTER. DOES THIS MEAN THAT THE DRUG ISN'T WORKING FOR ME?
In the clinical trials of the disease-modifying therapies—Avonex, Betaseron, Copaxone, and Rebif—no evidence suggested that the drugs made the treatment groups "feel better." Betaseron was found to reduce the frequency and severity of exacerbations in RRMS. Avonex reduced the frequency of relapses and slowed disease progression. Copaxone reduced the frequency of exacerbations. Rebif was found to reduce attack frequency and slow progression of disability. And all five drugs showed a reduction in new or active lesions on MRI. Although a significant effort has been made to inform people about the possible benefits and limitations of these treatments, it is clear that many people harbor a hope that they will feel better as a result of taking one of these treatments. This is not particularly surprising, since most people's life experience with medical treatment in general, and medication in particular, is that it is designed to make a person feel better.

In a study of 100 individuals eligible for Betaseron (funded by the National MS Society and conducted at the University of California, San Francisco), a significant proportion of those surveyed had misconceptions about the drug's potential effects. More than 80 percent expected that the drug would reduce their level of physical discomfort and improve their overall quality of life. Unfortunately, misconceptions such as these may cause people to become disappointed or dissatisfied with the effects of the drug they are taking and stop it prematurely, even if the drug is working for them in ways they cannot readily see or feel.

Because it is not possible to evaluate the extent to which any of these drugs is working for any one individual at any particular time, it is advisable for you to remain on the drug unless you are having frequent attacks, rapid disease progression, or severe side effects.

WHAT WILL HAPPEN IF I LOSE TRACK OF THE DATE AND FORGET TO TAKE MY MEDICATION?

Injectable Medications

Missing an occasional injection of is not thought to be harmful. If you miss a dose of Betaseron, Copaxone, Extavia, or Rebif, just give yourself the injection at the next reasonable opportunity and continue the appropriate schedule from that point. Do not, however, take two injections in one day. If you miss a dose of Avonex, take it as soon as you remember and continue on a weekly schedule. Do not, however, take two doses within two days of each other.

Oral Medication

If you miss a dose of Gilenya, resume the regular schedule on the following day. If, for any reason, you stop the medication for a couple of weeks, you will need to restart it in your doctor's office so that you can be monitored again for changes in your heart rate.

Infused Medications

If for some reason you are unable to keep the appointment for a scheduled infusion of either Novantrone or Tysabri, contact your physician or nurse to reschedule it as soon as possible.

I HAVE RECENTLY BEEN DIAGNOSED WITH MS AND HAVE NO APPARENT SYMPTOMS AT THIS TIME. SHOULD I START TAKING A DISEASE-MODIFYING MEDICATION RIGHT AWAY?
The decision to begin one of these medications should be made with your physician, taking into account your history, current symptoms, exacerbation rate, and any evidence on MRI of new lesion development. In general, the person whose disease shows signs of relatively recent activity—either clinically or on MRI—is the likeliest candidate to benefit from the treatment. Although people who are feeling and doing relatively well may see little reason to begin one of these medications, the fact is that MS is a very unpredictable disease. These medications are designed to reduce the number and severity of attacks in the hope that they will slow disease progression over the long term.

Particularly in light of the data indicating irreversible *axonal damage*, and brain *atrophy* even in the early stages of the disease, it is important to consider these medications carefully. Most MS experts now believe that treatment with a disease-modifying agent should be started early in the course of the disease, before significant, permanent damage occurs. Thus, if there are clear signs on clinical examination or on MRI that the disease process is active, even if you are not currently experiencing significant symptoms, most experts would favor initiating treatment. The

National MS Society has published a Disease Management Consensus Statement of the National Clinical Advisory Board advocating early and sustained treatment with one of these medications for individuals with relapsing forms of MS.

I HAVE BEEN HEARING ABOUT AXONAL DAMAGE AND BRAIN ATROPHY THAT CAN OCCUR EVEN IN THE EARLY STAGES OF MS. CAN YOU TELL ME WHAT THESE TERMS MEAN?

It is generally believed that the inflammatory process in MS causes damage primarily to the myelin sheath surrounding the **nerve** fibers in the CNS. Since the earliest descriptions of MS pathology, however, it has been known that the nerve fibers (axons) themselves also sustain damage. While inflammation is probably responsible for this phenomenon as well, the details of how axonal damage occurs remain unclear. Recent research has confirmed that nerve fibers can be affected or even severed in MS, and that this damage can occur very early in the disease. There is some speculation that this damage to the axons may be responsible for the permanent symptoms or **impairments** that can occur in MS.

Damage to nerve fibers and their loss may be partly responsible for the recently confirmed "atrophy" or brain shrinkage that occurs in MS. Loss of myelin and changes in brain fluids are also likely contributors. While myelin has the potential capacity to regenerate, at least early in the disease, the regrowth of nerve fibers is much more problematic.

Perhaps the greatest significance of these findings lies in the fact that these irrevocable changes can occur early in the disease. In part because of these findings, MS experts are advocating early treatment, with one of the disease-modifying agents for anyone with a confirmed diagnosis of relapsing MS. The goal is to slow the progression of the disease and prevent as much of this early, irreversible damage as possible.

I HAVE HAD ONE ATTACK, AND MY NEUROLOGIST IS RECOMMENDING THAT I BEGIN TREATMENT EVEN THOUGH THE DIAGNOSIS OF MS HASN'T BEEN CONFIRMED. HE SAYS I HAVE A "CIS." WHAT DOES THAT MEAN?

A CIS is a single clinical episode, lasting at least 24 hours, which seems to indicate inflammation in the CNS. The event can be *monofocal*, meaning that a single lesion produces a single symptom such as an episode of *optic neuritis*. Or, the event can be *multifocal*, meaning that lesions in more than one area cause multiple symptoms at the same time—for example, an episode of optic neuritis accompanied by weakness on the right side. Studies have shown that when CIS occurs in someone who also has MRI-detected lesions in the CNS that are similar to those seen in MS, a high risk exists for a second clinical episode, which would confirm the diagnosis of clinically definite MS. The goal of treatment in CIS is to delay that second episode or attack and thereby delay the onset of clinically definite MS; all of the injectable medications have demonstrated their ability to delay the onset of clinically definite MS:

● In the CHAMPS study (Controlled High-Risk Subjects Avonex MS Prevention Study), Avonex was shown to delay the onset of clinically definite MS. The patients in this study also had a significantly smaller increase in the number of new lesions and the total volume of brain lesions. Based on this study, the FDA extended the labeling of Avonex to include individuals who have experienced their first clinical episode and have MRI-detected brain lesions that are similar to those seen in MS.

- In a similar study (the ETOMS [Early Treatment of MS] trial), Rebif was also found to delay the onset of clinically definite MS and reduce the number of new lesions and the total lesion volume in the treatment group. The data from the ETOMS trial are now under review by the FDA.

- In the BENEFIT study (Betaseron in Newly Emerging MS for Initial Treatment), Betaseron was shown to reduce the risk of progression to clinically definite MS in people with CIS, as well as delaying the time to the second clinical event. Based on these results, the FDA extended the labeling of Betaseron to include those people who have experienced a single clinical episode and have lesions on MRI that are similar to those seen in MS. Because Extavia is the same formulation as Betaseron, it is also approved for this use.

- In the PreCISe trial, early treatment with Copaxone is found to be effective in delaying conversation to clinically definite MS in people with CIS and brain lesions detected on MRI. Based on these results, the FDA extended the labeling of Copaxone to include those people who have experienced a single clinical episode and have lesions on MRI that are similar to those seen in MS.

The decision to start treatment for CIS can be difficult, particularly if you are feeling fine and do not feel ready to begin an injectable medication. The best strategy is for you to work with your physician to figure out what would be your best course of action given your symptoms, history, and MRI findings, as well as your lifestyle and personal preferences.

MY MS USED TO BE RELAPSING-REMITTING. NOW THAT IT SEEMS TO BE SECONDARY-PROGRESSIVE, WOULD ANY OF THE INJECTABLE MEDICATIONS STILL BE APPROPRIATE TREATMENT FOR ME?

Although these drugs were originally tested on people with RRMS, subsequent studies have demonstrated the efficacy of Avonex, Betaseron, Extavia, and Rebif in people with all relapsing forms of the disease. According to the FDA, each of these drugs is now approved for any individuals who experience relapses, whether they have RRMS, PRMS (a course of MS that is progressive from onset, with relapses superimposed along the way), or have transitioned from RRMS to secondary-progressive disease but continue to have occasional relapses.

Copaxone is approved only for RRMS. One small trial of Copaxone in progressive MS, done in the late 1980s, failed to show a statistically significant benefit, but the trial was too small to be conclusive. A recent large trial of Copaxone in patients with PPMS (PPMS) was terminated before its anticipated conclusion because the drug failed to achieve the degree of benefit targeted in the design of the study.

I HAVE PROGRESSIVE MS, AND I'M WONDERING WHAT TREATMENTS ARE AVAILABLE FOR ME.

The answer to your question depends, in part, on what you mean by "progressive MS." There are two recognized types of progressive MS: PPMS refers to a disease course characterized by progression of disability from the outset, without an initial phase of ***acute attacks*** and ***remissions***. This course is seen in only 10 percent or so of people with MS. Unfortunately, no treatments are currently approved for PPMS. The primary focus of treatment for those with PPMS is symptom management and rehabilitation interventions to maintain and enhance function. The good news is that research is under way to find effective treatments for PPMS, including a clinical trial of the oral medication, Gilenya and another with a drug called ocrelizumab, which is administered by infrequent intravenous infusion.

SPMS refers to a disease course that is initially relapsing-remitting but subsequently becomes more consistently progressive. Data obtained before the advent of disease-modifying therapies indicated that of the 85 percent of people with MS who start out with relapsing-remitting disease, more than half will develop secondary-progressive disease within a period of 10 years, and 90 percent within 25 years. Avonex, Betaseron, Extavia, Gilenya, Rebif, and Tysabri are approved in the United States for all relapsing forms of MS, including SPMS, when the individual is still experiencing relapses. The only medication approved for SPMS with or without relapses is the immunosuppressant drug Novantrone (mitoxantrone for injection concentrate). As of the publication of this book, a trial of Tysabri in SPMS is anticipated to begin in the near future

ARE ANY OTHER MEDICATIONS USED TO TREAT PROGRESSIVE MS?

Various immunosuppressive agents—for example, Imuran (azathioprine), Cytoxan (cyclophosphamide), CellCept (mycophenolate mofetil), and Rheumatrex (methotrexate)—have been used by some MS physicians to treat progressive disease. Immunosuppressive medications dampen the body's natural immune response, which is designed to protect it from foreign substances. Many different immuno-suppressant agents are used to treat various types of cancer. In MS, we believe the immune system mistakenly attacks the person's own myelin as if it were foreign. By suppressing the immune system, such therapy may reduce the severity of the attack and thus reduce further damage to the myelin in the nervous system. Unfortunately, the clinical trials of these chemotherapeutic agents have not conclusively demonstrated their value for progressive MS, and none has been approved by the FDA for this use.

The benefits of Cytoxan have been controversial, and it has not gained widespread acceptance by physicians or their patients. Rheumatrex has been used in cancer treatment, for immunosuppression in organ transplantation, and for the treatment of rheumatoid arthritis. In relatively low doses, it was shown in one small study to slow the rate of progression in MS. However, Rheumatrex is potentially toxic to the liver, and treatment with this drug must be carefully monitored. It is not compatible with nonsteroidal anti-inflammatory drugs (such as aspirin or ibuprofen) or with alcohol, so its use involves a number of restrictions. Some evidence suggests that Imuran may slow progression in MS, but the effect, if it exists, is small and somewhat controversial.

All treatments currently available or in advanced stages of testing are designed to reduce further damage. Of course, individuals with MS often improve spontaneously. However, the longer symptoms of MS have been present, the lower the likelihood that this spontaneous improvement will occur.

MY MS SEEMS TO BE GETTING WORSE IN SPITE OF TREATMENT. NOW MY FAMILY IS SAYING IT MAY ALL BE BECAUSE OF CCSVI AND I SHOULD BE TREATED FOR IT. WHAT IS CCSVI AND WILL TREATING IT HELP MY MS?

CCSVI stands for chronic cerebrospinal venous insufficiency. Dr. Paolo Zamboni, a vascular surgeon in Italy and his colleagues coined this term in 2009 to describe possible abnormalities in major veins that drain blood from the brain and spinal cord to the heart in people with MS. Using advanced ultrasound techniques in a preliminary study, they reported evidence of slowed and obstructed blood drainage, as well as evidence of the opening of "substitute circles," where blood flow is diverted to smaller vessels in order to bypass obstructions in the veins. They also found that the diverted blood tended to reverse direction and flow back into the brain. Dr. Zamboni has hypothesized that this reverse blood flow might set off the inflammation and immune-mediated damage that is seen in MS. In other words, he believes that CCSVI—which he found in the majority of the MS patients he studied—may cause MS or be associated in some way with disease progression.

Dr. Zamboni and his colleagues have proposed treating CCSVI with an endovascular surgical procedure that involves inserting a tiny balloon or stent into the blocked veins, similar to what has been done for many years to treat blocked arteries. They published a small, ***open-label*** (see Chapter 5 for a description of the phases involved in clinical trials) study in 2009, in which they tested the safety and preliminary outcomes of vascular surgery in 35 people with RRMS, 20 with SPMS, and 10 with PPMS. Based on finding some positive effects—primarily in those with RRMS—the authors suggested that controlled trials were necessary in order to better determine the safety and benefits of this procedure.

Dr. Zamboni also suggested that if further evidence supports the link between MS and CCSVI, treatment of the venous abnormalities might become an additional treatment option for MS. He emphasized the need for more research on his hypothesis, and noted that people with MS should remain on their disease-modifying therapies while waiting for answers about CCSVI to emerge.

In an effort to help determine the validity of Dr. Zamboni's hypothesis, the National MS Society, in collaboration with the MS Society of Canada, funded seven research grants focusing on the possible role of CCSVI in the MS disease process. These studies are taking a comprehensive look at the structure and function of the veins draining the brain and spinal cord in a group of people whose MS varies in type, severity and duration, and comparing them to the structure and function of veins in people with other diseases and healthy volunteers. These studies will help to determine whether the CCSVI phenomenon originally described by Dr. Zamboni can be reproduced by other investigators, and answer questions about whether CCSVI is—or is not—a cause of MS or related to MS in some other manner. In addition, these studies will help to resolve some conflicting data that have emerged concerning how frequently CCSVI occurs in MS, and how often it occurs in people who do not have MS. If blockages are confirmed in people with MS, this will speed the way to determining whether therapeutic trials to correct them will be helpful in improving or altering MS disease process.

Until these other trials are completed, the value of the procedure for people with MS remains unclear. Endovascular surgery is not without risks, including infection at the puncture site; damage to the blood vessel, which could lead to the formation of clots; and internal or external bleeding if anticoagulants are used. Deaths have also been reported in some individuals who have undergone this treatment. If you are thinking about getting this treatment done, be sure to consult with your neurologist and family physician before making a decision.

WHY ARE THE DISEASE-MODIFYING MEDICATIONS SO EXPENSIVE, AND WILL THE COST OF THESE DRUGS EVER COME DOWN?

These drugs are expensive for several reasons. First, the technology to develop and produce them is highly specialized. Interferon beta-1b (Betaseron and Extavia) and interferon beta-1a (Avonex and Rebif) are not naturally occurring substances. They are produced in the laboratory—grown in, and harvested from, bacteria and mammalian cells respectively. Copaxone is synthesized in a complex process that is difficult to standardize and requires precise control to maintain standardization. A monoclonal antibody like Tysabri is produced by injecting an animal with a specific *antigen*, thereby inducing a correspondingly specific antibody response by the animal's immune cells. These antibody-producing cells are then extracted and fused with rapidly growing cells to produce a hybrid cell called a *hybridoma*, which is capable of producing large quantities of specific types of antibodies known as monoclonal antibodies. Thus, for all these drugs, manufacturing is complex and costly.

More importantly, however, the costs of developing the products are extremely high and are passed along to the consumer. It is important to realize that for every drug that does reach the marketplace, dozens of others have failed to achieve that goal. The costs of developing and testing those unsuccessful drugs must also be recouped through sales of those drugs that are successful.

Unfortunately for the public, pharmaceutical companies, like all other businesses, have a fiduciary obligation to their stockholders to try to maximize profits. Therefore, new drugs are generally quite expensive, especially those without similar competitive medications. With the approval of additional treatments, many people hope that competition may bring down the cost of these drugs.

ONE OF THE PEOPLE IN MY MS SUPPORT GROUP IS GETTING A TREATMENT CALLED IVIg. WHAT CAN YOU TELL ME ABOUT IT?

Intravenous *immunoglobulin* (IVIg) is a treatment that has been used in other autoimmune disorders, including neurologic diseases such as myasthenia gravis and Guillain-Barré syndrome, although the mechanism of action in any of these disorders is not known. IVIg, which consists of the antibody-containing portion of blood collected and fractionated from pools of donors, requires periodic intravenous administration. Several different treatment schedules have been employed, but most have involved monthly infusions.

Several earlier reports suggested a beneficial effect in MS, although the design of the trials was not ideal. All these studies evaluated the treatment with relapsing disease. A recent trial of IVIg in SPMS showed no benefit. In addition, a recently completed randomized, placebo-controlled trial in RRMS showed no advantage for

IVIg. Direct comparisons of the effectiveness of this treatment with those approved by the FDA —Avonex, Betaseron, Copaxone, Rebif, Tysabri, and Novantrone—are not available.

The treatment is generally well tolerated, although kidney problems may occur, and there is some concern about potential liver damage. Because IVIg is derived from natural blood products, there can be inconsistencies between batches and a potential risk from blood-borne viruses. For these reasons, as well as the lack of good evidence of benefit, IVIg is not considered by many North American experts in the field to be a treatment of choice for MS.

Insurance companies are likely to vary in their willingness to pay for the treatment, the costs of which tend to be higher than those for the other injectable medications.

IS IT POSSIBLE TO REPLACE OR REPAIR THE MYELIN THAT HAS BEEN DESTROYED BY MS?

It is not currently possible to enhance or improve myelin repair in MS. However, recent animal and laboratory investigations have shown that myelin repair occurs spontaneously in mammals and that this repair can be enhanced in animals. Some myelin repair occurs naturally in MS, particularly early in the disease, and this may be an important aspect of recovery from attacks. Further study is under way to try to find ways to enhance myelin repair in humans.

IS THERE A POTENTIAL ROLE FOR BONE MARROW TRANSPLANTATION IN MS TREATMENT?

Because MS is thought to be an ***autoimmune disease***, in which the person's immune system mistakenly attacks healthy tissues in the body, scientists are working to find out whether replacing the malfunctioning immune system could stop the disease process. Bone marrow transplantation (also called *hematopoietic stem cell* (HSC) *transplantation*), which has been used primarily to treat cancer, is currently being studied in clinical trials.

Bone marrow and blood contain HSCs. Stem cells are immature cells that are capable of developing into other blood components, such as red and white blood cells. The transplantation procedure involves several steps: (1) A drug called *granulocyte colony stimulating factor* is injected to increase the number of HSCs; (2) the stem cells are removed from the blood and stored; (3) the person undergoes high-dose chemotherapy and/or radiation therapy to destroy bone marrow cells, including those T cells that are thought to drive the immune attack in MS; and (4) the stored stem cells are transfused back into the person's blood, where they gradually mature and rebuild the immune system. This is referred to as *autologous transplantation* because the person's own stem cells are used in the process.

HSC transplantation is a radical therapy that has primarily been used in people with rapidly progressing MS that has not responded to other treatments. The procedure carries with it significant risks, including increased susceptibility to infection and bleeding during the period before the person's immune system is rebuilt—a side effect that can prove fatal. To date, more than 100 people have been treated with HSC transplantation. Most stabilize, at least temporarily following treatment (although recent studies have found renewed disease activity after a few years); some have shown modest improvement in symptoms; and between 5 and 10 percent have died. Because of the significant risks of the procedure, as well as the high cost, this treatment should be reserved—if used at all—for individuals with rapidly progressive disease who are being treated in carefully monitored clinical research settings. At the present time, HSC is being evaluated in Phase I, II, and III clinical trials in relapsing-remitting and SPMS.

WHAT OTHER KINDS OF STEM CELL TRANSPLANTATION ARE BEING STUDIED FOR POSSIBLE USE IN MS?

Many different kinds of stem cells could potentially provide benefit for people with MS. Although no stem cell therapies have yet been proven to be effective in MS, stem cells are being studied because of two unique characteristics they all share: First, all stem cells have the ability to multiple and reproduce themselves in greater numbers; second, they are able—in varying degrees—to develop into different types of cells that may be useful in preventing damage in the CNS or repairing damage that has already occurred. The following types of stem cells are currently being studied in MS:

- HSCs (see above)
- Mesenchymal stem cells (MSCs)—Adult stem cells, found in the bone marrow, skin, and fatty tissue. MSC produce cells that help other stem cells function correctly. They may help prevent damage to *myelin* and possibly promote remyelination where damage has already occurred. Autologus MSCs are in early Phase I trials in SPMS.
- Neural stem cells (NSCs)—Cells that are responsible for repairing myelin in the brain, but do not function properly in the brains of people with MS. Based on results from studies in animal models of MS, researchers are beginning to look at ways to treat a person's NSCs so that they do their job more effectively, as well as at transplanting replacement NSCs.

Stem cell therapy is a rapidly changing area of MS research. To stay current with the progress being made, visit the National MS Society's Web site at www.nationalmssociety.org/research.

STEM CELL THERAPY CLINICS IN DIFFERENT PARTS OF THE WORLD ARE CLAIMING THAT THEY CAN SUCCESSFULLY TREAT AND/OR CURE PEOPLE WITH MS AND OTHER DISEASES. ARE THESE CLAIMS TRUE?

At the present time, there is no proven therapy for MS that uses stem cells. More research is needed to determine whether stem cell therapies might offer safe and effective options for people with MS. None of the stem cell therapy clinics that are promoting themselves online and in the media have provided scientific or medical evidence that their treatments work, either in the short- or long-term, or are safe. Several of the clinics have been closed down by local health authorities, but more continue to open, particularly in countries without effective oversight by health authorities. Specific concerns about these stem cell clinics include:

- Lack of strict sanitary guidelines
- Lack of information concerning the sources of the stem cells that are used
- Inadequate oversight and follow-up to ensure safety and address any complications that arise during and after the procedures

  Some clues to potential fraud include:

- Claims to cure MS—the bigger and broader the claim, the more likely it is to be false
- Demands for payment in advance
- Promotional materials that rely exclusively on personal testimonials rather than published data in medical journals

While progress may feel frustratingly slow for individuals and families affected by MS, it is encouraging to think about how far we have come since this book was first published in 1996. Today we have more than twice as many approved therapy options and many more in the research pipeline. In addition to efforts to slow the disease process, investigators are now looking at ways to stop the disease in its tracks, repair damage that has already occurred, and even prevent it from happening in the first place.

RECOMMENDED READINGS

Selected booklets available from the National MS Society (800-344-3867) or online at
   http://www.nationalmssociety.org/Brochures:
   - *Choosing the Right Healthcare Provider*
   - *Research Directions in MS*
   - *The Disease-Modifying Medications*
   - *Managing Progressive MS*
   - *So You Have Progressive MS?*

RECOMMENDED RESOURCES

References in this area become outdated very quickly. The most accurate, up-to-date information about treatments and drug trials is available from the following sources:

   National MS Society: A wealth of information and resources is available by calling 800-344-3867 or online at
   www.nationalmssociety.org/Treatments and www.nationalmssociety.org/ClinicalTrials

   Medline Plus (www.medlineplus.gov): A service of the National Library of Medicine and the National Institutes of Health, providing health news, drug information, clinical trials listing, a medical encyclopedia, a medical dictionary, links to other databases and resources.

   Multiple Sclerosis International Federation: An excellent source of information about clinical trials at
   www.msif.org/en

NARCOMS Registry: a research program that allows people with MS to expedite MS research by volunteering information about their experience with the disease. For information about how to participate in the registry, go to
http://narcoms.org

National Institutes of Health: The National Library of Medicine maintains a database of information on clinical trials being conducted in the United States at
www.clinicaltrials.gov

Complementary and Alternative Medicine

Allen Bowling, MD, PhD

Complementary and alternative medicine—familiarly known as CAM—includes the wide variety of health-promoting strategies that are considered to be outside the realm of conventional or mainstream medicine. In other words, they are therapies that are not typically provided by physicians and have generally *not* been tested in the kind of controlled *clinical trial* that is considered the "gold standard" for evaluating new medical treatments (see Chapter 5 for more information about clinical trials). CAM therapies are widely used, especially by people who are dissatisfied or impatient with what mainstream medicine has to offer. Particularly with a chronic disease like multiple sclerosis (MS)—which has no cure and causes a wide range of *symptoms* that can significantly impact quality of life—people look to treatments that promise health and relief from disease activity and discomfort. This chapter answers some of the most commonly asked questions about CAM and provides guidance in how to evaluate these interventions and the claims made about them.

WHAT TYPES OF TREATMENTS ARE CONSIDERED *ALTERNATIVE* OR *COMPLEMENTARY*?
The National Institutes of Health (NIH) classify CAM in the following way:

- Biologically based therapies
  - Diets and fatty acid supplements
  - Herbal medicine (herbs, marijuana, and aromatherapy)
  - Orthomolecular medicine (vitamins, minerals, and other nonherbal supplements)
  - Pharmacologic, biologic, and instrumental interventions (e.g., aspartame, bee venom therapy, candida treatment, chelation therapy, cooling therapy, dental amalgam removal, enzyme therapy, hyperbaric oxygen, procarin)
- Alternative medical systems
  - Acupuncture and traditional Chinese medicine
  - Ayurveda
  - Homeopathy
  - Tai chi

- Lifestyle and disease prevention
  - Exercise
- Mind–body medicine
  - Biofeedback
  - Hypnosis and guided imagery
  - Meditation
  - Music therapy
  - Pets
  - Prayer and spirituality
  - Yoga
- Manipulative and body-based systems
  - Body work (e.g., chiropractic, Feldenkrais, massage, Pilates, reflexology, Tragerwork)
  - Unconventional physical therapies (e.g., colon therapy, hippotherapy, and therapeutic horseback riding)
- Biofield medicine
  - Therapeutic touch
- Bioelectromagnetics
  - Magnets and electromagnetic therapy

For a thorough evaluation and discussion of individual CAM interventions, refer to the book by Bowling in the Recommended Reading list at the end of the chapter.

IF ALTERNATIVE TREATMENTS LIKE BEE STINGS AND COBRA VENOM SEEM TO WORK WELL FOR SOME PEOPLE, WHY AREN'T THEY MORE WIDELY PRESCRIBED?

Alternative treatments, such as bee sting therapy, are often touted as helping people with MS. The problem is that these reports are generally "anecdotal;" they consist mostly of individual claims of success, without any scientific study. It is well known that MS often undergoes spontaneous improvement or *remission*. Furthermore, as discussed in Chapter 5, virtually every study of MS indicates a significant *placebo effect*, whereby people taking a *placebo* (nonactive substance) do better than they would with no treatment. Therefore, claims of success with any therapy, including alternative treatments, must be regarded with considerable skepticism until they have been confirmed in placebo-controlled clinical trials. In addition, some of these treatments, such as bee stings, carry potentially severe risks. Specifically, fatal allergic reactions can occur in some individuals receiving bee stings. These comments are not to suggest that there might not be merit to some alternative treatments, but rather to emphasize the importance of proper scientific investigation under controlled and safe conditions.

In response to the ever-growing interest in alternative therapies in the United States, the National Center for Complementary and Alternative Medicine (NCCAM) was added to the 26 institutes and centers that make up the NIH. The NIH is one of eight agencies under the Public Health Service in the Department of Health and Human Services. Since its inception in 1999, the mission of NCCAM has been to support rigorous research on CAM and to disseminate information to the public and professionals about which CAM interventions are effective, which are not, and why.

In the event that particular CAM interventions are found to be a safe and effective treatment, they may eventually become part of conventional medicine—as has occurred with many forms of exercise.

WHAT IS THE DIFFERENCE BETWEEN *ALTERNATIVE* AND *COMPLEMENTARY MEDICINE*?
These terms refer to the way in which unconventional medical therapies are used. When these interventions are used in combination with—or as a complement to—conventional medical treatments, they are referred to as *complementary*. When they are used instead of mainstream medical treatments, they are considered *alternative*. Studies have shown that as many as two-thirds of people with MS use some form of CAM, with the vast majority of them using these interventions in addition to the conventional MS treatments described in the other chapters in Part II.

Unfortunately, many people choose not to tell their physician about their use of CAM—either because they are concerned that their physician will react negatively or because they think it isn't important information for their physician to know. It is critically important for your physician(s) to know all of the therapies you are using—whether prescribed by another physician or purchased over-the-counter. This will enable your doctor to alert you to possible negative interactions or dangerous side effects of which you might not be aware.

DOES THE *PLACEBO EFFECT* PLAY A DIFFERENT ROLE IN CAM THAN IN CONVENTIONAL MEDICINE?
In the days before physicians had much to offer in the way of effective treatments, they focused their efforts on enhancing the placebo effect of their interventions by developing more of a nurturing relationship with their patients. In other words, the relationship with the physician may have provided as much benefit as the treatments they could offer. As modern medicine has advanced and insurance reimbursement has declined, some practitioners of conventional medicine have less of an opportunity to develop or enhance the placebo effect. As described above, one purpose of controlled clinical trials is to ensure that the treatment effect of a new therapy is greater than the placebo effect seen, at least for a short time, with virtually any treatment. Many CAM practitioners, on the other hand, still offer the type of practitioner–patient relationship that may nurture the placebo effect. They may, in effect, put the placebo effect to work for their patients.

WHEN IS IT REASONABLE TO CONSIDER USING CAM TO TREAT MY MS?
There are some situations in which it might be reasonable to consider using CAM. For example, a person with mild symptoms of muscle stiffness or pain that do not require conventional medication might choose to try an intervention such as yoga, tai chi, or meditation. A person might also want to try a CAM intervention when conventional therapies have proved ineffective. For any severe symptom, or for the management of a complex disease process, however, CAM should never be used in place of conventional medicine. CAM should only be used as a complement to conventional medicine, and only after discussion with one's physician. CAM therapies to consider are those that have some potential to be effective, carry little or no risk,

and are of relatively low-cost. Those to avoid include interventions that are costly, potentially dangerous, and unlikely to provide benefit.

IF I DECIDE TO TRY SOME FORM OF CAM, WHAT ARE THE APPROPRIATE STEPS TO FOLLOW?

It is important to include a physician in your decision-making process. Most CAM practitioners do not have expertise in the diagnosis and treatment of medical conditions. Make every effort to obtain accurate information about the intervention you are considering—including its effectiveness, safety, and the cost and effort involved. If you are unable to obtain this kind of information easily, or the only information you can find comes from anecdotal reports (e.g., "This product cured my MS;" "After 20 years of being unable to walk, all my symptoms have disappeared.") or companies that are trying to sell you a product, proceed with caution.

HOW WILL I KNOW IF THE CLAIMS MADE ABOUT A PARTICULAR PRODUCT OR PROGRAM ARE VALID OR RELEVANT FOR A PERSON WITH MS?

There are several "red flags" to watch out for, including advertising that:

- Relies heavily on individual, anecdotal claims rather than large group data
- Promotes products that *strengthen* or *enhance* the *immune system* when, in fact, the immune system of a person with MS is already overactive and should not be further enhanced in any way
- Makes a product sound too good to be true—for example, it claims to cure MS, get rid of all symptoms, cure a wide variety of diseases, work miracles
- Talks about "secret ingredients" rather than providing full disclosure
- Provides little or no objective evidence for its claims
- Belittles or bad-mouths conventional medicine

ONE OF MY FRIENDS RECOMMENDED THAT I TRY MARIJUANA TO RELIEVE MY MS SYMPTOMS. IS MARIJUANA AN EFFECTIVE TREATMENT FOR MS?

Smoking marijuana has been reported by some individuals to benefit their MS symptoms, particularly **spasticity** and pain. Early, clinical trials of orally administered tetrahydrocannabinol (THC), one of the active chemicals in marijuana, had mixed results. While some treated individuals reported feeling "looser" and less stiff, objective evaluations by physicians could not always confirm any change. Effects lasted less than 3 hours, and side effects included weakness, dry mouth, dizziness, mental clouding, short-term memory impairment, space–time distortions, and incoordination. The toxic effects of smoked marijuana may exceed those associated with smoking tobacco.

In March 1999, the National Academy of Sciences/Institute of Medicine released their White House-commissioned report on medical uses of marijuana. The report stated that the medical benefits of marijuana are modest, and that, for most symptoms, more effective medicines are already available. The report did recommend, however, continued research on the biologic effects of cannabinoids, the active compounds in marijuana, to determine if it is possible to derive their benefits without their detrimental side effects.

A rigorous, large, placebo-controlled study comparing cannabis extract and THC for the treatment of spasticity was conducted in Great Britain. The results of the study, involving 657 patients at 33 clinical centers, indicated that, in comparison to placebo, treatment with oral cannabis oil or synthetic THC had no objective effect on muscle spasticity (as measured by a standardized measure of spasticity). Study participants reported, however, some improvement in their spasticity and pain. Whether the positive effects that patients reported resulted from a specific chemical effect of cannabinoids, or a heightened placebo effect, could not be determined because the side effects of the active drug made it possible for 77 percent of those on active therapy to identify their treatment group. In other words, the study was not sufficiently ***blinded***. In addition, the study did not provide sufficient information about the extent of pain relief experienced by patients to determine if the benefits outweighed the significant side effects (including dizziness/light-headedness, dry mouth, and gastrointestinal symptoms).

The National MS Society is currently funding a study that may help to address some of the problems encountered in the study in Great Britain. The study, which is being carried out at the University of California, Davis, is a placebo-controlled study to test the safety and effectiveness of inhaled cannabis and of oral THC for the treatment of spasticity in 60 persons with MS. The team has developed novel instruments to objectively test *muscle tone* and other measures of spasticity and is using them to compare these experimental therapies with inactive placebo. The Society also established a task force to examine the use of cannabis in MS and to review what is currently known about its potential. This task force made specific recommendations on the research that still needs to be done to answer pressing questions about the potential effectiveness and safety of marijuana and its derivatives in treating MS (www.nationalmssociety.org/marijuana).

In the United Kingdom, a study, known as CUPID ("Cannabinoid Use in Progressive Inflammatory Brain Disease"), is evaluating the effects of THC on disease progression in more than 600 people with progressive forms of MS. The results of this study are expected to be available in 2013.

In the meantime, Health Canada, the drug regulatory agency for Canada, has approved the use of Sativex—a drug derived from cannabis—to treat MS-related pain. The approval was based on a small, 4-week clinical trial in the United Kingdom that involved 66 people with MS. Sativex contains extracts from a specific variant of the marijuana plant and is administered as a spray into the mouth. This drug is not approved in the United States—and any use of marijuana or its derivatives for medical purposes continues to be illegal in this country. In fact, the Supreme Court ruled in 2005 that the federal government has the power to prohibit and prosecute the possession and use of marijuana for medical purposes, even in the 15 states (Alaska, Arizona, California, Colorado, Hawaii, Maine, Michigan, Montana, Nevada, New Jersey, New Mexico, Oregon, Rhode Island, Vermont, and Washington), and Washington, DC, that currently permit it.

I'VE SEEN A LOT OF INFORMATION ON THE INTERNET ABOUT LOW-DOSE NALTREXONE. IS THIS A RECOMMENDED TREATMENT FOR PEOPLE WITH MS?
Naltrexone is an opioid antagonist that has been approved by the FDA for the treatment of addictions to opioids and alcohol. At significantly lower doses than those

used for addictions, it has been prescribed as a treatment for a variety of diseases, including various types of cancers, HIV/AIDS, Parkinson's disease, Alzheimer's disease, amyotrophic lateral sclerosis, emphysema, as well as MS and other ***autoimmune diseases***. To date, however, there have been limited studies in MS. Preliminary studies in the animal model of MS have produced promising results. In addition, two relatively small clinical trials in people with MS have produced positive results. However, another clinical trial in people with MS did not demonstrate any therapeutic effects. Due to these variable results, further studies are needed to definitively determine whether low-dose naltrexone is safe and effective in MS.

THE INFORMATION ABOUT THE ROLE OF DIET AND FATTY ACIDS IN TREATING MS IS VERY CONTRADICTORY. WILL CHANGING MY DIET TO INCREASE POLYUNSATURATED FATTY ACIDS HELP MY MS OR NOT?

Many diets have been recommended for MS with little or no supportive evidence. If one chooses to follow a specific diet, however, it is important to maintain a well-balanced intake of nutrients, because some of the more extreme dietary regimens may actually cause problems by depriving the body of necessary nutrients. Those studies that have been done in this area are not conclusive, and the conventional medical literature tends to promote the same well-balanced, high-fiber, low-fat diet recommended by the American Heart Association and considered beneficial for everyone, with or without MS. A moderate unconventional approach, based on research done on the role of polyunsaturated fatty acids in MS, would advocate reducing the intake of saturated fat and adding moderate amounts of omega-three fatty acids (fish oil, cod liver oil, and flaxseed oil), omega-six fatty acids (sunflower seed [or other] oil and possibly evening primrose oil), and perhaps additional vitamin E, since the addition of polyunsaturated fatty acids to the diet tends to lower vitamin E levels. A more aggressive unconventional approach, advocated by some, involves a significant change in diet as well as high-level dietary supplementation (e.g., the Swank Diet, which remains somewhat controversial and is not generally advocated by physicians for people with MS).

I'VE HEARD THAT VITAMIN D MAY BE BENEFICIAL FOR MS. SHOULD I TAKE VITAMIN D SUPPLEMENTS?

There are several aspects of vitamin D that are potentially relevant to those with MS. First, it is known that vitamin D helps maintain normal bone density by promoting the absorption of calcium, and that people with MS appear to be at higher risk for decreased bone density because of reduced mobility and use of corticosteroids to treat MS relapses. In its severe form, reduced bone density is known as ***osteoporosis*** and in its mild form as ***osteopenia***. It is important to discuss bone health with your health care professional to ensure that you are receiving appropriate bone density screening as well as adequate amounts of calcium and vitamin D.

In addition, vitamin D might play a more direct role in the disease process of MS. There are multiple studies indicating that a relatively high intake of vitamin D and relatively high blood levels of vitamin D are associated with a decreased risk of developing MS. And in those who have MS, high intake and blood levels of vitamin D are associated with a decreased risk of MS attacks and progression of disability.

These studies only show an "association" or relationship—they do not prove that high vitamin D intake prevents MS or slows the disease course. To prove a causal connection between vitamin D intake and MS, more rigorous studies are needed. These types of studies are under way and should help to better define the role of vitamin D in MS.

Until the results of these studies are available, people with MS have several options. One option is to do nothing and wait until more definitive information is available. A somewhat more "aggressive" approach is to take modest amounts of vitamin D supplements, such as 1,000 to 2,000 international units (IU) daily. The most aggressive approach is to have a blood test done for vitamin D (known as a "25-hydroxy-vitamin D test") and, if the level is low, take supplements as needed to raise the blood level to the normal range. When considering vitamin D supplements, it is important to keep in mind that for adults in the general population the recommended daily amount (RDA) is 600 to 800 IU and the safe upper limit for daily use (known as the "UL" or "Tolerable Upper Intake Level") is 4,000 IU.

MY FRIENDS AND RELATIVES ARE ALWAYS PUSHING ME TO TRY DIFFERENT DIETARY SUPPLEMENTS. I'VE SEEN THEM IN THE HEALTH FOOD STORES, AND MANY ARE DESCRIBED AS "NATURAL." DOES THIS MEAN THEY ARE SAFE FOR ME TO TAKE?

With the exception of polyunsaturated fatty acids, very little research has actually been done on most of the dietary supplements promoted for use in MS. Here are some important points to remember about dietary supplements:

● The fact that a supplement is sold in a health food store and labeled as being "natural" does not necessarily mean that it is safe or beneficial; while some are healthy or benign, others are actually quite toxic (e.g., chaparral, comfrey, germanium, lobelia, skullcap, and yohimbe).

● Supplements, like prescription medications, are not side-effect free; any supplement that provides benefits contains chemicals that are likely to also produce some side effects. For example, many herbs have sedating effects and others can irritate the urinary tract.

● Combinations of supplements with conventional medications have not been fully investigated, and little is known about how the interactions might affect the safety or benefit of each one individually.

As with all CAM interventions, your best strategy is to investigate supplements carefully and discuss them with your physician.

RECOMMENDED READINGS

Bowling AC. *Complementary and Alternative Medicine and Multiple Sclerosis* (2nd ed.). New York: Demos Medical Publishing, 2007.

Selected materials available from the National Multiple Sclerosis Society, 800-FIGHT-MS (800-344-3867) or online at *www.nationalmssociety.org/Brochures*:
  • *Acupuncture: The Basic Facts*
  • *Clear Thinking About Alternative Therapies*

- *Exercise as Part of Everyday Life*
- *Food for Thought: MS and Nutrition*
- *Vitamins, Minerals, and Herbs in MS: An Introduction*

RECOMMENDED RESOURCES

Complementary and Alternative Medicine Web site: A website maintained by Dr. Allen Bowling that provides comprehensive information on CAM and MS (http://neurologycare.net).

Oregon Center for Complementary and Alternative Medicine in Neurological Disorders (ORCCAMIND): A "center without walls," committed to research in CAM in neurologic disorders (www.ohsu.edu/orccamind).

National Center for Complementary and Alternative Medicine (NCCAM): Online resource center for CAM, which was established in 1998 by Congress to bring rigorous science to the study of CAM (http://nccam.nih.gov).

Partnering with an MS Nurse
to Enhance Wellness:
Key Management Concepts

June Halper, MSN, ANP-C, FAAN, MSCN

Multiple sclerosis (MS) can affect many aspects of a person's functioning over its long and unpredictable course. Some of the problems caused by the illness, such as pain, fatigue, weakness, imbalance, *optic neuritis*, or bladder and bowel symptoms, are a direct result of *plaque* formation in the central nervous system. Others, including skin breakdown or *osteoporosis*, can result from the lack of mobility or altered nutrition status as consequences of MS. Much has been learned in recent years about the successful professional and self-management of these primary and secondary problems in MS. With education and support provided by the health care team, people can learn to control their symptoms and reduce unnecessary problems and complications.

The nurse can be a helpful ally in these management activities, whether as a member of an MS center's health care team, in the community's visiting nurse service, as part of a hospital inpatient service, in a *rehabilitation* facility, or in the home. A primary goal of nursing care in MS is to help people learn effective, preventive self-management in order to control minor problems before they become major ones. This chapter has as its focus three areas in which nursing plays a key role—elimination dysfunction, skin care, and important wellness strategies for maintaining an optimal level of health and well-being despite a chronic illness.

BLADDER FUNCTION

The neurologic changes in MS frequently interfere with bladder function. These changes can be distressing and occasionally disabling, but they are manageable with effective interventions that may include individualized education, targeted diagnostic testing, medications, and self-management activities. The first step toward successful bladder management is to talk with your health care providers about any changes in bladder function you may be experiencing. So, this section begins with an explanation about how the healthy urinary system functions.

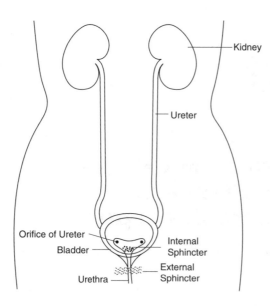

Kidney

Ureter

Orifice of Ureter

Bladder

Urethra

Internal
Sphincter

External
Sphincter

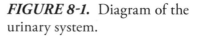

FIGURE 8-1. Diagram of the urinary system.

The urinary system (see Figure 8-1) includes the following:

- **Kidneys**, which filter impurities from the bloodstream and excrete them in the urine
- **Ureters**, the small tubes that transport urine from the kidneys to the bladder
- **Urinary bladder**, which stores urine until it is time to void (urinate)
- *Urethra*, which transports the urine out of the body

For normal urination to occur, the ***detrusor***, or bladder muscle, must contract to expel urine at the same time that the internal and external ***sphincters*** are relaxed to allow the urine to pass freely out of the body. In normal function, the urine is collected slowly, causing the bladder to expand. When approximately six to eight ounces (180–240 ml) of urine have accumulated, nerve endings in the bladder send a message to the voiding ***reflex*** area of the spinal cord, which, in turn, sends a message to the brain signaling the need to urinate. The brain then sends a message back to the spinal cord that signals the voiding reflex to contract the detrusor muscle and relax the urethral sphincter. Thus, a functional urinary system depends on an intact nervous system.

In MS, the excretion or elimination of urine can be altered in the following ways:

- *Inability to store urine.* This condition is usually seen in a small, spastic or tight bladder, resulting from ***demyelination*** of the pathways between the spinal cord and the brain. The bladder fills quickly and sends messages to the spinal cord, which, because of demyelination, is unable or slow to forward the message to the brain. As a result, voluntary control of urination is interrupted, and voiding becomes a reflex response to repeated signals from the spinal cord. Inability to store can result in symptoms of ***urinary urgency*** (having to get to the bathroom quickly), ***urinary frequency*** (feeling the urge to urinate even when urination has occurred very recently), dribbling small amounts of urine, ***urinary incontinence*** (wetting oneself), and nocturia (being awakened at night by the need to urinate).

- *Inability to empty.* This condition results when demyelination occurs in the voiding reflex area of the spinal cord. Even though the bladder fills with large amounts of urine, the spinal cord is unable to send the necessary messages—either to the brain that the bladder is full or to the bladder and sphincter. The resulting absence of either voluntary or reflexive voiding causes the bladder to overfill. Failure to empty results in a large, *flaccid* (atonic) bladder and symptoms of urgency, dribbling, hesitancy, and incontinence. This kind of bladder dysfunction also puts a person at significantly greater risk for urinary tract infections (UTIs), which can cause discomfort as well as a worsening of other MS symptoms.

   Combined dysfunction can result from a failure to store/failure to empty combination called ***detrusor-external sphincter dyssynergia (DESD)***. Combined dysfunction involves a lack of coordination between muscle groups, whereby the detrusor and external sphincter contract simultaneously, trapping urine within the bladder. Both urgency and hesitancy may occur, as well as dribbling or incontinence.

   It is important to remember that a particular symptom does not point to a specific type of bladder dysfunction. In fact, each of the primary urinary symptoms—urgency, frequency, hesitancy, incontinence, and nocturia—can be caused by any of the functional abnormalities described. Careful evaluation is needed to identify the cause of the problem and to select appropriate treatment measures.

I HAVE JUST BEEN DIAGNOSED WITH MS. WHAT ARE THE CHANCES THAT I WILL DEVELOP PROBLEMS CONTROLLING MY BLADDER OR BOWEL?

MS can affect the motor and sensory pathways from the brain and spinal cord that control both bladder and bowel function. Over the course of the disease, as many as 80 to 90 percent of people with MS develop transient or persistent urinary symptoms. Bladder symptoms can occur at the onset of the illness or at any time thereafter. They can usually be controlled with medications, self-care activities, and some possible modifications in lifestyle. Bowel problems occur somewhat less frequently, but are still common enough that everyone with MS must be aware of their relationship to the disease and be familiar with effective prevention and management strategies. The most important thing to remember about bladder and bowel symptoms in MS is that they can be helped. The MS health care team is familiar with these problems and their management. Although you may initially find it difficult or uncomfortable to discuss bladder and bowel questions with your doctor or nurse, the more open you are about any problems you are having, the more quickly and easily you can learn effective management techniques and avoid unnecessary complications and discomfort.

I HAVE RECENTLY BEGUN HAVING TROUBLE CONTROLLING MY URINE. ALL OF A SUDDEN, WITHOUT ANY WARNING, I HAVE TO GET TO THE BATHROOM IMMEDIATELY OR RISK WETTING MYSELF. WHAT IS THE TREATMENT FOR THIS PROBLEM?

The sudden sensation of having to urinate quickly is called urinary urgency. It usually results from the bladder's failure to store urine properly or from a failure to store/failure to empty combination (DESD). A careful evaluation is needed to determine the cause of the urgency.

   Urgency resulting from a failure to store can be managed in several different ways. An ***anticholinergic*** medication—such as Ditropan, Ditropan XL, or Oxytrol

Transdermal System (different forms of oxybutynin chloride), Enablex (darifenacin), and Vesicare (solifenacin)—will help to control spasms in the bladder and other smooth muscles of the body by inhibiting the transmission of parasympathetic nerve impulses (see Appendix B). Antimuscarinics, another class of medication, can also be used to decrease contractions of the bladder. Examples of antimuscarinic medications include Detrol (tolterodine) andToviaz (fesoteradine). Certain tricyclic antidepressants, most notably Tofranil (imipramine), share these anticholinergic properties and have also been found useful in controlling urinary muscle contractions (see Appendix B).

In addition to these oral medications, another type of medication was approved by the FDA in 2011 to treat this type of urinary urgency. Botox (onabotulinumtoxinA)—the same medication that can be used for cosmetic purposes to reduce wrinkles and to treat upper limb spasticity in MS—is injected into the bladder to relax the muscle and reduce episodes of incontinence (See Appendix B). Botox is approved for people who have not received sufficient benefit from an anticholinergic medication or are unable to tolerate the side effects. The effects of each injection last approximately 42–48 weeks.

Feelings of urgency resulting from the bladder's failure to empty or from DESD are best managed with a treatment regimen that includes an anticholinergic or antimuscarinic medication and ***intermittent self-catheterization (ISC)***.

WHAT IS INTERMITTENT SELF-CATHETERIZATION?
If the bladder fails to empty properly, or the bladder and sphincters do not work together in the proper rhythm, your physician may suggest that you do ISC on a scheduled basis—from one to five times a day. ISC can be thought of as physical therapy for your bladder, because it promotes regular filling and emptying (expanding and contracting) of the bladder muscle and may help restore normal function. You begin by emptying your bladder as thoroughly as you can. Then you drain the residual or remaining urine by passing a ***straight catheter*** (a very thin, hollow, plastic tube that resembles a straw) into your bladder through the urethra. The ***catheter*** stays in your bladder until the urine stops draining—no more than a minute or two—and is then removed. With a little practice, the procedure is easy, quick, and painless. ISC can be done while sitting on the toilet, lying on the bed, or even in the public restroom of your favorite restaurant. Your doctor or nurse can instruct you in the appropriate use, care, and cleaning of the urinary catheter. If you are unable to self-catheterize, the procedure may be carried out by your spouse, partner, or a visiting nurse. Typically, the nurse will stay involved only long enough to ensure that you or your spouse/partner has mastered the technique.

**WHAT KINDS OF TESTS WILL THE DOCTOR DO TO FIND OUT
WHY I AM HAVING PROBLEMS WITH URINATION?**
A number of tests are used to diagnose urinary problems. Your physician will first determine whether a UTI is causing your urinary symptoms. Infections in one or more of the structures of the urinary tract are caused by bacteria and can be detected by microscopic examination of a urine specimen. A test called a ***urine culture and sensitivity (C&S)*** will be used to identify the particular organism

(germ) that is present and the antibiotic to which it is sensitive. The bacteria from a midstream urine sample are allowed to grow for 3 days in a special laboratory medium and then tested for sensitivity to a variety of antibiotics. This allows your physician to prescribe the antibiotic most likely to kill the bacteria. An antibiotic that commonly cures UTI may be prescribed until the results of the C&S are known.

To determine whether your urinary symptoms are caused by the bladder's failure to empty, failure to store, or combined dysfunction, the doctor can evaluate your *postvoid residual (PVR)*. You will be asked to drink ample fluids for a day or two before the test and two glasses just prior to the PVR. As soon as you feel the need to urinate, you will do so and the amount of urine will be measured. After you have urinated, the nurse will pass a straight catheter into the bladder to drain and measure the urine remaining in the bladder. A completely noninvasive way of measuring *residual urine* that is now being used by many MS centers and *urologists* uses a bladder scanner. This scanner uses an external "wand" and a computer to determine the amount of urine remaining in your bladder after voiding. It is important to determine if urine is being retained in the bladder, because urine that is not voided can cause a UTI. Depending on the amount of urine found in your bladder after voiding, your health care provider may suggest a program of self-catheterization and/or medication to manage your symptoms.

In most instances, the results of either kind of PVR assessment, in combination with your body's response to the prescribed treatment regimen, will provide ample information about the source of your urinary symptoms. Further testing may be required if the physician is still unable to diagnose the problem. In the *intravenous pyelogram* test, dye is injected into your vein so that sequential x-ray pictures can be taken of the kidneys, ureters, and bladder. Ultrasound technology (using sound waves) can also be used to determine the presence of stones or other abnormalities in your bladder. A urinary *cystoscopy*—a somewhat more invasive test that can be done in a urologist's office or in the hospital—allows the physician to examine the inside of the bladder.

SOMETIMES, WHEN I FEEL THAT I HAVE TO URINATE, I FIND THAT I HAVE TROUBLE GETTING STARTED. I FEEL THE PRESSURE TO EMPTY MY BLADDER, BUT NOTHING COMES OUT. IS THERE ANYTHING I CAN DO ABOUT THIS?

The inability to initiate urination despite the sensation of a full bladder is called *urinary hesitancy* and usually results from the bladder's failure to empty properly. Patience almost always pays off; people find that the urinary stream usually starts within a minute or two. You can try running water in the sink to help relax the urinary sphincter. "Tickling" the opening to the urethra (the opening behind a woman's vagina or the tip of a man's penis) with a moist tissue may also promote relaxation. If these techniques do not produce results, you may tap lightly on the lower part of your abdomen. Do not press or hit yourself too forcefully, as this might worsen the problem.

Speak to your health care provider if you are unable to manage the hesitancy. A medication such as Lioresal (baclofen) will relax the sphincter to allow the bladder to empty more effectively (see Appendix B).

AFTER I FINISH URINATING, I SOMETIMES FEEL THAT MY BLADDER IS STILL FULL. NOTHING MORE COMES OUT, BUT I'M AFRAID TO LEAVE THE BATHROOM IN CASE OF AN ACCIDENT. HOW CAN I TELL IF THERE IS MORE URINE LEFT IN MY BLADDER?

The sensation of a full bladder after voiding can be caused by the bladder's failure either to empty or store properly. A PVR can be done to determine if you are retaining urine in your bladder and what treatment would be most beneficial. As indicated, it is important that you be able to empty your bladder fully, using whatever combination of medication and/or ISC is appropriate, both to maintain your personal comfort and to reduce your risk of bladder infections. Some individuals with MS find relief from this problem by "double-voiding"—urinating once, waiting a minute or more and perhaps changing position, and then voiding again.

I'M SO WORRIED I'LL HAVE A BLADDER ACCIDENT THAT I HARDLY DRINK ANYTHING ANYMORE. MY DOCTOR SAYS THAT I NEED TO DRINK FLUIDS SO THAT I WON'T GET BLADDER INFECTIONS. WHAT CAN I DO TO HANDLE THIS PROBLEM?

Urine, which consists of solid and liquid waste substances that are not needed by your body, is manufactured continuously by the kidneys. It is important for urine to be diluted with water, because urine that contains more solid particles than liquid will increase your risk of infection. Many people who experience ***urinary urgency*** or frequency restrict their intake of fluids in the hope of relieving their symptoms and freeing themselves from the bathroom. As a result, their urine becomes too highly concentrated with solid particles (resulting in a dark brownish appearance) and therefore more susceptible to infection. You should drink between six and eight glasses of fluid per day, early in the day if you prefer, to avoid having to go to the bathroom at night. You can also get fluids in such foods as soup, juices, Jell-O, fruits, and puddings. In addition to reducing your risk of bladder infections, adequate fluid intake will help you to maintain satisfactory bowel function. Identifying the cause of your bladder accidents will make it possible for your physician to design a bladder management program, possibly including medication and scheduled voiding, in an effort to "train" your bladder and help reduce the risk of accidents.

SOMETIMES I WET MYSELF WITHOUT EVEN KNOWING THAT IT IS HAPPENING— I CAN'T FEEL EITHER THE URGE TO URINATE OR THE URINE ITSELF. WHY IS THIS HAPPENING, AND IS THERE ANYTHING I CAN DO ABOUT IT?

Spontaneous voiding (urinary incontinence) can occur in MS for a number of reasons. Because either uninhibited bladder spasms or a weakened bladder muscle can cause urine to pass out of the bladder before the urge to urinate is felt, PVR testing is required to determine the cause of the problem. Diminished sensations in the genital area will reduce a person's awareness of the urge to void and perhaps even of the sensation of being wet. Usually, a treatment regimen consisting of ISC and/ or a trial of one of the medications described earlier will be sufficient to control the incontinence. If the bladder dysfunction that is causing the incontinence does not respond to this type of treatment regimen, your health care provider will probably refer you to a urologist for more extensive bladder studies to determine if some other problem is contributing to your symptoms.

I SEEM TO BE GETTING UP THREE OR FOUR TIMES DURING THE NIGHT TO URINATE. THIS IS VERY UNUSUAL FOR ME. IS THERE ANYTHING I CAN DO ABOUT THIS PROBLEM?

The first step in dealing with ***nocturia***, as this problem is called, is to make sure that you do not have a UTI. Then, your physician or nurse will do a PVR to determine the probable cause of the problem. Nocturia is most commonly caused by spasms in the bladder muscles that result in the bladder's failure to store urine properly. It can usually be treated very effectively with a bedtime dose of either Tofranil (imipramine) or DDAVP (desmopressin)—available as a nasal spray or in tablet form (see Appendix B).

I THINK I HAVE MEMORIZED THE LOCATION OF EVERY BATHROOM IN THE CITY. IS THERE ANYTHING I CAN DO WHEN I'M GOING OUT SO THAT I DON'T CONSTANTLY HAVE TO BE NEAR A TOILET?

The urinary symptoms of urgency and frequency, which sometimes make people feel as though their lives are controlled by the location of the nearest bathroom, can usually be treated and managed once they are properly diagnosed. Your health care team can diagnose the source of these symptoms and prescribe a course of medication and/ or ISC that will allow you to regain control of your bladder.

Once this sense of control is regained, you will feel more confident about venturing farther from the bathroom—especially if you take advantage of one of the available apps for your cell phone or other mobile device that identify nearby bathrooms wherever you happen to be. Most people still find that they feel more comfortable if, upon arriving at their destination, they check out the location of the bathroom so that they can get there without having to search for it.

Some people choose to wear a protective pad (e.g., Serenity or Depends) so that they do not have to panic about possible leakage. If you know that you have trouble controlling your bladder for long periods, and that you are going to be in a situation in which getting to a bathroom quickly is impossible (a football game, a wedding, or a long bus ride, for example), you can discuss with your health care provider the occasional use of a drug such as DDAVP (see Appendix B).

WHAT ARE THE SYMPTOMS OF A UTI, AND WHAT ARE THE TREATMENTS FOR IT?

UTIs can sometimes occur without any apparent symptoms or discomfort. More often, however, an infection causes symptoms such as urinary urgency and frequency, a burning sensation, abdominal pain, an elevated body temperature, increased ***spasticity***, and possibly foul-smelling, dark-colored urine. UTIs most commonly occur in the bladder and are usually treatable with oral antibiotics. An infection in the upper portion of the urinary tract, including the kidneys and ureters, is more serious and potentially more debilitating. Kidney infections are usually accompanied by a high fever and may require intravenous treatment with antibiotics. Both types of infection are treated by increased fluid intake and rest, as well as close medical monitoring.

Individuals who are particularly prone to UTIs may be prescribed an antiseptic, such as Hiprex (methenamine), to use on a routine basis to "cleanse" the urine and reduce the number of bacteria (see Appendix B). In addition, maintaining the acidity of your urine will help in the prevention of UTIs because the organisms that cause infections do not grow as easily in an acidic environment. You can make your urine more acidic by following certain dietary guidelines. These include an increase in your daily intake of (1) protein, such as that found in meat, fish, fowl, eggs, and gelatin; and (2) cranberries (and their juice), plums, and prunes. The cranberry juice, which provides a replacement for the vitamin C found in citrus fruits, should be taken at frequent intervals throughout the day, because vitamin C is processed and excreted very rapidly by the body. Decrease your intake of (1) citrus fruits and juices (grape-fruit, oranges, lemons, and tomatoes); (2) milk and milk products; (3) beverages or antacids containing sodium carbonate or sodium bicarbonate (use Gelusil or any other aluminum-type antacid in their place); and (4) potatoes.

To treat chronic, recurrent UTIs, your physician may prescribe long-term, low-dose antibiotics such as Bactrim (sulfamethoxazole) in an effort to suppress bacterial activity and reduce the risk of infection (see Appendix B).

**I FEEL VERY WEAK WHEN I HAVE A BLADDER (URINARY TRACT) INFECTION
EVEN THOUGH I NEVER SEEM TO RUN A VERY HIGH FEVER.
DOES THIS MEAN THAT THE INFECTION IS MAKING MY MS WORSE?**

Any type of infection—especially one that causes an elevation in body temperature—is likely to cause a feeling of weakness and an apparent *exacerbation* of symptoms. This is referred to as a *pseudoexacerbation* because it is caused by the underlying infec-tion and not by an actual progression of the disease. The important strategy when this occurs is to treat the infection promptly, thus removing the trigger for this temporary worsening of the symptoms. A pseudoexacerbation and accompanying weakness typi-cally remit or disappear once the infection is brought under control.

IS A UTI EVER LIFE-THREATENING?

A UTI can be life-threatening if left untreated and allowed to spread into the kid-neys. Since all blood is filtered through the kidneys, the infection can pass into the bloodstream and cause serious problems.

**ARE THERE DIFFERENT TYPES OF URINARY CATHETERS?
HOW DO I KNOW WHAT TYPE OF CATHETER IS BEST FOR ME?**

The type of catheter used for ISC resembles a straw and is called a *straight cath-eter*. One end is tapered and has a small hole called a *port*. This end is inserted into the bladder for urinary drainage. The other end has a larger opening that allows the urine to flow into the toilet or a collecting device.

A *condom catheter*, which is used only by males, consists of a tube connected to a very thin, flexible sheath worn over the penis. This type of catheter allows urine to drain into a collection bag.

A *Foley catheter* is an *indwelling catheter* that remains in the bladder for longer periods of time, allowing continuous drainage into a collection bag. The tapered end has a balloon that is inflated when the catheter is placed into the bladder. The bal-loon is filled with sterile water while in the bladder and emptied when the catheter is withdrawn, but cannot be felt by the person at any time. A Foley catheter is used for continuous drainage of urine when bladder function cannot be improved by the other means discussed in this chapter, or if a person is experiencing skin breakdown *(pressure sores)* because of chronic wetness that cannot be otherwise managed.

MY DOCTOR WANTS ME TO DO INTERMITTENT SELF-CATHETERIZATION. WHY CAN'T I JUST USE A FOLEY CATHETER ALL THE TIME SO I DON'T HAVE TO BE BOTHERED?

ISC is a strategy to maintain and sometimes improve bladder tone and bladder function. It prevents infections, reduces symptoms, and prevents the long-term complications of chronic UTIs. People may find that their bladder symptoms are more problematic at some times than others; they may need to do ISC for a period, and then find it unnecessary for a while. A Foley catheter is used by people who are unable to manage their bladder function any other way—either because their urinary symptoms have not been successfully controlled by medications or self-care strategies, or because their other symptoms (e.g., severe *spasticity*, tremor, weakness, **cognitive impairment**) interfere with their ability to do ISC. The urinary system is normally closed to the outside environment, even when a person self-catheterizes. Once an indwelling catheter is inserted into the bladder, this closed system remains open at all times, making the person susceptible to ongoing infections, the development of bladder stones, and other complications of the urinary system. Foley catheters are the last resort when other treatments are not viable.

IS IT POSSIBLE TO USE A FOLEY CATHETER FOR SOME SITUATIONS AND CATHETERIZE MYSELF THE REST OF THE TIME?

Some people who self-catheterize regularly can insert Foley catheters for situations when ISC is not possible. Airline flights or long car trips, for example, make ISC somewhat problematic. The Foley catheter is inserted prior to the journey and then removed. Because of the increased risk of infection with an indwelling catheter, it is very important to discuss the advisability of this strategy with your health care provider; it may be reasonable for some individuals but not for others. Anyone using a Foley catheter must increase fluid intake to minimize the risk of infection. You can resume your normal ISC bladder routine once the Foley catheter is removed.

WILL MY BLADDER SYMPTOMS EVER GET BETTER OR GO AWAY?

This is not an easy question to answer. Many people report that their bladder symptoms improve or disappear, at least temporarily, with the appropriate use of medications and ISC. Others report that their bladder dysfunction waxes and wanes but never fully disappears. As with other symptoms of MS, bladder symptoms vary from person to person and from one period of time to another. The key to bladder management is accurate knowledge about what is causing the problem followed by appropriate action to minimize complaints and control symptoms.

ARE THERE ANY OTHER PROCEDURES THAT MIGHT HELP MY BLADDER SYMPTOMS?

There are no interventions that completely resolve bladder problems caused by neurologic changes. In certain instances, when none of the medications or self-care techniques described have successfully relieved urinary symptoms, other procedures may be used to help bladder management. These procedures are not routine and should be discussed with your health care provider. You would need to follow up with a urologist—a physician who specializes in bladder problems.

Injection options **include the following:**

- Botox (botulinum toxin) has demonstrated its usefulness in the management of certain types of urinary symptoms. Injected into the external urinary sphincter, Botox helps to relieve the urinary urgency, frequency, dribbling, retention, and infections that can be caused by failure of the sphincter to relax and permit urine to drain. Treatment benefits, which typically last a minimum of 3 months, can relieve voiding problems and reduce a person's need for ISC or an indwelling catheter in the urethra. No significant complications or side effects have been reported. The manufacturers of Botox have applied to the Food and Drug Administration (FDA) for approval of this use of the medication.
- Collagen (or other biocompatible material) injections into the urethra can relieve the incontinence that occurs when the urethra is too weak to hold urine in the bladder. The collagen serves as a bulking agent to improve urethral function. This procedure, which may need to be repeated periodically, has been shown to work more effectively in women than in men.

Surgical options **include—but are not limited to—the following:**

- Sacral nerve stimulation (InterStim therapy for urinary control) is a treatment for people with urge incontinence caused by failure to store. InterStim uses an implanted neurostimulation system to send mild electrical pulses to the sacral nerve. The sacral nerve, located near the tailbone in the lower back, influences the bladder control muscles.
- Continent vesicostomy/augmentation cystoplasty is a surgically created opening in the abdomen that is connected to the bladder by a *stoma,* which allows for intermittent catheterization. In some cases, a small, spastic bladder may need to be enlarged using a piece of the intestine to ensure that the bladder is large enough to hold sufficient amounts of urine between catheterizations.
- Suprapubic **cystostomy** is a surgically created opening in the abdominal wall directly into the bladder. A drainage tube carries urine out of the bladder into an external collection bag. This procedure avoids some of the potential complications of an indwelling catheter.
- Sphincterotomy is a permanent surgical enlargement of the urinary sphincter in a male whose spasticity is so severe that he cannot empty his bladder. Following the surgery, the man must use a condom catheter to collect the urine. Sphincterotomy, which is rarely used in MS, should not be used in females.

BOWEL FUNCTION

As with bladder function, neurologic changes can sometimes interfere with a person's normal bowel functioning. In this section, we describe the parts of your gastrointestinal system and how they are supposed to work, and then provide answers to the most common questions about how to manage changes in bowel function when they occur.

The gastrointestinal tract, which is responsible for the digestion and absorption of food and the elimination of waste, is composed of the following parts (see Figure 8-2):

- *Mouth*, in which digestion is initiated by the chewing process and the addition of saliva
- *Esophagus*, which connects the mouth to the stomach
- *Stomach*, which stores food and advances the digestive process
- *Small intestine*, where the digestive process is continued
- *Large intestine*, where stool is formed
- *Rectum*, in which the stool is stored just prior to defecation
- *Anal canal*, which contains the internal and external sphincters that normally remain closed to prevent leakage

Stool normally passes into the rectum just prior to a bowel movement. When the rectum becomes full, it sends nerve impulses to a critical area of the spinal cord. The stool then passes through the anal canal, where it encounters first the internal sphincter, which opens reflexively in response to signals from the spinal cord, and then the external sphincter, which responds to signals from both the spinal cord and brain. The external sphincter is under "voluntary control," which means that a person can consciously tighten it to prevent defecation until the time and place are convenient. As with the urinary system, a functional gastrointestinal system is dependent on a functional nervous system.

Changes in bowel function can be manifested as **constipation**, bowel urgency, or loss of bowel control (incontinence). People rarely complain about loose stools

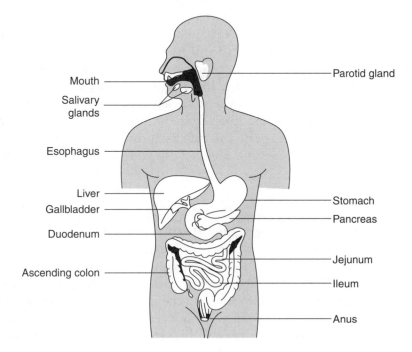

FIGURE 8-2. The gastrointestinal tract.

or diarrhea unless they have taken excessive amounts of laxatives or stool softeners. Constipation, by far the most frequent bowel complaint in MS, refers to infrequent, incomplete, or difficult bowel movements. The management of constipation in MS is important not only because of the abdominal discomfort it can cause, but also because of its potential for exacerbating other symptoms such as *spasticity* and urinary urgency and frequency.

Several factors conspire to produce MS-related constipation:

- *Demyelination* in the brain or spinal cord and reduced physical movement can each slow the passage of stool through the bowel. Because the body continuously draws moisture from the stool as it makes its way through the body, stool that remains in the intestine for extended periods of time becomes overly dry, hard, and difficult to pass.
- Dry, hardened stool can also result from decreased sensation in the rectal area. A person with decreased sensation may not experience the need to have a bowel movement, with the result that the stool remains in the rectum for an overly extended period of time.
- The same problem sometimes occurs because weakened abdominal muscles make it difficult to push the stool out of the rectum.
- A reduced fluid intake (usually in response to anxiety over bladder problems) will also cause the body to absorb more water from the stool.
- Certain medications slow bowel function and therefore contribute to the stool's loss of moisture.

Bowel changes in MS can be successfully managed with a self-care program that starts with a thorough evaluation of your dietary habits, medications, past and present bowel habits, and physical requirements for safe and comfortable toileting. If needed, an individualized bowel management program can be initiated with the help of the physician and nurse; successful bowel management then depends on the patience and time required to find the right combination of dietary changes, medications, and a consistent routine. In general, a healthy bowel program consists of adequate fluid intake, a high-fiber diet, adequate exercise, and a consistent, relaxed time for bowel evacuation, preferably 30 minutes after a meal, when the *gastrocolic reflex* is at its strongest. This reflex controls movement or peristalsis of the gastrointestinal tract. It is responsible for the urge to move your bowels after a meal.

ARE THE BOWEL AND BLADDER SYMPTOMS I HAVE RELATED? SOME OF MY FRIENDS WITH MS HAVE ONE OR THE OTHER SYMPTOM BUT NOT BOTH.

Bowel and bladder symptoms in MS may be related to one another, but they do not necessarily have to be. Spasms resulting from impaired neurologic function can cause symptoms of urgency and frequency in both the bladder and bowel systems. Weakened musculature can also interfere with the emptying process in either system. A full bowel can press on the bladder, causing symptoms of urinary urgency and frequency. Individual factors, such as your diet, amount of exercise, and pre-illness bowel patterns, are likely to have the biggest impact on your bowel functioning, independent of what is occurring with your bladder.

MY DOCTOR SAYS THAT DRINKING MORE FLUIDS WILL HELP WITH MY CONSTIPATION, BUT WHEN I DRINK I HAVE DIFFICULTY CONTROLLING MY URINE. I CAN'T DECIDE WHICH PROBLEM IS WORSE!

Increasing your fluid intake is certainly one important method for improving bowel function. It is generally recommended that you drink two quarts of fluid every day. Be sure to discuss any problems you are having with urinary control with your physician or nurse so that they can recommend appropriate management techniques. The dilemma, of course, is that both problems are annoying and uncomfortable. Bladder problems must be addressed first so that you can manage the high fluid intake needed for satisfactory bowel function. It may take some time and patience on your part to balance your bladder and bowel management, but it can be accomplished in ways that will reduce your symptoms, make you more comfortable, and avoid future complications.

ARE THERE SPECIAL DIETS THAT CAN HELP ME WITH MY BOWEL PROBLEMS?

In addition to increased fluid intake, it is very important to add fiber to your diet, usually in the form of bran, grains, fresh fruits and vegetables, and prunes and prune juice. Fiber increases the moisture-retaining bulk of the stool, allowing it to pass more quickly and easily through the intestinal tract. Also be sure that you engage in some form of physical exercise each day to help promote regular bowel function.

WHAT SHOULD I DO IF INCREASING MY INTAKE OF FLUIDS AND FIBER DOESN'T RELIEVE THE CONSTIPATION?

In addition to the high-fiber diet and increased intake of fluids, you can take a natural bulk supplement (made from the psyllium seed), such as Metamucil, on a daily basis, as well as a stool softener, such as Colace. These over-the-counter products will help to keep the stool soft enough to pass easily through your system. Regular adherence to this type of high-fiber regimen will be sufficient for most people to control constipation. If the problem continues, your physician will probably recommend that you use a mild laxative, such as milk of magnesia, every other night or so, and perhaps a glycerin suppository 30 minutes before you plan to move your bowels. Dulcolax (bisacodyl) suppositories can also be tried if the glycerin suppository is ineffective. Those who are unable to move their bowels even with these additional measures may require an Enemeez or Fleet enema to move the bowels. The Enemeez is generally preferred because it is the size of a suppository and therefore much easier to use. Two medications—Amitiza (lubiprostone) and Miralax (polyethylene glycol)—have also been found to be helpful in managing constipation secondary to MS. However, these medications should be used only for a limited period of time or until your bowel program becomes regularized unless recommended otherwise by your physician or nurse.

As you can see, a variety of steps can be taken to control constipation and create a comfortable bowel regimen. The goal is to maintain a consistent schedule of bowel evacuation using the mildest form of intervention that will encourage your body to function on a regular and comfortable basis.

WHY CAN'T I JUST USE A LAXATIVE OR ENEMA WHENEVER I NEED TO MOVE MY BOWELS?

Laxatives and enemas should ideally be used only to help evacuate impacted stool that has remained in your bowel for a prolonged period. You might need a laxative or suppository to empty the bowel if you have not moved your bowels in more than four or five days, and the stool has become too dry and difficult to pass. These products should be used only on an intermittent, as-needed basis because their chronic use can actually slow the bowel and increase constipation. As noted, the more effective technique for treating constipation is a management regimen that prevents it in the first place.

IF I'M SO CONSTIPATED MOST OF THE TIME, WHY DO I SOMETIMES SEEM TO HAVE DIARRHEA AT THE SAME TIME?

Occasionally, people who become severely constipated will find that looser stool from higher in the intestinal tract leaks around the impacted (dry and hard) stool. The solution to this problem is to remove the impacted stool with either a laxative or enema, and then begin a structured bowel program to retrain the bowel.

SOMETIMES I HAVE BOWEL ACCIDENTS EVEN THOUGH MY STOMACH IS NOT UPSET AND I DON'T HAVE DIARRHEA. I LOSE CONTROL OF MY BOWELS WITHOUT EVEN REALIZING THAT IT IS GOING TO HAPPEN. WHAT IS CAUSING THIS, AND IS THERE ANYTHING I CAN DO ABOUT IT?

Neurologic impairment in MS can cause spasms in the involuntary muscles of the bladder and bowel just as it does in the voluntary muscles of the legs and arms. These spasms can lead to involuntary loss of bowel control. In addition, full or partial loss of sensation in the rectum allows it to fill with stool without your being aware of this fullness. The rectum stretches beyond normal capacity and then empties unexpectedly in response to an involuntary relaxation of the anal sphincter.

The most effective management of this infrequent but distressing problem is to retrain your bowel by establishing a bowel regimen. This regimen should include the dietary changes already discussed, as well as having a consistent time for moving your bowels. The frequency of evacuation matters less than the regularity of the interval and particular time of day that you choose. After breakfast every other day would be appropriate for one person; every day after lunch might be more comfortable for someone else—it does not matter, as long as you stick with a consistent schedule. Whichever time you choose, make sure to allow yourself a quiet, relaxed period of time in the bathroom. Some people find that hot liquids such as coffee or tea help to stimulate the urge to defecate. If necessary, your physician may supplement this bowel regimen with an anticholinergic medication to relieve the spasms. Bowel retraining can take several weeks or even months, but it will help you to avoid bowel accidents and feel more in control of your body.

IT HAS BECOME INCREASINGLY DIFFICULT FOR ME TO MOVE MY BOWELS, EVEN WITH THE USE OF LAXATIVES AND SUPPOSITORIES. I HAVE NOT HAD A BOWEL MOVEMENT IN MORE THAN A WEEK AND DON'T KNOW WHAT TO DO.

A week is too long for most people to go without a bowel movement. In general, a person should take measures to have a bowel movement once 3 or 4 days have passed. You should notify your physician or nurse so that you can receive assistance emptying your bowel. In all likelihood, your bowel has become impacted with hard-ened stool that you will not be able to pass without help. Once your bowel has been emptied, the doctor or nurse will help you to establish a regimen to retrain your bowel and thus avoid the prolonged use of laxatives and/or laxative suppositories. Chronic use of these products results in "tolerance" to them so that the bowel will no longer respond to the medications in them.

SKIN CARE

The skin is the largest organ of the body. An intact skin protects the organs by main-taining body structure and preventing infections. The risk of skin changes and skin breakdown is increased when people who are severely disabled with MS become less active, sitting or lying for longer periods. Continuous pressure on any area of skin decreases the flow of blood to that area. Without the flow of blood to bring oxygen and other nutrients, the skin can become damaged or die in a process referred to as ulceration. ***Pressure sores*** (also known as bed sores) occur most frequently in areas where the skin is thin and lies over protruding bones that cause pressure (the base of the spine and around the elbows, heels, and ankles) (see Figure 8-3). In addi-tion, a person who has increased ***muscle tone*** and spasticity is at greater risk of skin breakdown because the skin has a tendency to rub against supporting surfaces and become irritated. Bowel and bladder incontinence can also increase the risk of skin

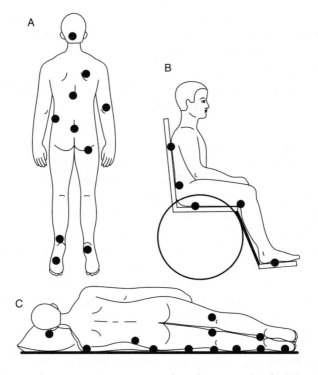

FIGURE 8-3. Dots show pressure points when lying on back (A), when sitting (B), and when lying on side (C).

breakdown because the accumulation of moisture can cause ulcers around the genital region.

Good skin care requires an adequate intake of nutritious foods and fluids as well as frequent changes of position, comfortable seating with even weight distribution, skin cleanliness and moisturizing, and frequent skin checks to identify current and potential problems. Once skin breakdown occurs, it requires prompt medical and nursing attention. Pressure sores are very slow to heal, and the most effective treatment is prevention.

NOW THAT I USE A WHEELCHAIR MUCH OF THE TIME, MY DOCTOR HAS ORDERED A SPECIAL SEAT CUSHION. HOW IS THIS CUSHION GOING TO HELP MY SKIN?
A good cushion for your wheelchair helps to distribute your weight evenly and prevent any single area of skin from being under constant pressure. In addition to using this specially designed cushion, it is important for you to shift your weight regularly, either by yourself or with someone else's assistance. This will periodically relieve pressure on the skin of your lower back, buttocks, and thighs, and allow the blood to circulate freely. A physical therapist can teach you wheelchair activities that are specially designed to relieve pressure on the skin and prevent pressure sores.

HOW CAN I TELL IF I AM DEVELOPING A PROBLEM WITH MY SKIN?
The best way to determine if you are developing skin problems is to be on the lookout for changes in skin coloring. Because it is difficult for you to get a clear view of the areas that are most prone to irritation, you may want to use a mirror for self-examination of at-risk areas. It is also advisable for you to be given a fairly regular "once over" by a nurse or family member. This is particularly important if you have experienced any loss of sensation, since this loss would probably prevent you from becoming aware of the sore. The earliest sign of a pressure sore is usually a reddening of the skin, which gradually becomes blistered and then opens. Sometimes the first sign is a soft, blackened area under the skin. If the sore is allowed to progress, fluid will begin to ooze from the opening, which gradually becomes wider and deeper.

SINCE MY MOST RECENT MS EXACERBATION I HAVE SPENT MANY HOURS OF THE DAY IN BED. SHOULD I BE USING A SPECIAL TYPE OF BED OR MATTRESS?
Anyone who spends many hours of the day in bed should be evaluated by a nurse familiar with skin care. The nurse will examine your skin, paying particular attention to the areas over bony projections (e.g., base of the spine, hips, heels), and evaluate your body alignment in bed. This type of examination will enable the nurse to identify current and potential skin problems and make any necessary recommendations about the use of appropriate bedding, including a special air mattress, mattress overlay, or other products designed to prevent skin breakdown. In addition to appropriate bedding, it is important for you to turn and reposition yourself at least every 2 hours throughout the day *and* night.

WHY IS SKIN BREAKDOWN A SERIOUS PROBLEM FOR SOMEONE WITH MS?
Skin breakdown is a serious problem for anyone. A pressure sore can develop in a few hours, but take several months to heal. Once a sore has formed, long periods of

immobility are required to relieve pressure and provide adequate air to the affected area. Such periods of immobility can easily cause troublesome secondary problems. Untreated sores can lead to an infection of the underlying bone (osteomyelitis), which is difficult to treat. Since the skin protects the body from outside infections, its breakdown can allow the tissues underneath to become infected. This type of infection might ultimately lead to septicemia (blood poisoning), which can be life-threatening.

I RECENTLY DEVELOPED A PRESSURE SORE ON MY BUTTOCKS. WHAT IS THE TREATMENT FOR THIS TYPE OF SORE?

Any area of the skin that has become reddened should be massaged regularly with a skin lotion. You should change your position frequently so that the area has plenty of exposure to the air. Be sure to notify your doctor or nurse immediately if you have already developed a small opening in the skin. Your physician will start you on a treatment regimen that involves keeping the area clean (with soap and water and/or a povidone iodine solution such as Betadine), dry, and pressure-free. If the sore has gone below the surface of the skin, the wound will be kept dry and open until the deeper area has healed. The nurse will monitor the status of the sore on a regular and frequent basis and keep your physician informed. Since the sore is on your buttocks, you will need to remain in bed and on your side or stomach for fairly long periods each day for it to heal. If the pressure sore continues to grow deeper or wider, you will probably need to go into the hospital for further treatment involving antibiotics to prevent infection and immersion in a whirlpool-type bath for deep cleansing of the area. While in the hospital, you may also be given a special Clinitron bed that promotes healing of the skin. A flotation effect, created by tiny, constantly moving, silicone balls, relieves pressure on your skin without your having to move or turn.

MY DOCTOR HAS SAID THAT I MAY NEED SURGERY FOR A PRESSURE SORE. WHY WOULD SURGERY BE NEEDED, AND HOW IS THE PROCEDURE DONE?

Occasionally, pressure sores do not respond to the measures already described. The blood circulation in the area of the sore may simply be too impaired for the healing process to proceed. If your sore has continued to worsen in spite of all treatment efforts, surgery may be required to close it. During surgery, any dead (necrotic) tissue in the area will be removed. A piece (flap) of skin from another area of your body that has better circulation may then be grafted onto the area of the sore. In the rare instances in which this type of surgery is required, healing of both the grafted skin and the area from which it was taken is generally quite successful.

DOES MY DIET HAVE ANYTHING TO DO WITH THE CONDITION OF MY SKIN? ARE THERE ANY FOODS THAT WILL PROTECT ME FROM SKIN BREAKDOWN?

Skin integrity depends on activity and exercise, your general state of health, and adequate nutrition. While one factor alone is unlikely to cause skin breakdown, a combination of deficits in any of these areas can certainly lead to problems. No specific food or diet will protect your skin from breaking down. Your best strategy for avoiding skin breakdown is to keep your skin clean, free of urine and other irritants, and moisturized; learn the exercises you need to know to enhance circulation and relieve areas of pressure on your body; and maintain a healthy diet.

I KNOW THAT LYING CONSTANTLY IN ONE POSITION CAN BE HARMFUL TO MY SKIN, BUT IT IS VERY DIFFICULT FOR ME TO TURN MYSELF OVER. IS THERE ANYTHING I CAN DO TO MAKE THE TURNING EASIER SO THAT I DON'T HAVE TO ASK MY HUSBAND (OR AIDE) TO HELP ME TURN?

Your physician can refer you to a ***physical therapist*** or ***occupational therapist*** for a home evaluation of this problem. Depending on your physical abilities and the type of bed you have, you can be taught to move and change position. Modifications such as an overbed trapeze, a pulley, or side rails can help you move and position yourself.

PROMOTING GENERAL WELLNESS

WHAT CAN I DO TO KEEP MYSELF AS HEALTHY AS POSSIBLE DESPITE MY MS?

This is a very important question because the evidence indicates that people with a chronic illness like MS often neglect their general health care needs. They begin to think of their neurologist (or other specialist) as their primary doctor, forgoing visits to their internist or general medical doctor. The result is that medical checkups and preventive health screening measures tend to go by the wayside. Because people with MS can face the same ***acute*** and ***chronic*** medical problems as anyone else, regular preventive health care is as important for those who have MS as it is for the general population. The strategies for protecting and enhancing your overall health and well-being, whether or not you have MS, include the following:

- Maintaining a healthy diet that:
  - contains a variety of foods, as shown in the food guide pyramid of the United States Department of Agriculture (www.MyPyramid.gov)
  - is high in fiber (grain products, vegetables, and fruits)
  - is low in fat, saturated fat, and cholesterol
  - is moderate in salt
  - contains an adequate amount of calcium and vitamin D
- Protecting your heart by:
  - not smoking
  - maintaining a healthy cholesterol level (less than 200 for the total and above 45 for the high-density lipoprotein [good cholesterol])
  - engaging in some form of aerobic exercise (as recommended by your physician) for 30 minutes, three to five times a week
  - following your doctor's recommended schedule for regular health screenings
- Obtaining periodic health appraisals and screening tests:
  - General physical (20–40 years old—every 5 years; 40–50 years old— every 3 years; 50–65 years old—every 2 years; over age 65—yearly). The evaluation should include a history, physical examination, blood and urine laboratory tests, and a chest x-ray and electrocardiogram, depending on age and history. Women should have pelvic and breast examinations on an annual basis. A bone density scan is recommended for women older than 65 years and for any

person with limited mobility or weight-bearing capacity and/or a treatment history that includes frequent treatment with **corticosteroids**.

■ Annual cancer screening, depending on the person's age (breast or testicular examination by the health care provider; Pap smear for women of reproductive age; mammogram for women older than 40 years of age; rectal examination for men and women after 40 years of age; stool blood testing and other colon cancer testing for men and women after age 50).

● Learning to manage stress by:
  ■ examining your priorities
  ■ eliminating the unnecessary stresses in your life while identifying more effective ways to manage those that are unavoidable
  ■ finding activities that provide you with regular periods of relaxation, enjoyment, and "down-time" (e.g., deep-muscle relaxation exercises, meditation, listening to music, socializing with friends, watching television, yoga)
  ■ consulting with a psychotherapist, if you feel the need, for help in identifying the sources of stress in your life and developing effective stress-management strategies

RECOMMENDED READINGS

Holland N, Halper J. (eds.). *Multiple Sclerosis: A Self-Care Guide to Wellness.* 2nd ed. New York: Demos Medical Publishing, 2005.

Kalb R, Holland N, Giesser B. *Multiple Sclerosis for Dummies.* Hoboken, NJ: Wiley Publishing Co., 2007.

Schapiro R. *Symptom Management in Multiple Sclerosis.* 5th ed. New York: Demos Medical Publishing, 2007.

Selected materials available from the National Multiple Sclerosis Society (800-344-3867) or online at www.nationalmssociety.org/Brochures:
  • *Choosing the Right Health-Care Provider*
  • *Bowel Problems: The Basic Facts*
  • *Urinary Dysfunction and MS*
  • *Food for Thought: MS and Nutrition*
  • *Vitamins, Minerals, and Herbs in MS: An Introduction*
  • *Fatigue: What You Should Know*
  • *Sleep Disorders and MS: The Basic Facts*
  • *Preventive Care Recommendations for Adults with MS*
  • *Dental Health: The Basic Facts*

RECOMMENDED RESOURCES

Medline Plus (www.medlineplus.gov): A service of the National Library of Medicine and the National Institutes of Health, providing health news, drug information, **clinical trials** listing, a medical encyclopedia, a medical dictionary, links to other databases and resources.

U.S. Department of Agriculture Food Pyramid (www.mypyramid.gov): A personalized food pyramid that allows you to determine the types and amounts of foods that meet your particular needs.

The Role of Physical Therapy: Strategies to Enhance Mobility and Safety and Conserve Energy

Matthew Sutliff, PT, MSCS, and Francois Bethoux, MD*

The *physical therapist* is a health care professional trained to evaluate and improve the movement and function of the body, with particular emphasis on physical mobility, balance, posture, fatigue, and pain. Many factors affect the abilities of people with multiple sclerosis (MS) to be as physically active as they would like to be. Physical therapy (PT) has as its goal to help people meet the mobility challenges and physical demands of their family, work, and social lives while accommodating the physical changes brought about by the disease.

In PT, the therapist and person with MS work as a team to minimize the limitations imposed by MS, maximize functional ability and overall quality of life, and prevent debilitating injuries and complications. The therapist recommends various treatment strategies following a thorough physical and functional evaluation. The individual provides the determination and commitment to follow through with the treatment regimen, as well as valuable feedback to the therapist. This feedback, along with assessment of daily functional tasks, allows the therapist to accurately determine if the treatment is working effectively and make any necessary revisions in the treatment plan. There are four important components to a successful PT program:

- Education for people with MS and their family members about the physical **symptoms** caused by the disease, and the steps that can be taken to alleviate current problems and prevent unnecessary complications
- An individualized exercise program designed to deal with these problems and maximize health and function
- Mobility enhancement and energy conservation through the use of a variety of mobility aids, adaptive equipment for the home, office, and automobile, and education about community resources
- Interventions specifically designed to address impairments or functional mobility limitations

*With grateful acknowledgment of materials from the previous editions written by Angela Chan, BPT, MHSc, and Brian Hutchinson, PT, MSCS.

WHAT IS THE DIFFERENCE BETWEEN A PHYSICAL THERAPIST AND A PHYSIATRIST?
A physiatrist is a physician specialized in rehabilitation. Physiatrists usually work in rehabilitation centers and clinics. When somebody is admitted to a rehabilitation facility, for example, after a severe exacerbation of MS, the attending physician is likely to be a physiatrist. Some MS centers also have physiatrists on staff. It is not mandatory to see a physiatrist to start physical or occupational therapy, since any physician can make the referral. However, when symptom management (see Chapter 4) and functional issues are complex, a physiatrist can help maximize your functional potential by prescribing medications (e.g., dalfampridine [Ampyra] to improve walking or baclofen [Lioresal] or tizanidine [Zanaflex] to relieve *spasticity*) and performing procedures (e.g., botulinum toxin injections to relieve spasticity), and by coordinating interventions provided by other rehabilitation professionals.

EVALUATION

HOW WILL I KNOW IF I NEED TO BE SEEN BY A PHYSICAL THERAPIST?
Your first contact with a physical therapist is likely to be initiated by your physician. Typically, the physician refers a person with MS to PT for help in managing one or more symptoms. If your physician has not yet recommended PT to you, you can ask whether it would be beneficial for you and if it is available in your area. It is never too early in the course of MS to have a consultation with a physical therapist since PT can help you maintain your comfort and flexibility, reduce the impact of MS-related fatigue, make exercise recommendations, and prevent unnecessary injury and complications. Many people maintain intermittent contact with their physical therapist over the course of their MS, consulting the therapist for treatment recommendations as specific physical problems become bothersome and affect their ability to engage in daily activities. Periodic evaluation by a physical therapist is helpful not only in managing current problems but also in identifying and preventing potential ones.

HOW DO I GET IN TOUCH WITH A PHYSICAL THERAPIST?
When referring you for PT, your physician will probably select a therapist in your area and tell you how to make contact. Many physical therapists work in health care facilities such as hospitals, community health centers, and *rehabilitation* centers. Others have a private practice, seeing patients in their office or in the patients' homes. Depending on where the therapist works, most PT services are covered, at least in part, by Medicare, Medicaid, or a private insurance plan. In Canada, PT is covered by the provincial health-care plan or private insurance plans. Some private practitioners who work in an outpatient center or in the home are available only on a fee-for-service basis.

Even though all physical therapists are qualified to provide rehabilitation treatment, MS poses unique challenges due to the complexity and variability of symptoms and functional limitations. It is a good idea to inquire if a therapist with experience in MS, or other neurologic conditions, is available in your area. Sometimes, a physical therapist with MS experience performs the first evaluation and helps design the treatment plan, while the PT sessions are carried out by another therapist closer to your home.

HOW WILL THE PHYSICAL THERAPIST EVALUATE MY PROBLEMS?
The physical therapist will perform a thorough interview along with a physical and functional assessment of:

- Posture, balance, and body movements
- Muscle strength
- Muscle, tendon, and joint flexibility
- Ability to discriminate sensations such as heat and cold, pain, pressure, touch, and movement
- Fatigue level and endurance
- Safety and mobility at work, at home, and in the community

Improving your ability to get around is often the therapist's primary objective. Mobility includes movement in bed, ambulation (walking), and transfers (e.g., from wheelchair to bed or from wheelchair to toilet seat). For individuals who are ambulatory, the therapist performs a gait analysis to assess quality and ease of walking. This analysis involves observing how the person walks and identifying causes of change in his or her normal walking pattern. The therapist will also note the type of assistance (e.g., cane, walker, leg brace), if any, a person is using to walk and under what circumstances. And, the physical therapist will take into consideration the effect of a person's symptoms on overall mobility. All of these factors then allow the therapist to form a plan of care that may include exercises, bracing, or assistive devices that can help improve a person's walking ability.

The goals of therapy established by you and the physical therapist will typically involve improving your mobility at home and at work, as well as your overall quality of life. Family members, friends, and caregivers can provide useful background information and share their perspectives on the impact of MS on your daily life. However, each individual with MS is unique in being able to describe his or her own frustrations and limitations and in setting personal goals for physical therapy, so your input will be critically important to the success of the treatment plan.

THE ROLE OF EXERCISE

ARE THERE DIFFERENT TYPES OF EXERCISE?
A physical therapist may recommend any of a wide variety of exercises:

- *Strengthening exercises* are designed to improve and/or maintain strength. Weights, elastic bands/tubing, or machines may be used to provide resistance so that your muscles have to work harder. Regular workouts are designed to improve muscle strength and endurance. The exercises should be directed toward improving function. Using strengthening exercises to the point of excessive fatigue, however, is generally not recommended for people with MS. The physical therapist will design an exercise program to strengthen specific muscles that may have become weakened by disuse.
- *Range-of-motion exercises* are performed to ensure that each joint is moved throughout the full range of available movement, with the objective being to maintain or increase joint flexibility. Tightness of the joint capsule, ligaments, and tendons may individually or in combination restrict joint movements. Joint stiffness may

also occur when swelling is present or after an injury. If movement of the joint does not occur on a regular basis, joint stiffness may become permanent and interfere with normal movement.

- *Stretching exercises* are recommended for muscles and tendons that have lost their elasticity or stretchability. When muscles and tendons around a joint lose this elasticity, the person feels stiff and finds it difficult to move. These exercises help to maintain the elasticity of tissues and prevent **contractures**.
- *Aerobic or cardiorespiratory exercises* are designed to improve endurance and aerobic function, which can, in turn, reduce fatigue.
- A physical therapist may also recommend specific exercises to improve balance and **coordination** or activities directed toward improvement of mobility.

The exercises prescribed by the physical therapist can also be divided according to the degree of assistance required by the person performing them: *Active exercises* are performed completely independently; *active assisted exercises* require some assistance by another person or machine; *passive exercises* are performed by a helper (therapist or caregiver) or a machine if a person is unable to perform them independently.

IN WHAT WAYS WILL EXERCISE HELP MY MS?

Different types of exercise provide different kinds of benefits:

- Exercises can help by developing and strengthening those muscles that continue to have adequate motor control and by helping to maintain the strength and endurance of those with inadequate motor control. Exercise will train your muscles to work better individually and together and may thereby improve coordination in your arms and legs. Thus, an exercise program can help you learn ways of walking and moving that compensate somewhat for the neurologic changes caused by MS.
- Exercises are also used to improve range of motion and to help relieve the effects of mild **spasticity**, balance problems, and some types of pain.
- Regular aerobic exercise—tailored to your individual abilities and limitations—has been shown to reduce fatigue and depression, promote strength and fitness, and help control weight. And some newer evidence suggests that regular aerobic exercise may even help lessen the decline of cognitive function that can occur in people with MS (see Chapter 14).
- Weight-bearing exercise can reduce the risk of **osteoporosis** in those who have become less mobile.

I WAS RECENTLY DIAGNOSED WITH MS. SHOULD I CONTINUE TO PARTICIPATE IN THE AEROBIC EXERCISE CLASS THAT I ALWAYS ATTENDED?

Research in MS has shown that a regular aerobic exercise program can reduce fatigue and depression and increase cardiovascular fitness. Therefore, you should try to maintain your current activity level unless you find it too tiring or uncomfortable. Your physician or physical therapist will be able to guide you in determining the amount of exercise (duration and intensity) that is appropriate. Since MS symptoms can be temporarily worsened by external heat and/or elevated body temperature, it is important to exercise in a cool environment; drink plenty of fluids before, during, and after exercise; and work at a pace that does not allow you to become extremely overheated.

HOW CAN I FIND OUT WHAT TYPE OF EXERCISE IS BEST FOR ME?

Exercises designed to address your particular needs are best prescribed by your physician, **occupational therapist (OT)**, or **physical therapist**. Some general fitness exercises can be performed in a health club or an exercise class setting. Specific benefits of exercising outside the home include opportunities to socialize with others, the encouragement and feedback from the instructor and fellow participants, and the guidance of a structured program. Getting yourself out to participate can also enhance continuity and commitment. Trainers in a fitness or health club can develop a general fitness program for you, but keep in mind that they probably have not had significant training in MS and the ways in which neurologic changes can affect your body. So be sure to consult with your physician before beginning any exercise program. If you require an exercise program that is more appropriate to your physical symptoms, your physician will refer you to a physical therapist.

ARE THERE ANY TYPES OF EXERCISE THAT ARE HARMFUL TO ME NOW THAT I HAVE MS?

No specific exercises are harmful to individuals with MS, however you should consult your doctor before starting something new. Common sense will be your best ally here. In general, your body will tell you how it is responding to exercise and will certainly let you know if it cannot tolerate the exercise program you have chosen. Be careful not to exert yourself to the point of exhaustion or raise your body temperature so much that you activate your MS symptoms. Although these momentary symptoms are indicative of being overheated rather than of any kind of disease activity or progression, they can be uncomfortable and unnerving. Exercises that challenge your balance (e.g., walking on a treadmill at a high speed) may also pose a risk of fall and injury. Regular, moderate exercise in a cool environment, with periodic rest breaks, will enable you to get maximum benefit from your exercise program and avoid unnecessary discomfort.

IS WEIGHT TRAINING HELPFUL FOR THE WEAKNESS THAT I FEEL IN MY ARMS AND LEGS?

In some cases weight training can be helpful, but not for all people. The weakness you are experiencing in your arms and legs may be the result of impaired nerve conduction to the muscles involved, rather than any weakness of the muscles themselves. Weight training is good for developing and strengthening muscles that do have adequate nerve conduction, and for toning muscles that have been weakened by disuse. Muscles that are relatively strong and can lift against gravity and some resistance typically benefit the most from weight training, particularly when it is performed in moderation. Weaker muscles that have difficulty moving a limb against gravity are typically *not* strengthened with weights, as the weights overpower these muscles and add to their fatigue. In those cases, assistive exercises are typically more beneficial, and resistance may be added later if the muscle strength improves. A physical therapist can design a fitness program that specifically addresses the types of weakness you are experiencing.

HOW CAN I EXERCISE EFFECTIVELY NOW THAT I HAVE LOST SO MUCH STRENGTH IN MY ARMS AND LEGS?

If you are unable to perform active exercise because of problems with weakness, spasticity, or imbalance, the physical therapist can work with you on assisted and passive exercises that are more appropriate for your needs. It is important to remember that not all exercise programs are designed to increase strength or endurance; exercise is equally important for maintaining flexibility, range of motion, posture, and muscle integrity. However, if your loss of strength is due to disuse, then a structured exercise program can improve your muscle strength and endurance.

I FEEL SO FATIGUED MOST OF THE TIME THAT MY REGULAR DAILY ACTIVITIES USE UP ALL THE ENERGY I HAVE. HOW CAN I POSSIBLY EXERCISE WHEN I FEEL SO TIRED?

Reduced energy level and endurance are common problems for people with MS. The fatigue that is so common in MS can have a variety of causes. The physical therapist can help you understand the various causes of your fatigue and explore with you ways of optimizing your energy and reducing fatigue. You may be able to conserve energy and minimize tiredness by doing various activities in a slightly different way, making more effective use of tools or strategies to save time and reduce unnecessary effort, and/or creating small rest periods in your day. Mobility aids are sometimes prescribed to increase a person's ability to cover greater distances with less fatigue. In addition, the physical therapist can teach you types of exercise—or modifications of current exercises—that are less physically strenuous and demanding than ones you might have done in the past. Regular aerobic exercise has been shown to reduce fatigue in MS. Keep in mind that exercise does not have to be fast or vigorous to provide you with substantial benefit. In fact, an important benefit of some exercises is increased relaxation.

IS SWIMMING A GOOD EXERCISE FOR ME?

Water is an excellent medium for exercise. It allows weakened muscles to move more easily while providing sufficient resistance to help strengthen other muscles. Water also helps to stabilize a person who has balance problems. Because swimming is a highly coordinated physical activity involving the whole body, it helps to regulate breathing and build endurance. In addition, your physical therapist can develop a personalized exercise program for you to do in the water, even if you do not like or know how to swim. Water-walking, as well as other types of exercises for the arms and legs, can be very beneficial. Specialized hydrotherapy techniques can also be helpful in maintaining flexibility and promoting relaxation.

It is advisable to gather some information before you go to a swimming pool. How far is it from the changing room and the toilet to the pool? Is someone available to provide assistance in and out of the pool if necessary? What is the temperature of the water? Although people react differently to water temperature, a water temperature of 80°F to 84°F seems to be the most comfortable for individuals with MS. The temperature of a "therapeutic pool" is frequently too hot. If you are experiencing any MS-related bowel or bladder symptoms that might interfere with your comfort in the swimming pool, talk them over with your physician or nurse before beginning a swimming program.

IS THERE ANY REASON FOR ME TO STOP PLAYING THE RECREATIONAL SPORTS THAT I ENJOY?
The answer to this question depends on the symptoms of MS that you are experiencing and their impact on your enjoyment of any particular sport. If you can physically play the sport, even if not as well as before, then you should probably continue to do so. Too many people stop playing sports as soon as they are diagnosed, or because they can't play as well as they did in the past. There is no reason to stop playing your sport unless you feel that you are putting yourself (or someone else) at risk of injury. Stopping prematurely will deny you recreation and enjoyment, as well as the benefits of exercise and the continued challenge to your body. The point is to adapt to change, not to stop living because of it.

MANY TYPES OF EXERCISE EQUIPMENT ARE ADVERTISED AND SOLD IN SPORT STORES. HOW CAN I FIGURE OUT WHICH EQUIPMENT IS RIGHT FOR ME?
It is important to check with your doctor and/or physical therapist before starting any type of exercise program or purchasing any exercise equipment. They can work with you to identify your particular needs and goals and find the programs and equipment most suited to your physical condition. The pieces of exercise equipment differ not only in their uses, but in the demands they make on your stamina, coordination, and balance. For example, you can increase endurance and heart fitness by using either a treadmill or a recumbent bicycle, but one type of equipment may be more appropriate for you than another, depending on your particular symptoms and degree of mobility.

Keep in mind that, when you exercise certain parts of your body (e.g., your legs to pedal a bicycle), those body parts do not work in isolation. Muscles from other parts of your body (e.g., heart and trunk) work in tandem to provide support for your efforts. Because greater exertion also increases the demand for oxygen to all those muscles, you will breathe more deeply and rapidly. This will expand your lungs and increase oxygen in your blood. Due to the pumping of the heart, an increase in blood circulation occurs throughout the body. Thus, most types of physical exercise will help to improve heart health, blood circulation, and general fitness. Expensive equipment is not necessary for exercising or fitness training. Walking at a moderate pace or similar aerobic exercise can achieve similar results.

I RECENTLY SAW AN ADVERTISEMENT FOR A MOTORIZED BICYCLE. WILL THIS TYPE OF BICYCLE KEEP MY MUSCLES FROM GETTING WEAKER?
In the motorized bicycle, the motor is driving the bicycle movement, which in turn moves your legs. Therefore, your own muscles are not required to work. Since your own muscles are not providing the power for movement, you will not derive the same benefits as you would from active muscle work on a regular or recumbent bicycle. For

the motorized bicycle to have any impact on your muscle strength, you would need to turn this passive exercise into a more active one by making your muscles work along with the bicycle.

Some people use the motorized bicycle for passive range-of-motion exercise. The movement of the pedals causes bending and extending movements at the hips and knees, and some movements at the ankles. Because the movements generated by the bicycle are generally not the full range of possible movements at these joints, it is important to supplement this activity with other flexibility exercises. Also, if you have stiffness or spasms (spasticity) in your legs, you may find that your legs have difficulty following the movement of the motorized bicycle.

Although some individuals find the movements from the machine relaxing, this side benefit does not occur for everyone who uses the machine. You must balance the possible benefits gained from the machine with the cost of purchasing the machine, and of any assistance you might need to get on and off the machine and secure your feet to the pedals.

BECAUSE OF MS, I'M NOT GETTING AS MUCH EXERCISE AS I USED TO, AND I'M PUTTING ON WEIGHT. WHAT SHOULD I DO?

Weight control is an issue of concern for almost everyone, and it becomes more challenging when symptoms of MS make a person less mobile and more fatigued. In turn, excess weight can further limit your mobility and lead to other medical complications. Increasing overall physical activity has been shown to promote strength and fitness, help control weight, and reduce fatigue and depression in MS. Therefore, increasing your activity by adding an extra day of exercise or slowly increasing the duration of your exercise session(s) can be helpful. With the help of your physician or physical therapist, choose the type of exercise that meets your needs and interests. If your endurance and ability are limited, you might consider a senior's fitness program, water-walking, yoga, or tai chi as other options. Keep in mind as well that certain types of hobbies, such as gardening, can also provide very beneficial exercise. In addition, it may be necessary to adjust your diet to compensate for your decreased activity level. You can discuss this with your physician and nurse, or with a dietician.

MY POSTURE SEEMS TO HAVE CHANGED SINCE I'VE HAD MS. ARE THERE EXERCISES THAT WILL IMPROVE MY POSTURE?

Posture is a key area in the PT assessment. Maintaining good posture is important not only for the sake of your appearance but also to prevent uncomfortable muscle and joint strain that can arise from standing, sitting, and moving improperly. For example, *repetitive strain injury* refers to chronic pain caused by doing certain types of muscle work on a repetitive and prolonged basis, without any single incident of injury. Wrist pain due to prolonged computer work is a common example of a repetitive strain injury. People who spend a lot of time at a computer must be alert to the way they are sitting in relation to the desk and keypad, and to the positioning of their backs, legs, wrists, and forearms. The resulting pain may be similar to MS symptoms, but have nothing to do with MS. Similarly, people who use various types of mobility aids for walking must be sure that the devices are measured and designed accurately, and that they are being used appropriately. For example, pain or injury can result from using a cane that is too short or too long because a cane of improper length can distort a person's posture and gait. A person who sits in a wheelchair that does not provide proper back, leg, and foot support will also begin to experience neck, back, and leg pain.

The therapist will observe the position of your head, neck, shoulders, torso, pelvis, hips, knees, ankles, and feet. Standing posture and seated posture, as well as posture during movement, are noted. The physical therapist is able to identify areas of muscle insufficiency and/or stiffness and develop corrective movements targeting these areas. Postural muscles are primarily endurance muscles, which require specific training and/or proper support.

ARE YOGA AND TAI CHI GOOD FORMS OF EXERCISE FOR SOMEONE WITH MS?
Yoga and tai chi are excellent forms of exercise for people with MS. They involve mental discipline and controlled breathing, which promote relaxation of the mind and body, and help people feel more in tune with their body. Yoga, which can be adapted for people who use a wheelchair, involves a lot of stretching exercises for the whole body. It has been shown in controlled research to reduce MS fatigue. Tai chi movements are slow and controlled, with periodic changes in position. Many of the movements in tai chi require good balance, so it is important to perform your exercise routine close to a grab bar or railing in case you need to steady yourself. In one study, people with MS who participated in a tai chi program demonstrated improved walking ability and enhanced quality of life. As with any other form of exercise, it is important that the yoga and tai chi exercises be tailored to your particular physical needs and limitations.

I HAVE BEEN EXPERIENCING A LOT OF PAIN WITH MY MS. CAN PHYSICAL THERAPY HELP ME TO MANAGE THIS PAIN? HOW CAN EXERCISES HELP WITHOUT CAUSING ME MORE PAIN THAN I'M ALREADY HAVING?
Several types of pain can be associated with MS (see Chapter 4). In addition to primary (***neurogenic***) pain resulting directly from demyelinating lesions in the central nervous system (CNS), a person can experience pain secondary to other symptoms such as spasticity, weakness, and abnormal movement. The initial step in pain management, therefore, is to consult with your physician and/or physical therapist to identify the source(s) of the pain you are experiencing.

Physical therapists use a variety of strategies to help reduce pain, including the application of localized heat or ice, exercise, and teaching proper positioning and support for the body. Problems with balance and ambulation often cause changes in posture, and these postural changes can gradually result in secondary pain in the lower back, hips, and knees. The use of ambulation aids such as crutches or walkers can also contribute to secondary pain in the shoulders and upper back if they are used incorrectly. If the pain is a result of changes in your posture, balance, or gait (i.e., if you have begun to sit or walk differently because of weakness or spasticity), the therapist may design a treatment regimen that involves education about the mechanics of your problem as well as exercises designed to improve the impaired functions contributing to the pain. Rather than giving you additional pain, the exercises involved will actually reduce pain by alleviating its causes. In addition, the therapist may recommend the use of a new or different mechanical aid, such as a cane, walker, leg brace, or wheelchair, if any of these would contribute to a reduction in the pain you are experiencing. If the pain is a result of spasticity and the inactivity resulting from it, the physical therapist will prescribe a daily regimen of range-of-motion or stretching exercises designed to reduce stiffness and enhance flexibility.

CAN EXERCISE HELP ME WITH MY BALANCE PROBLEMS?

Loss of balance and risk of falling are areas of primary concern for the physical therapist and common problems for many with MS. Impaired balance in MS can result from *plaques* in the areas of the CNS that control equilibrium, and from a variety of other problems, such as weakness, stiffness, loss of sensation, and loss of coordination in the legs. Even vision impairment may contribute to poor equilibrium. The physical therapist can recommend particular exercises designed to maximize your ability to maintain your balance. The therapist may also recommend *assistive equipment* such as a walking aid, grab bars, or transfer device. Safety is a primary concern, because impaired balance can lead to falls resulting in bruising, swelling, pain, and even fractures.

SINCE MY LAST EXACERBATION, I HAVE BEEN UNABLE TO WALK. WILL EXERCISING MY LEGS HELP ME TO WALK AGAIN?

Walking is a complex motor activity that depends on many functions working in a coordinated fashion. Exercising your legs will maintain flexibility of the joints and muscles, encourage the muscles to work to their best potential, and prevent further muscle deterioration. Therefore, depending on the degree and location of *demyelination* that occurred during your last *relapse*, and the amount of spontaneous recovery you experience, leg exercises might facilitate your efforts to walk again. However, there is no guarantee, because exercise does not correct the neurologic damage done by the disease. Even if walking is not possible, exercising your legs will help you to sit properly and thereby prevent the pain and stiffness that can result from prolonged sitting.

CAN EXERCISE HELP A PERSON WHO IS UNABLE TO WALK AND SPENDS MOST OF THE TIME IN A WHEELCHAIR?

Exercise is extremely important for the person who is no longer able to walk. In its various forms, exercise enhances flexibility, posture, strength, and endurance, each of which contributes to comfort and physical well-being.

- Stiffness in the legs affects a person's ability to sit upright with proper foot positioning. Passive range-of-motion and stretching exercises can help relieve this type of stiffness.
- Exercises for the arms, upper body, and trunk are very important for maintaining good posture, which, in turn, reduces the risk of back and hip strain.
- Weight training to maintain upper body strength also facilitates transfers in and out of the wheelchair or bed and promotes cardiac health. In addition, upper body exercises can strengthen the neck or torso and thereby increase a person's ability to sit comfortably for longer periods of time.

● Any exercise regimen that enhances the mobility of the person in a wheelchair also reduces the risk of skin breakdown (see Chapter 8) and blood clots in the legs. People who spend long periods in a wheelchair are taught specific exercises designed to shift their weight and thus relieve pressure on areas of the body that are particularly prone to skin breakdown. They are also taught to stand (if possible) for brief periods of time each day to allow the force of gravity to slow the reduction in bone density (osteoporosis) that can result from reduced mobility and inadequate amounts of weight-bearing exercise. This is critically important, since a reduction in bone density contributes to the risk of bone fractures. Standing activities can also help with digestion, and bowel and bladder functions.

SHOULD I CONSIDER BREATHING EXERCISES?

MS can cause progressive weakening of the muscles of respiration, in much the same manner as it causes weakening of muscles in the legs or arms. For this reason, decreased respiratory capacity and respiratory complications (such as pneumonia) are a significant problem in individuals with advanced MS and limited mobility. There is also evidence to suggest that ventilation is impaired in persons at earlier stages of MS who remain able to walk and have minimal disability. For this reason, it is now suggested that respiratory training be incorporated in a regular exercise program, through techniques such as tai chi, deep breathing, diaphragmatic breathing, or incentive spirometry exercises.

SINCE I HAVE BEGUN TO SPEND MUCH MORE TIME SITTING DOWN, I HAVE SWELLING IN MY FEET AND ANKLES, ESPECIALLY BY LATE AFTERNOON. WHAT CAN I DO ABOUT IT?

Because leg swelling can result from a variety of causes, it is important to consult with your physician to make sure that no other medical conditions need to be addressed. Once other causes have been ruled out, you can utilize various strategies to reduce any swelling that results from reduced mobility. During walking and standing, the activity of the muscles in the legs helps to pump the blood in the legs back up to the heart. In the sitting position, the force of gravity draws the blood down toward the feet. With prolonged sitting, insufficient muscle activity occurs in the legs to counteract the force of gravity and pump the blood back up to the heart.

Try, if possible, to stand up for at least 5 minutes of every hour. If you are unable to stand independently, you might consider using a standing device to support you—and some models can even help you rise from a sitting to a standing position. Short periods of standing will relieve the prolonged pressure on your buttocks and allow the leg muscles to pump some of the blood back to your heart. If standing is very difficult, raise your legs after every 2 hours of sitting, and rest them on a chair or a stool that is at least as high as your hips. While your feet are elevated, try to do some foot and ankle exercises to help pump the blood back to your heart. Keep your feet elevated above the level of your hips for at least 30 minutes.

For severe swelling, it may be necessary to lie down for some portion of each day with your feet elevated above the level of your heart. An additional strategy to control lower leg swelling involves wearing pressure stockings that must be prescribed and specially fitted for you.

WHAT EXERCISES CAN I DO TO RELIEVE THE STIFFNESS I FEEL IN MY BODY?
Stiffness in MS is often related to spasticity, which is caused by abnormal regulation of **nerve** impulses in the spinal cord (see Chapter 4). In addition to stiffness, spasticity can cause involuntary movements such as spasms (jerky movements) and clonus (repetitive movement, usually at the ankle/foot). Mild spasticity in MS can often be managed effectively with a regimen of stretching and range-of-motion exercises. These exercises are very important for maintaining flexibility of the muscles and tendons and thereby reducing further stiffness and other complications.

For example, the foot may "turn in" when the muscles and tendons on the inside of the foot become shortened—and the muscles turning the foot out are weakened by disuse. Without exercise, the ankle joint can become stiff. Passive and active exercises for the muscles controlling ankle movements are vitally important in this situation. The physician or physical therapist may also suggest a special type of leg brace to help with this problem. The key is to begin the treatment regimen before changes to the muscles and joints become permanent.

In addition, regular cardiorespiratory exercise is beneficial for generalized stiffness. Keep in mind, however, that exercises alone may not be sufficient to treat your spasticity. If the stiffness continues or worsens, or if the exercises become too difficult or uncomfortable for you to do, your physician may recommend that you use medication or injections in combination with exercise to manage the spasticity.

WALKING AND MOBILITY AIDS

I'VE BEGUN TO STAGGER SO MUCH WHEN I WALK THAT PEOPLE THINK I'M DRUNK. WHAT CAN I DO ABOUT THIS PROBLEM?
Staggering is a symptom of poor balance or loss of coordination in the legs. There are two major consequences of impaired balance: the first is the risk of potentially dangerous falls; the second, unfortunately, is that others often perceive the person who staggers to have a drinking problem. Depending on the cause and extent of your balance problems, your physician or physical therapist may recommend a mobility aid such as a cane (see Figure 9-1), **forearm (Lofstrand) crutch** (see Figure 9-2), or walker. The use of a mobility aid will provide you with extra stability and will also send a clear signal to any observer that your staggering is the result of a disability, rather than drinking.

The physical therapist will determine which type of aid is most beneficial for you by evaluating how much additional stability you need. A single cane, for example, adds a point of stability only on one side of your body. A **quad cane** (see Figure 9-3), which has four short legs attached to a small platform at its end, provides greater stability by giving you a broader base on which to lean. The therapist may recommend that you use two canes or crutches if you would benefit from a stabilizing point on each side of your body.

Devices such as walking sticks or Trekker Poles can be considered also, and they provide the stability of a cane (or 2 canes), without the "stigma" that some people associate with a cane.

If these aids do not provide sufficient stability, the therapist may recommend a standard walker or a 3- or 4-wheeled rollator walker (see Figure 9-4).

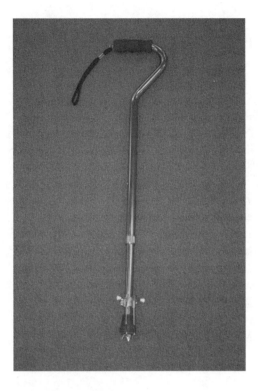

FIGURE 9-1. Cane.

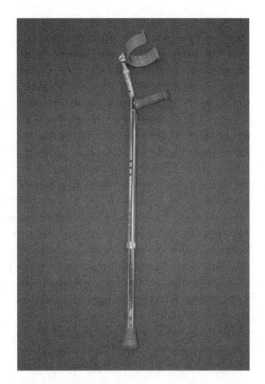

FIGURE 9-2. Forearm crutch.

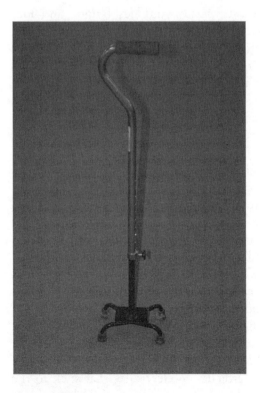

FIGURE 9-3. Quad cane.

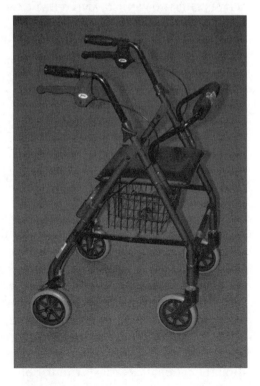

FIGURE 9-4. Four-wheeled rollator walker.

Because a walker moves directly in front of you, it provides greater stability and also reduces fatigue. The standard walker (without wheels) is effective, but can be tiresome because it must be lifted to move it forward. Wheels on the front of the walker can be added to enhance the movement of the walker and make it easier to maneuver. Three-wheeled rollators are handy in tight areas, such as homes with narrow doorways and hallways. However, the 3-wheeler is not as stable as a 4-wheeled rollator, and the 4-wheeler has added benefits, including a built-in seat for those times when you need a rest but are too far from a chair, hand brakes, and a basket for carrying things. Rollators come in a variety of sizes and styles, all made for different needs. If you will be walking on gravel or grass, then larger wheels may be needed. If you will be lifting it in and out of your car, then a lightweight version may be most useful. These factors should all be discussed with your PT when considering an assistive device.

Bear in mind that as your needs change, the type of aid that is recommended for you will change as well. You may also find that a particular type of equipment works best for you in one situation, while another type of aid is more useful in a different situation; the major objectives are to maintain stability and safety, conserve energy, and walk safely. Be sure to consult the therapist if you are experiencing difficulty in spite of using a walking aid. In addition to choosing the proper ambulation aid, it is important to be properly trained in its use by your physical therapist to maximize safety and efficiency of use.

I SEEM TO TRIP A LOT, AND I'VE EVEN HAD A FEW FALLS. WHY IS THIS HAPPENING, AND WHAT CAN BE DONE ABOUT IT?

Weakness of your foot, ankle, or hip muscles, stiffness in your legs, fatigue, and poor balance could, individually or in combination, contribute to tripping and falling. Since falls can have major consequences, the first step in the management of this problem is to identify its source. Having diagnosed the problem, your physician will provide the necessary treatment and/or make the appropriate referral. If tripping is primarily the result of leg weakness, you will probably be referred to a physical therapist for a treatment regimen of exercises, possible bracing recommendations, and evaluation for a mobility aid such as a cane or walker. If the tripping and falling occur primarily when you are already tired from overexertion, the physical therapist may recommend that you use a mobility aid, such as a motorized scooter, when you need to cover longer distances.

If your falls are primarily the result of foot drop, you will probably be referred to an *orthotist* or physical therapist for an ankle–foot orthosis (AFO) (see Figures 9-5 and 9-6). The AFO is a plastic or carbon fiber brace that supports a weakened ankle so that you can walk with a heel-to-toe motion and avoid catching your toe on the ground. These braces come in various styles; some are solid plastic, others have moveable joints. The newer carbon fiber AFOs are very light and provide a gentle "spring effect" as you step. Your therapist can help you assess the advantages and disadvantages of each.

Functional electrical stimulation devices are another type of walking aid. These devices utilize electrical stimulation to assist in lifting the foot and decreasing foot drop. Functional electrical stimulation (FES) utilizes a small device that is strapped to the leg, just below the knee. The device attaches to electrodes that stick to the skin. These electrodes stimulate a nerve in the leg that helps to lift the foot up

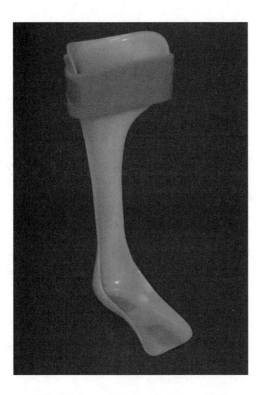

FIGURE 9-5. Post leaf spring AFO.

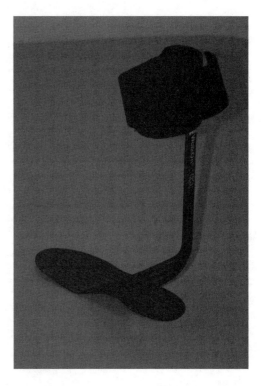

FIGURE 9-6. Carbon AFO.

when walking. FES devices have different mechanisms to turn the stimulation on and off; one device measures the "tilt" of the shinbone as the person walks, others use a heel "pressure sensor" in the shoe to activate the stimulation. In either case, the stimulation causes the foot to lift as the leg bends, and lifts the heel off the floor to make a step. The stimulation then turns off when the heel touches down to the floor at the completion of the step. This on/off cycle continues for as long as the person continues to walk. FES devices are very useful for some people with MS whose weakness is fairly isolated to the foot and ankle. The devices are expensive, however (typically $4,800–$6,200 initially, plus electrode costs), and they are rarely covered by insurance for people with MS. The best advice is to "try before you buy" with any device that you may consider.

The Hip Flexion Assist Device (HFAD, see Figure 9-7) was recently developed for people with not only ankle weakness and foot drop but also weakness at the hip and knee. The HFAD uses elastic bands to help lift the entire leg when walking. A simple test can be done to determine if there is weakness of the hip flexors: while sitting, try to lift each leg (with the knee bent) straight up. If lifting is difficult in one or both legs, the HFAD may be beneficial to assist with walking.

**IF I USE A LEG SPLINT OR BRACE, WILL MY LEG MUSCLES
BECOME WEAK OR USELESS?**

A foot or leg splint is generally prescribed because of muscle weakness. In other words, the splint does not cause weakness; rather it substitutes for muscles that are

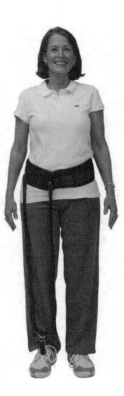

FIGURE 9-7. Hip flexion device.

already weakened due to lack of adequate nerve innervation. Since it is true that certain muscles in the foot are not required to work as hard when a splint is used, the physical therapist may prescribe stretching and active exercises to be done during the hours when the splint is off. This will help to promote normal range of motion of the joints and improve the muscle action in the legs.

ALTHOUGH I CAN WALK AROUND THE HOUSE, I CAN'T WALK MORE THAN A BLOCK WITHOUT GETTING WEAK. WHAT SHOULD I DO? I DON'T WANT TO BE STUCK AT HOME ALL THE TIME.

Weakness and fatigue are most likely limiting your ability to walk distances. If some of the assistive devices mentioned previously do not adequately solve this problem, then a mobility aid such as a wheelchair or motorized scooter could greatly enhance your mobility and ability to enjoy life outside your home. People often believe that as long as they can walk at all, they have no use for this type of equipment. As a result, they use all their available energy just getting from point A to B, and then have no energy left to enjoy themselves or get back again! A scooter is actually designed for use by a person who is independent, ambulatory, and on the go. By using a scooter to get from place to place, you conserve your energy and also get more things accomplished once you arrive at your destination.

You will probably find that your family and friends are very supportive of your decision to use a mobility aid. You will once again be able to participate with them in a variety of activities that previously felt too difficult, too tiring, and too slow, including trips to restaurants, the shopping mall, the zoo, a museum—and even Disney World.

Since there are restrictions on insurance coverage of powered mobility devices, do not buy any piece of equipment without first consulting with a health care professional. If your needs can be met with a mobility aid, a physical or occupational therapist can help you choose the type of equipment that would best meet your current and future needs. A salesperson does not understand your medical condition and the potential changes you may experience in the future and, therefore, cannot and should not advise you on what is the best equipment for you.

WHAT IS THE DIFFERENCE BETWEEN A MANUAL WHEELCHAIR, A MOTORIZED SCOOTER, AND AN ELECTRIC WHEELCHAIR? HOW DO I KNOW WHICH IS BEST FOR ME? DOES INSURANCE PAY FOR ANY OF THEM?

A manual wheelchair is a nonmotorized mobility device (see Figure 9-8). A person who wants to use this type of wheelchair without assistance from another person must have sufficient upper body strength to propel the chair. If you have significant upper body weakness or fatigue, another person will need to assist you. The advantage of this type of mobility aid is that it is collapsible and hence easy to transport. Some people who are able to walk most of the time keep a lightweight, portable wheelchair in the trunk of the car for use in places like shopping malls, where they need to cover large distances.

A motorized scooter is a vehicle that resembles a golf cart (see Figure 9-9). It typically has three or four wheels, runs on rechargeable batteries, and is driven by a thumb-push mechanism. To use a scooter effectively, you must be able to stand and transfer into the seat safely and independently. Electric scooters can be disassembled and put into your car. Depending on the size and style of your car, it is possible to install an electric lift that will raise the heaviest parts of the scooter into the trunk. Some scooters are designed primarily for indoor use, while others can travel very well

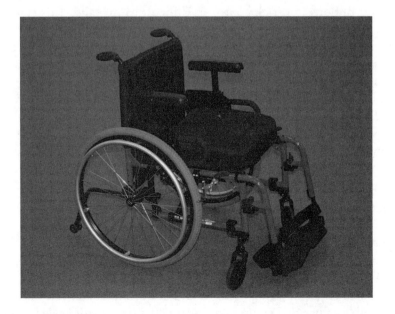

FIGURE 9-8. Manual wheelchair.

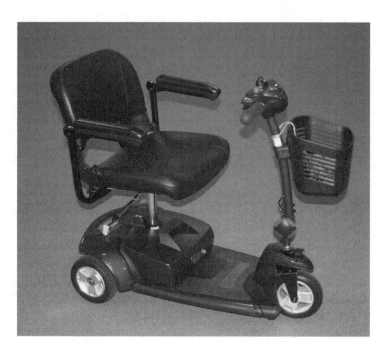

FIGURE 9-9. Motorized scooter.

over outdoor terrain. All can be taken on an airplane as checked baggage. The major limitation is that the seating system does not provide adequate support if there are postural changes.

A motorized wheelchair (see Figure 9-10) has a battery and is typically driven with a stick control by the person sitting in the wheelchair. However, there are many different drive options if a stick control is difficult to manage. This type of chair is useful for the person who has difficulty standing and transferring independently, and needs more seating support than is provided by the seat of an electric scooter. Its major limitation is that it is generally not collapsible or easily transportable. The person who wants to use a power wheelchair independently within the community will probably need a wheelchair-equipped van for transportation.

Many factors must be considered before deciding what equipment is best for you. Your physician and physical or occupational therapist can evaluate your physical requirements and tell you which option(s) would be best for you. Once you know which types of equipment meet your needs safely, the therapist will help you to think through the following questions:

- Where do I want to be able to use this equipment? It is important to know that many insurers require that a wheelchair or mobility device be used *in the home*, at least part time, for them to consider it for payment.
- Where will I store the equipment when I am not using it?
- How will I transport it from one place to another?
- Will I be able to get the equipment in and out of my home? Do I need a ramp?
- Will I be able to use this equipment independently, or will I need someone else's help?

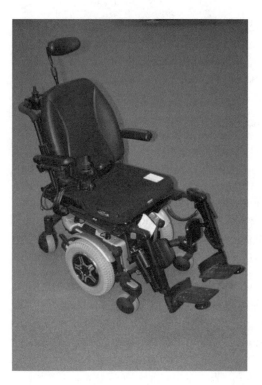

FIGURE 9-10. Motorized wheelchair.

- Do I need specific features to accommodate physical changes like posture or loss of flexibility?

Answering these questions will help you to select the particular equipment that meets your needs most effectively. Some government agencies and insurance plans pay the entire cost or a portion of the cost of mobility equipment. Since physical therapists are aware of the different funding sources and their requirements, they may be able to help you to apply for funding.

IF I START TO USE A WHEELCHAIR TO GO LONG DISTANCES, WILL I LOSE THE ABILITY TO WALK?

No. Inability to walk is caused by demyelination and/or damage to the *axons*, not by using a wheelchair. Due to increased fatigue or diminishing endurance, you may wish to use a wheelchair or scooter to increase your mobility at work or in the community. Or, you may begin to use a mobility aid for high-energy outings such as trips to malls, museums, or the zoo. Using the mobility equipment to enhance your life and broaden your scope of activities will not cause your symptoms to worsen. A mobility aid is not the cause of weakness or fatigue—it is the solution to these two common problems.

SHOULD I PURCHASE A SECONDHAND WHEELCHAIR?

In the event that a wheelchair is not approved by insurance, a secondhand chair may be an option. For example, the common requirement of using the wheelchair "in the home" may not be met if the chair will only be used for long distances. In these cases, relatively inexpensive scooters, folding wheelchairs, or secondhand wheelchairs may be an option. If the wheelchair will be a primary mode of mobility, however, the equipment should be customized. The therapist can help guide you in this decision and help to determine the best mobility option for you.

IT IS DIFFICULT FOR ME TO GET AROUND TOWN TO DO MY ERRANDS AND TAKE CARE OF HOUSEHOLD BUSINESS WITHOUT HAVING SOMEONE TO HELP ME. CAN A PHYSICAL THERAPIST BE OF HELP WITH THIS PROBLEM?

In addition to recommending the appropriate mobility equipment, the physical therapist is one of several possible sources of information (including MS Care Centers, the National MS Society, and other members of your health care team) about transportation in your community. The therapist may recommend obtaining a disabled license plate from the local motor vehicle department, which will enable you to make use of handicapped parking spaces. The therapist can also show you how to apply for access to any available public transit programs for the disabled, or for a designated disabled parking spot near your home, school, or workplace. This is only a sample of the questions commonly asked of physical therapists. Questions more specific to your own situation should be directed to your own therapist. Although two individuals with MS may seem to have the same symptoms, the underlying causes of these symptoms may be quite different. It is best to get an individual assessment of your particular situation.

RECOMMENDED READINGS

Bowling AC. *Complementary and Alternative Medicine and Multiple Sclerosis.* New York: Demos Medical Publishing, 2007.

Holland N, Halper J. *Multiple Sclerosis: A Self-Care Guide to Wellness* (2nd ed.). Washington, DC: Paralyzed Veterans of America, 2005.

Iezzoni LI. *When Walking Fails: Mobility Problems of Adults with Chronic Illnesses.* Berkeley, CA: University of California Press, 2003.

Fishman LM, Small E. *Yoga and Multiple Sclerosis.* New York: Demos Medical Publishing, 2007.

Schapiro R. *Symptom Management in Multiple Sclerosis* (5th ed.). New York: Demos Medical Publishing, 2007.

Selected publications from the National MS Society (800-344-4867) or online at www. nationalmssociety.org/Brochures:
- *Managing MS Through Rehabilitation*
- *Exercise as Part of Everyday Life*
- *At Home with MS: Adapting Your Environment*
- *Stretching for People with MS*
- *Stretching with a Helper for People with MS*
- *Gait or Walking Problems: The Basic Facts*
- *Pain: The Basic Facts*
- *Spasticity: The Basic Facts*
- *Fatigue: What You Should Know*
- *Pulmonary Function and Rehabilitation in MS.* A Clinical Bulletin by Donna Fry PT, available at www.nationalmssociety.org/ClinicalBulletins

The Role of Occupational Therapy: Strategies to Enhance Independence and Productivity at Home and at Work

*Cindy Gackle, OTR/L, MSCS**

Due to the nature of the disease process, the ***symptoms*** of multiple sclerosis (MS) can vary greatly from one individual to another. For some, the symptoms may be slight, such as tingling in the hands or mild ***spasticity***. For others, the symptoms may be more severe, including problems such as weakness (***paresis***), balance problems, pain, fatigue, difficulty with ***coordination***, vision changes, speech disturbances, and ***cognitive impairment***.

In addition to the variety of symptoms caused by MS, a person can also experience variation in the progression of symptoms. Many people experience fluctuations between periods of ***relapses*** and periods of ***remission***. Others experience increasingly severe symptoms over the course of time with little or no remission (see Chapter 2).

Occupational therapy (OT) assists individuals to manage both the variety of symptoms and the variations in symptom progression. Therapy focuses on improving and preserving one's ability to perform everyday skills that are essential for productive independent living, such as dressing, bathing, grooming, meal preparation, writing/computer access, and driving. Energy management training to combat the disabling effect of MS fatigue is also an integral part of treatment by OT. The ***occupational therapist*** tailors treatment to an individual's specific needs and deficits. From the time of diagnosis, the goal of treatment is to develop and support specific abilities and adaptations that promote functional independence in everyday living and enhance quality of life. The occupational therapist addresses four major areas that are essential to maintaining independence:

● Upper body strength, movement, and coordination
● ADL (activities of daily living) training, which may also include use of various kinds of adaptive equipment to improve one's independence and safety, as well as

*With grateful acknowledgment of materials from the first and second editions written by Jean Hietpas, OTR, LCSW.

training in *assistive technology* (AT) for the home and office, and computer and environmental modifications for greater accessibility

- Compensatory strategies for cognitive impairments, sensation problems, or vision loss (see Chapter 14 for information about the role of OT in the assessment and management of MS-related cognitive changes)
- Energy management education and specific task training to use one's energy more efficiently in order to minimize the impact of fatigue while performing daily activities

The occupational therapist uses both assessment and treatment tools to manage MS-related problems and to teach specific skills that will optimize independence. Assessment, which is an ongoing process over the course of the disease, involves the expertise of the occupational therapist and the active participation of the person with MS. As part of the assessment process, you will be asked about your ability to perform your daily activities, and your physical abilities (such as upper body strength and function, and standing/sitting balance, etc.). Cognitive skills will be assessed, as well as how fatigue may be impacting you and your ability to perform your tasks. Also included is how you are able to access and maneuver around your home and work environments, such as the bathroom, bedroom, kitchen, and work space.

Once problem areas have been identified, the occupational therapist will work with you to develop a treatment plan to correct or manage these problems.

HAND FUNCTION

I'M EXPERIENCING INCREASING WEAKNESS IN MY HANDS AND FINGERS. WILL EXERCISE MAKE MY HANDS STRONG AGAIN? WHAT EXERCISES ARE BEST FOR THIS PROBLEM?

Our hands are the "doing" centers for many of our everyday tasks. Many of the jobs we need to do become frustrating and difficult when hand strength and coordination decrease. The hand weakness you experience as a result of MS is due to reduced *nerve* conduction rather than weakened muscles. Therefore, the primary goal is not necessarily to increase hand strength (although for some people the hands do become stronger), but to preserve existing dexterity and muscle strength and, to the extent possible, prevent further deterioration. Your occupational therapist will prescribe a personalized set of exercises, including active range-of-motion, coordination, and mild resistive exercises (such as therapy putty). The exercise program will be individualized in order to involve all appropriate muscles and prevent overfatigue.

MY HANDS FEEL WEAK AND CLUMSY MOST OF THE TIME. IS THERE ANYTHING TO HELP TIE MY SHOES AND BUTTON MY SHIRT?

A variety of products are available to help with frustrating tasks such as tying shoes and buttoning shirts. Several options include the following:

- Slip-on shoes, using a long-handled shoehorn if you are unable to bend over and reach your feet

- Elastic shoelaces will turn your tie shoes into slip-ons. Lace your shoes while they are on your feet, tightening them just enough to allow you to slip them on/off easily while still getting adequate support for walking. Once you have the correct tension, tie a knot and then the bow, so that the tension will be maintained even if the bow becomes untied.
- Lace locks are another alternative to secure shoes. These spring-loaded lace tighteners can often be found in the "notions" section at fabric stores.
- Velcro closure-style shoes.
- A shoemaker can stitch the tongue of the shoe in place so that it won't move around and get in the way, or sew a loop on the backs of your shoes so you can pull them on with a long-handled hook.
- A *stocking aid* can be helpful if you are finding it difficult to reach your feet to put on socks. The stocking is positioned on the aid, as you would put your sock on your foot, with the heel side facing down. The rope handles are used to "toss" the aid to your foot, and then you pull on the rope to position the stocking on your foot.
- *Reacher*s can be helpful to extend your reach when putting on pants as well as picking up shoes off the floor.
- Buttoning is made simpler with a *buttonhook*, which is used to pull the button through the buttonhole with a minimum of strength and dexterity.
- Shirt cuff buttons can be made more manageable by replacing the cotton thread with elastic thread—the elasticity will allow you to slide your hand through without undoing the buttons.
- Another strategy is to remove the buttons, close the buttonholes, and reattach the buttons on top of the buttonholes. Velcro pieces can then be sewn behind the buttonholes and on the original button sites for easy closure.
- Some people prefer to wear shirts with large, easy to grasp buttons, pullovers, or polo-type shirts that have very few buttons.

Mail-order catalogs and Internet Web sites containing these and other products are available for consumers (see Recommended Resources list at the end of the chapter). As you begin to look for ways to make it easier to dress yourself, you will discover numerous ways to simplify many aspects of your daily routine, conserve energy, and save time.

I'VE BELONGED TO A BRIDGE GROUP FOR YEARS. LATELY, I HAVEN'T GONE TO THE GROUP BECAUSE I'M AFRAID OF DROPPING THE CARDS. DO I HAVE TO GIVE UP CARD PLAYING?

It is important not to give up the things that you love to do. Card holders (see Figure 10-1) come in a variety of shapes and sizes for different kinds of card games.

Playing cards with large numbers and symbols are readily available, and a card shuffler may be helpful as well. A rubber fingertip can make it easier to grip the cards, as can a fingertip moistener, which leaves your fingers tacky and makes it easier to hold playing cards (and turn pages). Both are available at most office supply stores.

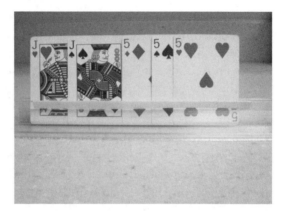

FIGURE 10-1. Card holder.

NUMBNESS AND TINGLING IN ONE OF MY HANDS CAUSES ME TO DROP THINGS. IS THERE ANYTHING I CAN DO ABOUT THIS PROBLEM?

Sensory symptoms that include numbness and tingling have a tendency to come and go intermittently in MS (see Chapter 2). At present, no available treatment is likely to have any lasting impact on the numbness and tingling that you are experiencing. The best approach is to learn how to accommodate to these symptoms to protect yourself from burns or other injuries, and prevent your possessions from unnecessary breakage.

The decreased sensation and dexterity that often accompany numbness and tingling are the likely cause of your tendency to drop things. You drop something because you are less able to feel it in your hand. Visual contact with the object near your hands, or while holding it, is very important to compensate for this decreased sensation and dexterity—so try to keep an eye on what you are doing. Use cups with large handles that accommodate your whole hand rather than one or two fingers. Also, using a coffee mug with a lid, such as the kind used for travel, will help avoid painful burns. Try using a pen that has a thicker body with a textured surface. Slow down enough to make sure that you have a good grip on dishes and other breakable items, and consider purchasing a set of unbreakable dinnerware. You may find that you need to carry each item with two hands to ensure its safety and yours. Some people have found that rubber gloves help improve their grip and compensate for sensation loss.

I HAVE A SIGNIFICANT TREMOR IN BOTH OF MY HANDS, WHICH MAKES IT DIFFICULT FOR ME TO WRITE LEGIBLY OR EAT WITHOUT MAKING A MESS. IT'S VERY IMPORTANT TO ME TO BE ABLE TO CONTINUE DOING THESE THINGS INDEPENDENTLY. ARE THERE ANY GADGETS THAT WOULD HELP WITH THIS PROBLEM?

Tremor is one of the most difficult and frustrating of MS symptoms (see Chapter 4). Fortunately, a number of well-designed writing and eating aids can alleviate some of the problems it can cause in your daily life. Some helpful strategies and adaptive equipment include the following:

- Position yourself close to your work, and with your arms closer to body; this will help provide some stability to counteract the instability from the tremors. Use the table to stabilize your arms while eating. Although many of us learned that it was not good etiquette to have our arms rest on the table when eating, this is a very helpful strategy to manage the tremors, and it is not a sign of poor etiquette.

- Weighted utensils can be very helpful, such as silverware and cups (see Recommended Resources list at the end of the chapter).
- "Knork Flatware" is a brand of silverware that has a heavier weight to it, which can dampen the tremor—and, it looks like everyday silverware (see Figure 10-2). The modifications to a standard fork give it a unique design that allows you to both cut and spear the food without changing utensils.

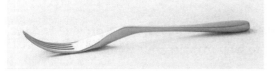

FIGURE 10-2. Knork Flatware.

- Dinner plates with a curved edge, or a plate guard, will contain the food and prevent it from scattering onto the table. Drinking glasses are available with lids to prevent spillage.
- Weighted gloves or light wrist weights may be helpful. However, this strategy may not be particularly useful if your arms are extremely weak, or if you fatigue easily.
- Larger diameter pens with a textured surface are easier and less tiring to hold. Because they are less fatiguing for the small muscles of the hand, they may also reduce hand tremor. Weighted pen holders can also be helpful; however, they may cause excess muscle fatigue.
- A signature stamp can be made for signing letters and documents. It is recommended that you communicate with your bank before using this strategy for writing checks. Online banking/checking is another good alternative.
- There are a variety of different pen holders that may be helpful. The Writing Bird by Norco (see Figure 10-3) resembles a rounded paperweight with a hole for your pen and grooves for your fingers. You write by grasping the molded holder with your entire hand and moving it along the page.

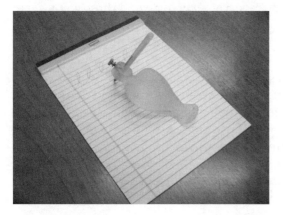

FIGURE 10-3. Writing Bird.

- Plastic writing "guides" are also available to help you write in straighter, more legible lines.
- The Smart Pen manufactured by Livescribe (www.livescribe.com) is a unique and quite effective record and playback system. It is a pen with a built-in digital

recorder that can record conversations, meetings, and lectures, while you take handwritten notes. Using specially designed paper (called "dot paper"), the pen lets you tap your notes to play back the recording. The notes can be shared with others, as well as loaded on to your computer, iPad, iPhone, or the Internet.

- Digital recorders are another technological means of recording information without writing. There are a variety of styles and features to consider when deciding which recorder would be most useful for you, including ease of managing the controls, the recording quality, and so on.

An occupational therapist can work with you to identify and provide training with specific devices and teach strategies to help manage your tremors.

I FEEL TIGHTNESS IN MY NECK AND ARM MUSCLES. ARE THERE STRETCHES OR OTHER EXERCISES THAT MIGHT HELP ME WITH THIS?
Maintaining flexibility and range of motion in the neck and arms is very important for easing discomfort and preventing tightness. Stretching and range-of-motion exercises are the best strategy for enhancing arm mobility and comfort. An occupational therapist or physical therapist can assist you in creating the right program for your particular needs.

Exercise can be fun, and may include activities such as swimming, yoga, tai chi, and exercise groups. It is very important to create a program that you enjoy and can commit to do on a regular basis (see Chapter 9).

FATIGUE

IT SEEMS TO TAKE SO MUCH EFFORT JUST TO GET UP IN THE MORNING AND DEAL WITH BATHING, DRESSING, AND BREAKFAST. IS THERE SOMETHING I CAN DO TO MAKE THOSE TASKS EASIER AND LESS TIRING?
When MS fatigue interferes with your ability to perform basic physical tasks, take time to think about your routine. The primary goal is to continue to participate in what is meaningful for you, including the tasks you *have* to do and those you *want* to do. So it is important to look at how you spend your energy. Experiment with ways to simplify and reorganize your routine to conserve your energy and spend it on the activities that really matter.

Examples of different ways to manage your tasks, and subsequently your energy, might include such simple changes as taking a shower in the evening so that you have less to do in the morning. Plan brief (2-to-3–minute) rests into your schedule to pace your energy and avoid becoming exhausted. If you are heat-sensitive, consider taking a cool or lukewarm shower rather than a fatigue-producing hot shower. Use a fan in the bathroom to keep cool and for air circulation. A shower chair to sit, instead of standing, can minimize the amount of energy used when showering. Consider selecting your clothes for the next day and putting them on a bedside chair before you go to bed in the evening.

As you purchase clothes now and in the future, try to select items that are easy to take on and off and require a minimum of energy to maintain. Generally, slightly larger clothes and shirts/blouses with large buttons down the front are easier to get on and off. Likewise, loose-fitting slacks with an elastic waist are comfortable and easy to pull on and off. Women can add a scarf or jewelry to almost any kind of pullover shirt or sweater to enhance it. Men may find it useful to wear clip-on ties or to leave their neckties tied so that they need only be slipped over the head and tightened. Dress shirts can remain permanently buttoned except for the top buttons, allowing you to pull the shirt over your head. Sit when dressing; a stable chair is often easier than sitting on the edge of the bed.

Adaptive aids such as dressing sticks, sock aids, elastic shoelaces, and long-handled shoehorns can be helpful. An occupational therapist can assess what equipment would be most beneficial for you, and provide training in its use.

Plan your breakfast the night before, and leave the nonperishable items and dishes on the counter or table so that they are ready to use in the morning.

I ENJOY MY WORK, BUT AM FINDING IT INCREASINGLY DIFFICULT TO MANEUVER AROUND MY OFFICE AND MANAGE MY FATIGUE OVER THE COURSE OF THE WORKING DAY. I'M AFRAID I WON'T BE ABLE TO STAY AT THIS JOB IF IT GETS ANY WORSE.

Work simplification and work efficiency are key to enhancing comfort and productivity on the job:

- Make sure that your work space, furniture, and office equipment are designed and correctly positioned to promote correct body mechanics/ergonomics and physical comfort, thus reducing fatigue.
- Organize your workspace to eliminate unnecessary reaching, lifting, and walking.
- Reexamine your approach to tasks to ensure that you are doing them in the simplest, most energy-efficient, and least time-consuming way.
- Become familiar with the tools and/or adaptive devices available to simplify your tasks, including computer modifications.
- Plan your schedule to make the best use of high-energy times, prioritizing tasks and delegating as appropriate. Build in short rest periods.
- Get a good night's sleep, and eat regular nutritious meals.
- If you are not using any assistive devices to walk, consider a physical therapy evaluation to learn about the variety of options that can increase your mobility and reduce your fatigue (see Chapter 9).

You can schedule an appointment with an occupational therapist to evaluate your work situation and recommend ways to simplify your tasks and help you be more comfortable and efficient on the job. Many of the adaptations he or she might suggest are considered "reasonable accommodations" under the Americans with Disabilities Act (ADA; see Chapter 20). The occupational therapist can help you formulate your requests for accommodations from your employer.

I FEEL SO HELPLESS WHEN FATIGUE TAKES OVER AND INTERFERES WITH MY PLANS FOR THE DAY. WHAT CAN I DO TO MANAGE MY ENERGY AND FEEL MORE IN CONTROL OF MY TIME AND PLANS?

It is important to discuss the fatigue with your physician so that he or she can work with you to identify its cause(s). There are medications (e.g., Symmetrel [amantadine], Provigil [modafinil], Nuvigil [armodafinil]—see Appendix B) that can be used to manage the primary fatigue of MS, which is often referred to as *lassitude*. Other factors that can contribute to fatigue must be identified and addressed as well, including depression, medication side effects, poor nutrition, sleep disturbances caused by spasticity, pain, **nocturia**, or other MS symptoms, and deconditioning caused by lack of mobility and exercise. These are all common in MS. A proactive approach to managing your energy will contribute to feeling more empowered and in control.

The concept of managing energy can easily be compared to the way you manage finances. "Banking" energy involves *making deposits* into your "energy bank" by by resting when you need to and getting enough sleep at night, and *saving* by using your energy only for the things that are most important to you. "Budgeting" involves planning and choosing how to spend your energy. Once your energy is "banked," you can "budget" it so that you can accomplish what you need and want:

- Plan and prioritize your day, alternating activities with rest. Resting *before* you feel exhausted is most effective.
- Pace yourself, alternating low-energy activities with high-energy activities, and spread them out during the day and week. Plan your schedule so you have energy for your high priority activities.
- Analyze how you do your tasks so you can simplify and/or modify for more efficient use of your energy. Are there steps that can be combined or eliminated? What can be changed to make the task easier?
- Use energy conservation techniques and/or assistive devices to help you be more efficient with your tasks.
- Pay attention to how you position yourself with your work; good body mechanics and ergonomic adaptations help conserve energy.
- Communicate about your needs; ask others for assistance or delegate tasks.
- A regular exercise routine will increase your overall physical conditioning and reduce your fatigue (see Chapter 9).
- Regular nutritious meals will help to fuel your "energy bank."
- Assess the expectations you place on yourself for how you perform an activity. The amount of energy you spend will vary depending on the standards you set, so try to be realistic.
- Make active decisions about how to spend your energy; plan your day with your priorities in mind to help ensure adequate time for the most important activities as well as adequate time for rest, leisure, and self-care.

"Banking" and "budgeting" strategies can be helpful tools for energy management and achieving a balanced lifestyle. With increased awareness and attention to priorities, you know how much energy you can spend on the tasks that need to be done, as well as those activities that you enjoy.

Obtaining a referral from your doctor for treatment with an occupational therapist can be helpful to address your specific needs and teach you methods that will enhance learning and the use of energy management techniques.

BATHROOM SAFETY AND PERSONAL HYGIENE

GETTING ON AND (ESPECIALLY) OFF THE TOILET HAS BECOME DIFFICULT. ARE THERE ANY MODIFICATIONS I CAN MAKE THAT WILL EASE THIS PROBLEM?
Several modifications can be made with your body mechanics and the use of adaptive equipment. It is important to pay attention to the placement of both your arms

and feet when changing from the seated to the standing position and vice versa. To go from a standing to a sitting position, place yourself squarely in front of the toilet seat, bend your knees until you can touch each side of the toilet seat with your hands, and then lower yourself slowly to the seat. Then, with your feet placed firmly in front of you, use your hands and arms to push off from the toilet seat.

The simplest assistive device to help you get on and off the toilet is a secure grab bar on the wall next to the toilet. Obviously, this is only effective if the toilet is adjacent to a wall. Drop-down bars can be mounted to the back wall if no side wall is available. Another alternative is to place a commode over the toilet, which allows for adjustment of the seat height and provides bilateral armrests to assist you in lowering and raising your body.

There are a number of other medical equipment items, such as a raised toilet seat, with or without armrests, or a toilet safety frame, that can be helpful (see Figure 10-4). When leg strength is significantly weakened, a toilet lift that mechanically helps with safe sitting and standing may be helpful.

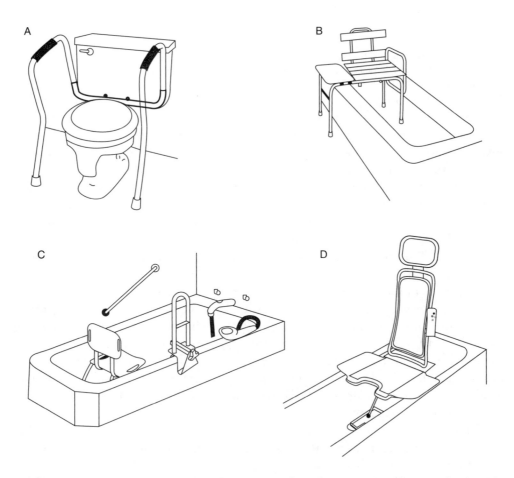

FIGURE 10-4. Bathroom aids. (A) toilet safety frame, (B) tub transfer bench, (C) shower chair, clamp-on tub grab bar—vertical style, diagonal wall grab bar, and handheld shower hose, and (D) bathtub lift.

An occupational therapist can help you determine which piece of equipment best suits your needs, and provide the necessary training for your optimal safety and comfort.

I'M CONCERNED THAT I'M NOT ADEQUATELY CLEANING MYSELF AFTER TOILETING. ARE THERE WAYS TO DO THIS MORE EFFECTIVELY?

Independence in toileting is a very personal matter, yet one that can be problematic because of poor sitting balance or limited use of the hands. Try using a wet washcloth or flushable moist wipe to clean yourself, or have a squeeze bottle with lukewarm water to rinse yourself after toileting. Several toileting aids, such as toilet tongs, are available through ADL equipment suppliers. If you have diminished hand dexterity, the tongs may not be advisable. An alternative is the Bottom Buddy Toilet Aid, which is designed for use when reaching is difficult. It has a soft, flexible head to grip tissue or premoistened wipe securely and releases the paper with the push of a button on an easy-to-use handle.

Also available are portable or permanently installed bidets that rinse and, in some models, dry the genital area.

GETTING IN AND OUT OF THE SHOWER-TUB COMBINATION HAS BECOME DIFFICULT FOR ME. DO YOU HAVE ANY SUGGESTIONS FOR MAKING THIS TASK EASIER AND SAFER?

It is important to make sure that your transfer in and out of the shower stall or tub-shower is safe. Adequate balance and a certain amount of strength are both necessary for safe transfers. If your balance is in question, the easiest solution is to install a grab bar to hold onto during the transfer. Grab bars should be permanently mounted to a stud in the wall (your local hardware store may be able to recommend a handyman to install them). An occupational therapist can assess your ability to transfer and recommend the appropriate bathroom equipment to optimize your safety and independence, and minimize your fatigue. If your upper body strength is not sufficient, or if your lower body is too weak, an occupational therapist may recommend a tub transfer bench for a seated transfer in and out of the tub-shower (see Figure 10-4).

A height-adjustable shower chair or tub transfer bench is also the answer if your standing balance and endurance are not sufficient to allow you to stand confidently during your shower. Equipment use will also maximize safety and use less energy (see Figure 10-4). A handheld shower hose, mounted on a height-adjustable, wall-mounted rod, will make a seated shower more enjoyable. A nonslip mat in the tub or shower stall will help prevent a fall. This type of equipment is available through a local medical supply company. Resources can usually be found in the Yellow Pages under Medical Equipment and Supplies.

Modifying your bathtub with a Walk-Thru Insert (See Figure 10-5) can make it more accessible and safer. This tub-to-shower conversion lowers the tub wall entrance making it much easier to access.

It is also possible that a standard tub can be removed to create a barrier-free shower, removing the lip and the need to lift your leg to step up and over into the shower. For

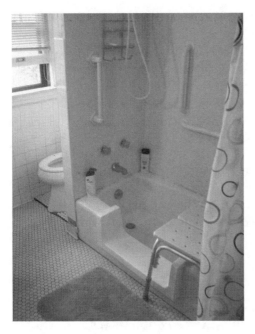

FIGURE 10-5. Walk-Thru Insert.

those who prefer to take baths, an option is a walk-in bathtub, which allows the user to easily enter and leave through a watertight door that swings open when the tub is empty of water and a door-release lever is opened.

The Internet site, www.abledata.com, is a great resource for more information about these options, including educational literature about remodeling the bathroom for increased accessibility and safety.

MOBILITY

GETTING UP AND OUT OF A CHAIR IS BECOMING HARDER FOR ME. WHAT IS THE BEST TYPE OF CHAIR FOR ME TO SIT IN, AND ARE THERE ANY RECOMMENDED TECHNIQUES OR GADGETS THAT WILL MAKE IT EASIER FOR ME TO GET UP AGAIN?

The easiest type of chair is one that has a relatively high seat and solid arms. The height of the chair is critical because it is always more difficult to get out of low, soft chairs than high, firm ones. You can add a 2-to-3–inch dense foam cushion to raise the height of your chair, or add leg extenders to raise the overall height of the chair.

It will be easier to get up from the seat if you scoot forward first and then use your hands to push up from the arms of the chair. If these adaptations are not sufficient, portable lifter cushions that are placed on the chair will gently lower and assist you out of a seated position (for example, UpEasy Seat Assist). There are also chairs and recliners with a mechanical lift system (see Recommended Resource list; and your local medical equipment stores may also be a good resource).

MY BED IS SO LOW THAT I HAVE A HARD TIME GETTING OUT OF IT. ARE THERE WAYS TO MODIFY MY BED THAT WILL SOLVE THIS PROBLEM?

Getting up from low surfaces can be difficult. First, pay attention to your body mechanics: Try rolling onto your side, facing the edge of the bed, and pushing yourself up with your bottom arm while swinging your legs over the side of the bed. If you have trouble rolling over onto your side, you can purchase bed rail bars that can be attached to the sides of your mattress.

Once in a sitting position on the edge of the bed, try to push yourself up with your hands. If the bed is too low or too soft for you to be able to push yourself upright, you can raise the height of the bed by placing it on wood blocks or commercially available bed risers, which are available from a variety of retailers, such as Bed, Bath, and Beyond. A strategically placed grab bar on the wall next to your bed, a bed rail, or a floor-to-ceiling pole next to the bed can allow you to pull yourself from a sitting position to a standing position.

HOME CHORES

WE EAT A LOT OF FRESH VEGETABLES AND MAKE SALADS FOR OUR MEALS, BUT PEELING, CHOPPING, AND CUTTING HAVE BECOME DIFFICULT. ARE THERE ANY TECHNIQUES OR GADGETS THAT WILL MAKE THIS TASK LESS DIFFICULT?

Many types of blenders and food processors are available at your local hardware or department store. These devices save on the effort and time needed to prepare vegetables. Select kitchen knives and other utensils that have a good solid grip and are easy to maneuver. Good Grips utensils, for example, have a built-up handle with a nonslip surface. Rocker-handle knives and knives with L-shaped handles are also easier to maneuver (see Figure 10-6).

Dycem is a nonslip material designed to stabilize bowls and cutting boards while you work. The nonslip material that is often used as shelf and drawer liners is a less expensive option that will also provide stability. Some cutting boards are designed to hold or stabilize the item you are cutting.

You might also ask a family member to help you wash and cut a 2- or 3-day supply of vegetables at one time and store them in plastic containers or bags in the

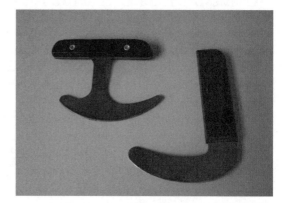

FIGURE 10-6. Rocker knives.

refrigerator. Another solution might be to take advantage of the convenience packs of ready-to-eat salad vegetables now carried by many grocery stores. Electric or battery-operated can openers can be helpful.

In addition to using proper utensils and convenience foods, try to conserve your energy by gathering all the items you need for the job in one place before starting food preparations. A wheeled cart can be helpful to transport the supplies. Plan ahead and pace yourself. Partial preparation the day before can be a helpful time and energy saver.

I ENJOY COOKING, BUT FIND THAT I GET WORN OUT FROM THE EFFORT AND WEAK-ENED BY THE HEAT. DO YOU HAVE ANY SUGGESTIONS FOR SOLVING THESE PROBLEMS?
Many nutritious and easy-to-prepare foods are now available that require less preparation time, and can often be prepared in the microwave. For example, traditional oatmeal provides a nutritious and tasty breakfast and is quick to prepare in the microwave; adding walnuts and dried cranberries can provide additional nutritional value. Instant foods such as oatmeal, rice, and potatoes are now easily available. Soups, and frozen foods such as vegetables and meals, are also easy to prepare.

A microwave, convection oven, or toaster oven creates little or no heat and reduces meal preparation time. If you are now using a standard oven or doing a lot of stove-top cooking that makes the kitchen overly warm, you might want to consider the use of a "cooling vest." This handy garment looks like an outdoor vest designed to hold frozen gel packs. Wearing this vest during cooking or any other uncomfortably warm activity can keep you cool and reduce the heat-induced fatigue that is so common in MS (www.bodycooler.com, www.polarsoftice.com, www.steelevest.com). It also helps to have a fan in the kitchen to keep the room and yourself cooler.

Make sure that the kitchen is organized, clean, and neat so that you have an open work area, and that tools/supplies are placed within a comfortable reach. Conserve your energy by having a stool in the kitchen to sit on during meal preparation and clean-up. Using a dishwasher for clean-up or recruiting family assistance for tasks that are difficult for you are also effective strategies. And for those days when you're too tired to even think about cooking, there are food services available that do the planning of nutritious meals, and also the cooking. (e.g., www.seattlesutton.com), All you have to do is heat and eat—and some meals don't even require heating.

WHEN I DO THE LAUNDRY, I HAVE TO CARRY IT UP AND DOWN FOURTEEN STEPS. IS THERE ANYTHING I CAN DO TO MAKE THIS PROCESS EASIER AND SAFER?
Carrying items can be dangerous if your standing balance is unstable. Break the task into small, light loads rather than carrying one large load, or put the laundry in a bag with a drawstring and pull it up and down the stairs behind you (holding on to the handrail with the other hand). A pop-up hamper has handles that make it easier to carry while still holding on to the handrail with one hand. Having handrails on both walls is most helpful. Depending on your staircase, you may be able to create a

simple pulley system that allows you to pull the laundry bag up and down the stairs with a minimum amount of strength and exertion.

Another solution might be for a family member or neighbor to carry the laundry up and down the stairs. Do not hesitate to recruit assistance for tasks that become too difficult or too dangerous for you to do alone. You might also want to consider relocating your laundry equipment to the main living area such as the kitchen or closet on the main floor. Another option is to put in a stair glide that would allow you to ride up and down the stairs with your laundry bag.

Some people find that the sorting and folding of laundry is time consuming and tiring. Ask family members to presort their own clothes into dark and light piles before bringing them to the washing machine, and to make sure that each item is turned right side out. You can also tell them that anything that is given to you turned inside out will be given back to them clean but still inside out. Depending on the ages of your family members, you might even ask each person to take care of his or her own laundry!

GOING TO THE GROCERY STORE IS A MAJOR ORDEAL. THE AISLES ARE CROWDED, I CAN'T REACH MANY OF THE ITEMS I NEED, AND GETTING THE GROCERY BAGS INTO MY HOUSE IS EXHAUSTING. THERE MUST BE AN EASIER WAY!

Grocery shopping can be a major ordeal for many people, and it is compounded for those with physical problems. Plan what you need, and make a list prior to going to the store. Photocopy a master grocery list and simply check the items you need for that shopping trip. Try to shop during off-peak times when the store is less crowded. Know your grocery store (some stores have printed maps indicating which products are stocked in each aisle) and bypass the aisles you do not need. Request shopping assistance at customer service for items that are out of your reach. A *reacher* can be a handy tool to assist with reaching some items, but take care when choosing items. You certainly do not want a soup can on an overhead shelf to fall on your head! Often an employee can accompany you while you shop, or the requested items will be waiting for you at customer service. Although you may initially feel reluctant to ask for this kind of help, most people find that store employees and other shoppers are more than happy to provide assistance.

A few grocery stores have power scooters available for public use, and some stores provide a delivery service. In most supermarkets, a store employee is available to carry the groceries to your car. When you return home, ask a family member to carry the groceries from the car, or carry the perishable items in a separate bag or back pack and leave the other items for later, when you have more energy. A fold-up, portable cart on wheels may help you to carry items more easily.

If getting to the grocery store becomes too energy expending or impossible, call your local stores and ask if they will take a telephone order for delivery. While it can be very frustrating to have to rely on someone at the store to pick out your items (particularly fresh fruits and vegetables), you will probably find that the process works fairly well once you and the store's employees have gone through it a few times. Online grocery shopping and delivery via the Internet has become more popular and prevalent across the United States (e.g., www.peapod.com). Local grocery chains are beginning to provide such a service, or may partner with a national company.

HOME ACCESS

WE ARE PLANNING TO REDO THE BATHROOM AND KITCHEN IN OUR HOME. WHAT KINDS OF MODIFICATIONS WOULD YOU RECOMMEND?

Accessibility and ease of use are the main factors to consider in making home modifications. Several good references to home modifications are available (see the section on Environmental Adaptations in Appendix F). When designing for accessibility in the bathroom, universal design features to consider include the following:

- Door width, 36″
- Adequacy of space in which to maneuver, including any ambulation device, such as crutches, walker, scooter, or wheelchair
- Height, shape, and mounting of the sink and toilet
- Accessibility of the medicine cabinet and other storage areas
- Access to the shower stall, or replacement of a tub with a walk-in shower
- Design of door handles and faucets—lever style are the easiest
- Design of light switches, and placement so that both the light switches and electric outlets are accessible from both a standing and a sitting position

Likewise, a well-designed kitchen can make meal preparation more pleasurable and less exhausting. Carefully placed appliances, counters, sinks, cabinets, and work areas should be considered and discussed when remodeling your kitchen. You will want to be able to reach the items you need without having to do a great deal of walking back and forth or reaching. As with any other long-term, expensive decisions and purchases, try to think not only about your present needs but also about your potential needs in the future. You might plan for your countertops to be lower than usual in case you want, or need, to do more of your cooking from a seated position. Similarly, you might want to consider overhanging countertops that would allow space for your legs if you were working from a seated position. You are well advised to consult with an occupational therapist, as well as a general contractor or architect who is knowledgeable about accessibility and universal design, before proceeding. Working with an accessibility specialist can be a very worthwhile investment toward creating a home that allows maximum mobility and independence (http://www.tcaging.org/downloads/homedesign.pdf; copy of brochure, "Practical Guide to Universal Home Design").

I WANT TO REMAIN IN MY CURRENT HOME, BUT I HAVE TO ADMIT THAT IT HAS BECOME DIFFICULT GETTING UP AND DOWN THE ENTRANCE STEPS.

Several options are available to provide safe access in and out of your home. Solidly mounted handrails on both sides of the stairs can help with getting up and down the stairs. A physical therapist can assess your ability to use stairs safely using the handrails for support. Modifying outdoor steps to long-tread, low-riser steps with handrails is another alternative that can make stair climbing easier (www.wheelchairramp.org; 651-646-8342). Ramps are another alternative, but may be more energy-draining for some people. Ramps are necessary for wheelchair access, and should have a slope no steeper than 1 to 12. This means that each inch of height requires at least 12 inches of slope and each foot of height needs 12 feet of slope. The steeper the ramp, the less safe it is for anyone using it. A mechanical lift or residential elevator are other alternatives that may be considered.

COMMUNICATION

**I ENJOY TALKING ON THE TELEPHONE, ESPECIALLY SINCE IT HAS BECOME MORE DIF-
FICULT FOR ME TO GET OUT AND SEE FAMILY AND FRIENDS. HOLDING THE PHONE
IS STARTING TO BECOME TIRING AND AWKWARD. IS THERE ANYTHING I CAN DO TO
MAKE MY TIME ON THE PHONE MORE COMFORTABLE?**

Several good telecommunication products and services are available that will make
talking on the phone easy and enjoyable. Speaker phones permit hands-free operation so that you can speak and listen without having to hold the receiver. If you wish
to have a more private conversation, try a hands-free telephone headset. Bluetooth
wireless and hands-free headsets have become very popular with a broad range of cell
phones. Video communication has become even more personal via the Internet with
Skype and a webcam.

Ask your telephone company if they offer an operator-assisted service for disabled individuals who are unable to dial a telephone number. Oftentimes you can be
exempt from charges with completion of the appropriate paperwork.

If you are experiencing problems with your hearing or vision that interfere
with independent phone use, your phone company has various no-charge services.
Contact your local phone service to find out if you would benefit from any of these
programs.

DRIVING

**I'M LOOKING FOR A NEW CAR. IS THERE ANYTHING IN PARTICULAR I SHOULD
TAKE INTO CONSIDERATION WHEN SELECTING ONE?**

Take your time when selecting a new car. Try to anticipate what your needs might
be in the future as well as thinking carefully about your present needs. For example,
a stick shift or standard transmission car might seem more appealing to you now,
but can cause future difficulties if you develop weakness or incoordination in your
left foot. Compare the ease with which you can get in and out of different models,
noting the height of the seat. Operate the door handles, gear shift, turn signal, wind-
shield wipers, horn, cruise control, radio, air conditioning, parking brake, and seat
adjustments to see how easy to manipulate and accessible they are. Always purchase
air conditioning in the automobile to prevent fatigue on a hot day. Consider a tilt
steering wheel and power seats to give you maximum adjustability and comfort.

CarFit is an educational program that offers older adults the opportunity to check
how well their personal vehicles "fit" them, and also provides information and materials on community-specific resources that could enhance their safety as drivers and/or
increase their mobility in the community. At a CarFit event, a team of trained techni-
cians and/or health professionals work with each participant to ensure they "fit" their
vehicle properly for maximum comfort and safety (http://www.car-fit.org/).

Try lifting packages in and out of the back seat and the trunk of the car. Large
parcels, grocery bags, a small child, and possibly a wheelchair or other piece of adaptive equipment are examples of the "cargo" that people often need to be able to
maneuver in their cars. Vehicles with a lower trunk opening allow you to take items
in and out without having to lift them as high off the ground. You may find that a
four-door sedan allows easier access to back-seat storage space for crutches or a wheelchair, or that a station wagon or hatchback vehicle better fits your needs. A minivan

or van is also an option to consider if you currently use a power mobility device, such as a scooter or power wheelchair, or anticipate using one in the future.

BEING ABLE TO DRIVE MY CAR IS VERY IMPORTANT TO ME, BUT MY RIGHT LEG DOESN'T MOVE AS QUICKLY AND RELIABLY BETWEEN PEDALS AS IT USED TO. I'VE HEARD ABOUT HAND CONTROLS, AND I'M WONDERING WHETHER THEY COULD WORK FOR ME.
Thousands of people operate vehicles with the use of hand controls. They work well for someone who has good upper body control but limited lower body function. Hand controls come in a variety of styles and configurations. They are usually attached to the steering column and look like additional handles protruding from it. Acceleration and braking are accomplished by pulling the control toward you or pushing it away from you.

Since safe driving depends on a variety of functions, including eye-hand coordination, head and neck flexibility, adequate vision, quick thinking, and reasonable reaction time, it would be well worth your while to seek a driving evaluation before investing in equipment for your car. Ask your physician, occupational therapist, or your chapter of the National Multiple Sclerosis Society for the name of the nearest driver evaluation program. Another valuable resource is www.aota.org; click on "Find a Driving Rehab Specialist," to find a listing for a driving specialist or program. This Web site also provides education data about driver safety. A certified driving rehabilitation specialist (CDRS) is able to evaluate what kind of adaptation would be most appropriate for your individual needs. Another resource for locating a CDRS is the Association for Driver Rehabilitation Specialists, which also has a full listing of driving evaluators state-by-state (www.driver-ed.org; 866-672-9466 Toll Free in the United States & Canada).

The major car companies may also offer listings of driver evaluation programs, as well as the names of companies that will perform adaptive modifications on your car. The National Mobility Equipment Dealers Association lists and rates mobility dealers across the country and can point you in the direction of a driver rehabilitation specialist (www.nmeda.org; 800-833-0427).

CHILD CARE

SHORTLY AFTER MY BABY WAS BORN, I BEGAN EXPERIENCING A GREAT DEAL OF FATIGUE AND WEAKNESS IN MY ARMS AND LEGS. I DON'T HAVE MUCH HELP AVAILABLE AND NEED TO LEARN HOW TO HANDLE MY DAUGHTER SAFELY, PARTICULARLY AS SHE BECOMES MORE ACTIVE. DO YOU HAVE ANY SUGGESTIONS?
Principles of energy conservation and good body mechanics will be important as you analyze the various tasks you must perform to take care of your daughter safely. Instead of carrying the baby in your arms, experiment with a sling or infant carrier that you can strap to your torso. If carrying your baby in this manner is too tiring, explore what options you have for child equipment with wheels, such as a bassinet, portable crib, high-chair on wheels, or stroller. Wash, change, and dress your baby at counter height, and use a safety belt on the changing table. Kneel while washing your baby in the bathtub and use an infant-size, lightweight tub with a nonslip surface inside the big tub when the child is young. Consider using disposable diapers as well as easy-on and easy-off clothing with few fasteners.

Learn to rest when your child rests. Prioritize tasks and spread out the more difficult jobs throughout the week. Remember to relax and take care of yourself as well as your new baby. Peer networking through your local chapter of the National Multiple Sclerosis Society can be a valuable resource for exchanging ideas with other parents of young infants. Another resource that may be of assistance, *Through the Looking Glass*, is a nationally recognized center that has pioneered research, training, and services for families in which a child, parent, or grandparent has a disability or medical issue (www.lookkingglass.org).

COMPUTERS

I'M THINKING OF BUYING A PERSONAL COMPUTER. WHAT DO I NEED TO CONSIDER WHEN MAKING THIS PURCHASE AND WHERE SHOULD I GO TO FIND THE ONE THAT BEST MEETS MY NEEDS?

It is best to start by asking yourself, "How could a computer be useful for me?" You might, for example, come up with a list of tasks that includes letter writing, filing information and creating mailing lists, bookkeeping and finances, electronic mail and online communication, drawing graphics, sending and receiving information via fax, and playing computer games. The next step is to try using a computer if you have not yet had the experience. Take a computer literacy course, and talk to friends about ways in which they use their computers. In other words, try to find out whether you are likely to be able to enjoy and make effective use of a computer before you go to the expense of purchasing one.

Now you are ready to go to a computer store and spend time with a salesperson who can explain the jargon and describe the various types of equipment and accessories available. It is very helpful to have a friend along, preferably someone who knows more about computers than you do. When talking with the salesperson, it is important that you be quite specific about your disability. A computer system can be adapted for many kinds of visual, sensory, and motor problems. If you find that the salesperson is simply trying to sell you a computer without taking time to understand your needs, try a different salesperson or a different store. Remember, however, that a salesperson does not necessarily have the skills necessary to assist you with identifying specific adaptations that can optimize your functional ability with a computer. There are a variety of adaptations that are possible to improve one's accessibility with a computer, such as screen magnification to help with decreased vision, and keyboard modifications as well as voice recognition to compensate for upper extremity incoordination.

Resources describing standard accessibility features and functions of the computer's operating systems include www.microsoft.com/enable/ for Microsoft products, and www.apple.com/accessibility/ for Apple products. Tools to make computer technology more manageable and accessible are available at www.nationalmssociety.org/AssistiveTechnology. Because technology options are expanding all the time—at a much faster rate than most of us can keep up with—it is good to know about helpful resources.

Your physician or the National Multiple Sclerosis Society can refer you to an occupational therapist and/or Assistive Technology Services Center for guidance.

An assistive technology professional (ATP) is specially trained in rehabilitative AT, and will be able to assess your needs and recommend technology options that enhance independence and match your abilities. To search for an ATP in your area, go to the Web site for RESNA (Rehabilitation Engineering and Assistive Technology Society of North America)—www.resna.org—and click on "member directory." Another source for AT information is AbleData (www.abledata.org; 800-227-0216).

SUMMARY

Including an occupational therapist on your rehab/health care team can help you to maximize your participation in your "job" of everyday living. Finding an OT does not have to be difficult. Sometimes it may take a bit of exploring. Some OTs have additional training and are certified as an MS specialist (MSCS). The National MS Society (800-344-4867) may be able to help you locate a therapist in your area.

RECOMMENDED READINGS

Holland N, Halper J. (eds.). *Multiple Sclerosis: A Self-Care Guide to Wellness.* 2nd ed. Washington, DC: Paralyzed Veterans of America, 2005.

Lowenstein N. *Fighting Fatigue in Multiple Sclerosis.* New York: Demos Health, 2009.

Peterman-Schwarz S. *300 Tips for Making Life with Multiple Sclerosis Easier.* 2nd ed. New York: Demos Medical Publishing, 2006.

Resources for Rehabilitation. *Living with Low Vision: A Resource Guide for People with Sight Loss.* 7th ed. Winchester, MA: Resources for Rehabilitation, 2001 (available by calling 781-368-9080 or online at http://www.rfr.org).

Rogers J. *The Disabled Woman's Guide to Pregnancy and Birth.* New York: Demos Medical Publishing, 2006.

Schapiro R. *Symptom Management in Multiple Sclerosis.* 5th ed. New York: Demos Medical Publishing, 2007.

Selected materials available from the National Multiple Sclerosis Society (800-344-4867) or online at http://www.nationalmssociety.org/Brochures:
- *At Home with MS: Adapting Your Environment*
- *Exercise as Part of Everyday Life*
- *Managing MS Through Rehabilitation*
- *Fatigue: What You Should Know*
- *Food for Thought: MS and Nutrition*
- *Tremor: The Basic Facts*
- *Vision: The Basic Facts*
- *A Place in the Workforce*
- *The Win-Win Approach to Reasonable Accommodations: Enhancing Productivity on Your Job*
- *ADA and People with MS*
- *Should I Work? Information for Employees*

RECOMMENDED RESOURCES

ADL ADAPTIVE DEVICES
Ableware: Independent Living from Maddak Inc.
Tel: 973-628-7600
Web site: http://www.ableware.com

Active Forever
Tel: 800-377-8033
Web site: http://www.activeforever.com

AliMed
Tel: 800-225-2610
Web site: http://www.alimed.com

North Coast Medical, Inc.
Consumer catalog—Functional Solutions
Tel: 800-821-9319
Web site: http://www.ncmedical.com

Sammons Preston Rolyan, Inc.
Consumer catalog—Enrichments
Tel: 800-323-5547
Web site: http://www.sammonspreston.com

Check the *Medical Equipment & Supplies* section of your local Yellow Pages.

How MS Affects Sexuality and Intimacy

Frederick W. Foley, PhD, and Michael A. Werner, MD

Multiple sclerosis (MS) can affect intimacy and sexuality in a variety of ways. People sometimes report feeling less sexual drive or interest, difficulties with arousal, orgasm, or difficulties communicating with their partner. These changes may be a direct result of neurologic changes or because of efforts to cope with the impact of these changes on their lives. The traditional way of evaluating sexual dysfunction is to classify problems according to aspects of the sexual response cycle, such as disorders of sexual interest or libido, arousal, and orgasm. However, because of the complex ways in which MS can affect sexuality, communication, and intimate behaviors, much of the MS literature has described primary, secondary, and tertiary types of sexual dysfunction.

- *Primary sexual dysfunction* is a direct result of neurologic changes that affect the sexual response. In both men and women, this can include a decrease or loss of sex drive, decreased or unpleasant genital sensations, and diminished capacity for orgasm. In addition, men may experience difficulty achieving or maintaining an erection and/or deceased ejaculatory force or retrograde ejaculation (see Chapter 18). Women may experience decreased vaginal lubrication, loss of vaginal **muscle tone**, and/or diminished clitoral engorgement.
- *Secondary sexual dysfunction* stems from symptoms that do not directly involve nervous pathways to the genital system, such as bladder and bowel problems, fatigue, **spasticity**, muscle weakness, body or hand tremors, impairments in attention and concentration, and nongenital sensory changes.
- *Tertiary sexual dysfunction* results from disability-related psychosocial and cultural issues that can interfere with one's sexual feelings and experiences. For example, some people find it difficult to reconcile the idea of having a disability with being fully sexually expressive. Changes in self-esteem—including the way one feels about one's body, demoralization, depression, or mood swings—can all interfere with intimacy and sexuality. The sexual partnership can be severely challenged by changes within a relationship, such as one person becoming the other's caregiver. Similarly, changes in employment status or role performance within the

household are often associated with emotional adjustments that can temporarily interfere with sexual expression.

Partners can easily misinterpret these sexual changes as a personal rejection or loss of interest in the relationship—and they may well be experiencing their own changes in sexual responsiveness in the face of the illness. Both members of the couple often find it difficult to communicate with one another about their changing sexual and intimacy needs.

The few studies on the *prevalence* of sexual problems in MS have relied primarily on the survey or questionnaire method. The largest study to be completed so far—and the first in North America—found that 69.7 percent of a large sample of persons with MS reported one or more sexual problems that interfered in sexual pleasure or performance most or all of the time. Similar to other studies, difficulty with orgasm, erectile difficulty, inadequate vaginal lubrication, and loss of libido were the most frequently reported symptoms.

A positive finding from the research is that sexual problems in MS can be successfully addressed. One treatment study of couples where one partner had MS found that sex education, cognitive behavior psychotherapy, and enhanced communication with medical providers significantly improved marital satisfaction, communication, problem solving, and sexual satisfaction (Foley et al, 2001). A recent, small, randomized study in women with MS found that reading educational materials (like this chapter, for example) and talking with an MS nurse helped to significantly reduce sexual difficulties (Christopherson et al, 2006).

I'VE NOTICED A LOT OF CHANGES IN MY BODY AND MY SEXUAL FEELINGS IN THE PAST FEW YEARS. MY DOCTOR HAS NEVER BROUGHT UP THE SUBJECT OF SEX, AND NEITHER HAVE I. WHERE IS THE BEST PLACE TO GET INFORMATION ABOUT SEXUAL PROBLEMS IN MS?

Changes in sexual feelings normally occur throughout the life span. However, the experience of MS can complicate the typical changes that occur. MS affects sexual feelings both directly and indirectly, as discussed previously. *Neurologists* and other health care providers often do not spontaneously bring up the subject of sexuality. Physicians and nurses may ignore sexuality because they perceive this line of questioning as an unwelcome intrusion into the private lives of their patients, because of personal discomfort in asking about sexuality, because of lack of professional training in this area, or because of time pressures on them to address mostly medical issues.

Although it can be difficult and potentially embarrassing, your sexuality is important enough to bring up with your primary MS physician. Discuss your changes in sexual feelings and ask directly about treatments that are available to enhance sexuality. Consult your physician for the ways in which your MS symptoms, and the medications used to treat them, may be affecting your sexual responses. Although the burden of opening the door to communication about sexuality may initially fall on you, taking this step with your health care team will ensure that this frequently untreated problem gets the attention it deserves.

To get information about literature on sexual problems in MS, begin by contacting the National Multiple Sclerosis Society (800-344-4867) or visit their Web site at http://www.nationalmssociety.org/sex. Refer also to the Recommended Readings and Resources at the end of this chapter.

HOW ARE SEXUAL PROBLEMS DIAGNOSED OR ASSESSED?
Diagnosis of sexual dysfunction is usually based on the self-report of the person with MS or the sexual partner. Sexual dysfunction can present as difficulties with libido (sex drive), sensory changes including numbness or pain in the genital area, physical arousal (ability to feel sexual excitement and have it manifested in an erection or clitoral engorgement and vaginal lubrication), and/or orgasm. Determining whether the problem(s) stems from primary, secondary, and/or tertiary sources requires a medical assessment by a health care professional who is knowledgeable about MS and sexual function. The diagnostic process may include a physical and neurologic examination, sexual history interview, and review of all medications taken. Screening for depression and other contributing tertiary factors may be done.

Occasionally, additional medical tests may be used. The sensation of the penis or clitoris can be measured with a biothesiometer, which checks the threshold for sensation. Nocturnal erections can be measured with a device (RigiScan) that is worn at night. A penile Doppler may be done to measure blood flow in and out the penis during an erection. For both women and men, it is very important that a full hormonal profile be done, including testosterone, serum hormone binding globulin, estradiol, DHEA, prolactin, and thyroid hormone.

Proper assessment of the contributing factors to the problem sets the stage for effective clinical management. Using measures that have been properly standardized with an MS population can allow for a clear understanding of the nature of problems or the impact of treatments on sexual function. The Multiple Sclerosis Intimacy and Sexuality Questionnaire-19 is a measure standardized on an MS population that assesses primary, secondary, and tertiary sexuality (Sanders et al., 2000). This 19-item, self-report instrument requires a few minutes to complete, and provides an overall score and primary, secondary, and tertiary subscale scores.

MY WIFE STILL SEEMS TO ENJOY HAVING SEX AS MUCH AS SHE ALWAYS DID, BUT SHE DOESN'T HAVE AN ORGASM ANY MORE. SHE SAYS IT'S NOT MY FAULT, BUT I DON'T UNDERSTAND WHAT THE PROBLEM IS.
MS can interfere directly or indirectly with orgasm. *Primary orgasmic dysfunction* stems from MS **plaques** (also called lesions) in the spinal cord or brain that directly interfere with orgasm. Orgasm depends on intact **nervous system** pathways originating in the brain (the center of emotion and fantasy during masturbation or intercourse) and pathways in the upper, middle, and lower parts of the spinal cord (which control sensations from erogenous zones such as lips, nipples, clitoris, etc.). Sensation and orgasmic response can be diminished or absent if these pathways are disrupted by plaques. Orgasm can also be inhibited by secondary or indirect symptoms, such as sensory **paresthesias**, cognitive problems, and other MS-related changes. In addition, anxiety, depression, and loss of sexual self-confidence or sexual self-esteem are tertiary problems that can interfere with one's ability to enjoy the sexual experience, and thus inhibit orgasm. Finally, some of the medications used to treat depression may significantly decrease a woman or man's ability to reach an orgasm. Selective serotonin reuptake inhibitors (SSRIs) are the most commonly used antidepressants today. Buproprion (Welbutrin), which can also be used to treat depression, actually has a positive effect on orgasmic ability, and is sometimes used in combination with the SSRIs or in some instances as a replacement for them.

Treatment of orgasmic loss in MS depends on developing an understanding of what factors are contributing to the loss. If sensation is disturbed in the clitoris and lower body areas, the orgasmic response can sometimes be enhanced by increasing stimulation to other erogenous zones, such as breasts, ears, and lips. Similarly, increasing cerebral stimulation by watching sexually oriented videos, exploring fantasies, and introducing new kinds of sexual play into sexual activities, can help trigger orgasms.

It can be both intimate and informative for the person with MS to develop a sensory "body map" by exploring the exact locations of pleasant, decreased, or altered sensations on his or her own body. To develop a "body map," the person begins by systematically touching him- or herself from head to toe (or all those places that are within comfortable reach), varying the rate, rhythm, and pressure of touch. It is helpful to allow approximately 15 or 20 minutes for the exercise, paying attention to areas of sensual pleasure, discomfort, or sensory change, and altering the pattern of touch to maximize the pleasure. The next step is for the person to share the "body map" information with his or her partner, instructing the partner on how to touch in similar fashion. This information can set the stage for the rediscovery of sensual and erotic pleasure.

Increasing stimulation through vigorous oral stimulation or via mechanical vibrators can help if decreased sensation in the genitals is a factor. Strap-on clitoral vibrators (available by mail order) do not interfere with intercourse and require little manipulation once in place. Vibrators that attach to the base of the penis provide direct clitoral stimulation when vaginal penetration is complete and can help stimulate erections in some men as well. In general, AC electric plug-in vibrators have more powerful motors and are more stimulating than DC-powered battery-operated ones. However, some electric vibrators are quite powerful and can irritate vaginal or clitoral tissue if applied too vigorously.

MY SKIN FEELS VERY TINGLY ALL THE TIME. IT USED TO FEEL GOOD WHEN MY HUSBAND HUGGED ME OR RUBBED MY BACK, BUT NOW JUST BEING TOUCHED CAN FEEL UNCOMFORTABLE. I EVEN GET PINS AND NEEDLES IN MY VAGINAL AREA. I NEED TO DO SOMETHING ABOUT THIS PROBLEM BEFORE HE GIVES UP TRYING.

Painful or irritating genital or body sensations can sometimes be managed successfully with medications such as Elavil (amitriptyline), Tegretol (carbamazepine), and Dilantin (phenytoin) (see Chapter 4 and Appendix B). Even with pharmacologic management, however, conducting a variant of the sensory body-mapping exercises described earlier with one's partner is helpful for retaining a sensually pleasing relationship. To optimize the benefit of these exercises, it helps to be in a comfortable location where you can be undressed, and agree ahead of time to focus on the mapping exercise and not engage in sexual activities at the same time. Have your partner begin by gently stroking the top of your head, and slowly moving down your body from head to toe. Your partner should vary the rhythm and pressure of touch while you give frequent verbal and nonverbal feedback about the kinds of sensations produced in each area. Mutually exploring alternative touches in the context of good communication can set the stage for sensual pleasure both during and independent of sexual activity. As with the treatment of all sexual symptoms in MS, sexual experimentation and communication are the keys to enhancing sexuality.

I LOVE MY HUSBAND VERY MUCH, BUT I SEEM TO HAVE LOST ALL INTEREST IN HAVING SEX. HE'S WORRIED THAT I DON'T LOVE HIM ANYMORE, BUT I KEEP TELLING HIM THAT I WOULDN'T BE INTERESTED IN SEX WITH ANYBODY RIGHT NOW. WHAT'S HAPPENING TO MY BODY? WILL MY SEXUAL FEELINGS EVER COME BACK?

Decreased libido is much more common in women with MS than in men (Foley et al., 2007). The brain does not appear to have a specific, localized sexual center; rather, sexual interest and pleasure seem to be influenced by several different areas of the brain. Sexual interest normally waxes and wanes throughout the life span, and tends to decrease in general as we age. We know that "libido," or sexual drive and interest, can be directly affected by MS lesions. Changes in libido can also occur as secondary or tertiary symptoms. For example, a person who is experiencing severe fatigue as a result of MS, or is depressed or demoralized, is less likely to feel interested in sexual activity. The reduced libido can then be a cause for misunderstanding by the partner and anxiety for the person with MS. The misunderstandings and anxiety associated with this problem will further reduce the person's sexual feelings and interest. Therefore, assessing and treating secondary and tertiary sexual symptoms are important components to restoring libido.

- Significant progress has been made in the treatment of decreased desire. Because age-related hormonal changes can contribute to loss of sexual desire in everyone—with or without MS—a thorough endocrine evaluation is crucial. For those who have experienced hormonal changes, treatment with some combination of DHEA-S, testosterone, and estradiol can be very successful in enhancing sexual desire.

- To date, there are no published clinical trials of medications that restore libido in MS. However, there are a number of medicines in various stages of development that specifically target low sexual desire in women. Studies of more than 2,000 premenopausal women with low libido have been conducted with flibanserin. Although the preliminary findings are encouraging, the results have not yet been published, and the medicine has not yet been approved in the United States or Europe. It works in the central nervous system (CNS) by increasing dopamine (a chemical neurotransmitter) after several weeks. There are other medicines that can increase the amount of dopamine (e.g., bupropion, an antidepressant that is now available in generic form, can increase dopamine levels while simultaneously helping to treat the depression that is so common in MS—see Chapter 16 for more information about depression and MS). Bremelanotide is a compound that is undergoing preliminary clinical (Phase II) trials. It functions as a melanocortin receptor agonist (the melanocortins are hormones that stimulate various brain structures such as the pituitary gland) in the CNS. It is administered by subcutaneous injection, and may increase libido in both women and men. However, advanced clinical (Phase III) studies have not yet been conducted. Similar to flibanserin, it is not yet approved by the Food and Drug Administration (FDA).

- There are behavioral and counseling approaches that are used to enhance sexuality when sex drive has decreased. The woman or man who is involved in a sexual or intimate relationship with another person can begin by focusing on the "sensual" and the "special person" aspects of the relationship.
  - Sensual aspects include all physically and emotionally pleasing, nonerotic contact, such as back rubs, handholding, and gentle stroking of the face, arms,

and other nongenital body zones. Sex partners often neglect these sensual, nonsexual aspects of their physical relationship during periods of diminished sexual drive, in part because of the difficult emotions that may accompany loss of libido. Making a date for a nonsexual but sensual evening can enable partners to enjoy each other physically and to engage in enjoyable sensual exploration of their bodies without the pressure of working toward sexual intercourse. In essence, experiencing sexual pleasure has to be "relearned" when the CNS has compromised one's libido since sexual desire is most often linked to sexual behavior. Relearning one's sensual nature is a critical first step in the process. The "body-mapping" exercise described earlier in the chapter can help reestablish the relationship between sexual pleasure and sexual behavior, even in the absence of libido.

- The "special person" aspects of a relationship include all those behaviors that one engages in to show the other person that he or she is special and important. Loving gestures from an earlier, "romantic" phase of a relationship, such as unexpected flowers, a surprise note in a lunch bag, or a spontaneous, affectionate hug, tend to be forgotten amidst the pressures of raising children, developing careers, and coping with MS symptoms and disabilities. Restoring or increasing these special acts toward one another can set the stage for increasing intimacy that can, in turn, stimulate new libido or set the stage for sexual pleasure without libido.

- Exploration of one's sensual and erotic body zones is also an important step in restoring libido for the person without a current sexual partner. Combining enjoyable cerebral sexual stimulation (achieved via fantasy, sexually explicit videos, books, etc.) with masturbation or sensual, physical self-exploration is sometimes helpful. Using vibrators or other sexual toys may complement these efforts. Although beginning to work on restoring libido may feel like an unrewarding "chore" when there is little or no intrinsic sex drive, working toward rekindling this vital aspect of "self" can be an important aspect of coping with MS.

- *Kegel exercises* (also called pelvic floor exercises) are sometimes prescribed to enhance female sexual responsiveness, although they have not been tested in a clinical trial to determine whether they are helpful in MS. To perform the Kegel exercise, a woman alternately tightens and releases the pubococcygeus muscle (identifiable as the muscle that starts and stops the urine flow in midstream). Exercising this muscle several times when you urinate is recommended to help you identify which muscles are involved. After you identify the relevant muscle groups, flex them 20 times a day or more when you are not urinating, since incomplete emptying of the bladder may occur in MS. The rationale for these exercises is that sensation from the muscles around the vagina is an important part of erotic sensation, and female orgasm consists of contractions in several of them. Kegel exercises are directed at strengthening their tone and responsiveness. However, if there is either near or total loss of sensation in the genital area, pelvic floor biofeedback is required in order to teach the person how to contract the muscles correctly.

**SOMETIMES I HAVE TROUBLE GETTING AN ERECTION EVEN THOUGH I FEEL
SEXUALLY EXCITED. OTHER TIMES, I GET AN ERECTION BUT THEN LOSE IT
PARTIALLY OR COMPLETELY WHILE MY PARTNER AND I ARE TRYING TO
HAVE INTERCOURSE. WHY IS THIS HAPPENING?**

The first step in understanding MS-related erectile problems and their treatment is
to understand the normal erectile mechanism. Getting an erection is like filling a
balloon. Two things have to happen: one has to fill the balloon with air and then tie
the balloon to prevent the air from coming out. The arteries that lead to the penis are
lined with smooth muscle. When a man is excited, either psychologically or physically, his body releases transmitting substances that cause relaxation of the smooth
muscle. As the smooth muscle relaxes, the arteries become enlarged, allowing an
increased blood flow into the penis. This increased blood flow into the penis is what
causes an erection. As the penis becomes erect, the veins in the penis (that normally
return penile blood to the body) become compressed, causing the blood to remain
in the penis. This "trapping mechanism" allows an erection to be maintained until
orgasm occurs.

Normal erectile function depends on an intact nervous system. A complex series
of nerve impulses must travel between the brain, spinal cord, and penis in order for
an erection to be initiated and maintained. When nerve transmission is impaired
at any point along the way, a man's ability to achieve or maintain an erection can
be affected. The lower area of the spinal cord has nerve pathways traveling to and
from the genitals, which allow for *reflex erections*. If these pathways are intact, reflex
erections (that do not involve the middle or upper parts of the spinal cord or brain)
can usually be triggered by stimulating the penis directly. Therefore, some men with
impaired erectile function can obtain reflex erections by vigorously stimulating the
penis with a vibrator. Reflex erections can also result from "stuffing." To engage in
stuffing, the woman sits astride her partner and gently inserts the flaccid penis into
the (well-lubricated) vagina. It is important that the stuffing be done with some care
because the flaccid penis can fold back on itself and be squeezed or injured by the
pressure of the partner's weight. Internal damage to the penis could go undetected in
the presence of reduced sensation.

ARE THERE ORAL MEDICATIONS I CAN TAKE FOR ERECTION PROBLEMS?

A group of oral medicines known as phosphodiesterase type 5 inhibitors, or PDE-5
inhibitors, are used to help with erectile dysfunction. These include Viagra (sildenafil
citrate), Levitra (vardenafil), and Cialis (tadalafil). These medicines work by blocking
the action of an enzyme called PDE (type 5 phosphodiesterase enzyme). When PDE
is blocked, another chemical compound called cGMP (cyclic guanosine monophos-
phate) remains at higher concentrations in the erectile tissues of the penis. Since
cGMP mediates the erection response, blocking PDE allows for enhanced erections.
In controlled clinical trials, all three of these medicines were associated with significantly improved erectile function and greater frequency of intercourse among men
with impotence related to both physical and psychological causes. It is important to
note, however, that only Viagra, which was the first of these drugs to arrive on the
market, has been tried in a group of men with MS. In a placebo-controlled clinical
trial of Viagra in men with MS, Viagra was shown to have a positive impact on quality

of life—including sexual life, partnership relations, family life, social contacts, and overall satisfaction. The other PDE-5 inhibitors have yet to be studied in MS.

Since all PDE-5 inhibitors work with the same biochemical pathway, the side effects and effectiveness of these drugs are highly similar. However, men may have significantly different responses to the three drugs, and should try all three before deciding which offers the greatest benefit with the fewest side effects.

- Viagra has its maximum effect 1 hour after it is taken. Its half-life (the time it takes a medication to fall to half its original concentration in the blood) is 4 hours, and most of it is out of the bloodstream by 8 hours. It is available in doses of 25-, 50-, and 100-mg tablets, with the lowest effective dose suggested for use. It cannot be taken with a fatty meal, as it does not get absorbed. Ideally, it is taken on an empty stomach or a minimum of 2 to 3 hours after a heavy meal. Most men feel that in terms of efficacy, Viagra is the strongest; however, it often has the most side effects.

- Levitra has its maximum effect 45 minutes after it is taken. It has a similar half-life to Viagra. It does not need to be taken on an empty stomach. Levitra is available in 5-, 10-, and 20-mg doses. For most men, it has fewer side effects than Viagra. This combined with the fact that it can be taken with food, often makes it preferable to Viagra (for the men for which it is strong enough).

- Cialis has its maximum effect 2 hours after it is taken, but has a half-life of 18.5 hours—which is significantly longer than either Viagra or Levitra. Low levels remain in the body up to 36 hours later, potentially offering increased flexibility and spontaneity. For these reasons, Cialis is referred to in France as "le weekend" drug. Keep in mind, however, that whatever side effects it causes will last longer as well. Cialis is also available in 5-, 10-, and 20-mg doses. Cialis is also available in a box of 30 tablets for daily use, which cost about the same as seven or eight of the 20-mg pills. The advantage is that if it works for the man, then there is no "spontaneity" issue; he is always ready. However, one never gets as high a blood level as if one takes 20 mg 2 hours prior to relations.

For all three medications, it is important to remember that their maximum efficacy is when they are in the bloodstream at the highest levels (i.e., between 1 and 2 hours after being taken).

All three medications are relatively expensive (between $10 and $13 per pill), and some insurance companies in the United States will not reimburse for the costs of these medications. However, many plans will do so, if your physician gets "preauthorization." If you provide a prescription from your doctor, and it is not paid for by your plan, call your plan and find out whether they will pay for the drug with preauthorization, and how many they will pay for per month.

PDE-5 inhibitors are the first oral medications that have been scientifically shown to be successful in enhancing erectile function in men with organic (physically based) and/or psychogenic (emotionally based) erectile disturbance. However, PDE-5 inhibitors are not associated directly with improvement in sexual desire (although some men may experience increased desire when concerns about performance are alleviated by the medication). When significant conflict or distress is present in a relationship, counseling is necessary to restore intimacy and improve communication.

WHAT ARE THE SIDE EFFECTS OF PDE-5 INHIBITORS?

These medicines are not to be used by men who are taking nitrate-based medications, such as ISMO, Imdur, Nitro-Dur, Nitro-Paste, Nitrostat, Nitro-Bid, and the like. Men taking these or other nitrate medications in conjunction with PDE-5 inhibitors may experience a sudden and potentially dangerous reduction in blood pressure, even if they only take the nitrate medications occasionally. PDE-5 inhibitors cause a small transient decrease in blood pressure in most men. Coupled with the cardiovascular stress of intercourse, this side effect can cause heart attacks or strokes in men with preexisting vascular disease. Men with recent heart attacks, significant high blood pressure, and/or heart disease should have a cardiology evaluation prior to being started on one of these medications (although, the rule of thumb is that if a man is healthy enough to have intercourse, he can tolerate the PDE-5 inhibitors, unless told otherwise by his physician).

It is important to take PDE-5 inhibitors only when prescribed by a doctor who knows all the treatments and medications you are taking. Side effects of these medicines in the clinical trials were relatively infrequent, with headache, facial flushing, heartburn, nasal congestion, and blue-green visual aura being reported.

Priapism—a prolonged erection—is a very infrequent side effect of these medications. In a normal erection, the penis remains rigid because the trapping mechanism keeps blood from flowing out of the penis until ejaculation occurs. Since oxygen is delivered to body tissues via the circulating blood, the penis does not receive fresh oxygen for the period of time that the penis remains erect. Therefore, a man whose penis remains erect for too long a period of time risks irrevocable damage to the erectile mechanism and to the penis itself. If a man's erection lasts longer than 4 hours, he must seek immediate medical treatment, since an erection lasting longer than 4 hours will permanently damage penile tissue.

In the original Viagra clinical trials, only 15 percent of men reported any side effects.

ARE PDE-5 INHIBITORS EFFECTIVE WITH WOMEN?

Women have erectile tissue in the clitoris that has been found to function in a similar biochemical manner to penile erectile tissue. It is therefore possible that PDE-5 inhibitors may help to sustain or enhance blood flow to the genitals in women, which may be associated with increased vaginal lubrication and/or clitoral engorgement. To date, only one study of Viagra in women with MS has been conducted. It was a well-designed study but enrolled only 19 women, and Viagra enhanced lubrication but otherwise did not provide a clear benefit. Since Viagra does not enhance sexual desire in men, it would not be expected to impact this sexual symptom in women with MS. Pfizer, the drug's manufacturer, has stopped all studies of the drug in women, having concluded that it did not provide significant benefit. However, some doctors are prescribing it for their female patients who want to try it out for themselves.

ARE THERE OTHER ORAL MEDICATIONS OR HERBAL ALTERNATIVES AVAILABLE FOR DEALING WITH SEXUAL PROBLEMS?

Other oral medications are sometimes used for certain types of sexual problems, but their efficacy from a scientific standpoint is generally poor. Testosterone is a sex hormone that is associated with libido in both men and women. Testosterone supplements have been prescribed for men and women with testosterone deficiency to improve impaired libido or arousal. Although decreased testosterone has not been linked specifically to MS, testosterone levels do decrease significantly as men and women age. Oral testosterone is not suggested, nor available in the United States, as it can negatively affect the liver. Bioidentical testosterone, given through the skin or in the fatty tissue as a pellet are the safest and most biologically similar means of supplying increased quantities of testosterone.

Oxytocin is a hormone that acts as a neuromodulator in the CNS. It is sometimes called the "bonding" hormone, since it is produced during birth and breastfeeding, and is released during orgasm in both men and women. It is thought to be responsible for making people feel emotionally close and connected, as a nursing mother does to her child, or as in couples who want to "cuddle" after sex. It is available in a nasal spray or as a sublingual lozenge, and has been prescribed off-label to enhance orgasm. However, it has not been tested in clinical trials to see if it enhances sexual responsiveness. Largely driven by consumer demand, other oral agents are in the development phase at several pharmaceutical companies.

ARE THERE OTHER OPTIONS FOR DEALING WITH ERECTILE PROBLEMS?
Several other options are available to treat erectile problems caused by MS.

- One noninvasive device that readily aids in erections is the vacuum tube and constriction band, which can be purchased from a pharmacy with a prescription from a *urologist* or other physician. With this method, a plastic tube is fitted over the flaccid penis, and air is pumped out of the tube to create a vacuum around the penis. The pumping process may be done mechanically (via hand pump or squeeze bulb) or with a battery-operated, push-button mechanism. The vacuum draws blood into the erectile tissues and produces an erection. Once engorgement of the penis is achieved, a latex band is slipped from the base of the cylinder onto the base of the penis. Air is returned to the cylinder and the tube is removed. The band maintains engorgement of the penis by restricting venous return of blood to the body, thus allowing for intercourse or other sexual activity. However, the use of the band must be limited to 30 minutes or less to avoid any medical complications. Moderate hand sensation and dexterity are required for placing and removing the band in some models. Other models have assistor sleeves that permit hands-free placement of the constriction band. The constriction band alone can be used with satisfactory results by persons who can attain erections readily, but have difficulty maintaining them.
- To date, the best-studied treatment for erectile dysfunction in MS involves the injection into the penis of medications that activate the engorgement and trapping mechanisms. The medication stimulates relaxation of the smooth muscle of the arteries so that the penis can become erect, and similarly activates the necessary trapping mechanism that keeps the penis rigid until ejaculation. Injection therapy should be prescribed by an expert who can teach good (virtually painless) technique that maximizes effectiveness while minimizing discomfort. The needle used is a very fine gauge diabetic needle, which is put into a device (autoinjector), which does the injection for the patient. Prior to the PDE-5 inhibitors (Viagra,

Levitra, Cialis) this was the primary method used for erection issues and particularly with men with MS. It usually gives a much stronger erection than can be achieved with an oral medication, and works in the majority of men with MS.

● Men who have not responded to either oral or injectable therapies, and have been unsuccessful with sexual counseling, may find the surgically implanted penile prosthesis to be a better alternative. Although this technique is the most invasive alternative, men as a rule are very satisfied with a prosthesis, which is completely internal, inflates and deflates as needed, and is placed through a relatively small incision in the scrotum.

Following a careful evaluation of your history and presenting symptoms (medical, psychological, neurologic, and sexual), your physician will work with you to determine which type of treatment would be most beneficial for you.

HOW WOULD I USE THE PENILE INJECTIONS TO HELP ME WITH MY ERECTILE PROBLEMS?

Once you and your doctor have decided that penile injections are a reasonable treatment option, the doctor will teach you the injection techniques so that you can self-inject at those times when you wish to have an erection. The injection is done with a very fine needle into an area at the base of the penis that, although somewhat sensitive to pleasure, is relatively insensitive to pain. The doctor may recommend an "autoinjector" that works with a simple push-button mechanism. Most men report very little, if any, pain from this injection. The sensation is best described as similar to being flicked by a rubber band. Some men with neurologic impotence of the type caused by MS report an achiness caused by one of the medications (alprostadil) that is sometimes used in these injections. If this occurs, different medications can be substituted.

When you wish to achieve an erection, you can give yourself an injection (or be given one by your partner if you are unable to do it yourself). After the injection has been given, pressure needs to be applied to the penis for 5 minutes in order to stop any bleeding from within the penis. As you initiate foreplay or self-stimulation, you will develop an erection that will last for approximately an hour. Depending on your state of sexual arousal and the amount of medication you have been given, the erection may subside when you ejaculate or continue for some period of time beyond ejaculation. The penile injections can be used no more than once every 24-hour period.

WHAT MEDICATIONS ARE USED MOST COMMONLY IN PENILE INJECTIONS?

Injections for the management of erectile dysfunction have been available for more than 15 years. Three different medications are currently prescribed (see Appendix B). Caverject and Edex are two brand names for alprostadil (also called prostaglandin E1), which is the newest injectable drug and the one most commonly used by men with MS. Alprostadil is the natural substance released by the smooth muscle cells when a man is sexually excited. This medication has been found to be very effective with few side effects; however, it tends to cause significant aching in men with neurogenically based erectile dysfunction, including men with MS. Alprostodil has been approved by the FDA for the management of erectile problems and is therefore paid for by most prescription plans. Caverject is available in 10- and 20 mcg doses; Edex is available in 10-, 20-, and 40 mcg doses.

Alprostadil is also available in pellet form for insertion into the urethra of the penis (Muse), if penile injections are not desirable. In this form, the medication is inserted into the urethral opening with an applicator. Side effects may include urethral discomfort and burning. The medication may also cause a systemic drop in blood pressure. Muse comes in doses of 250, 500, and 1,000 mcg. In general, it is not as effective as the penile injections, as it is not given directly into the erection chambers themselves.

The original drug used for injections is a smooth muscle relaxant called papaverine. Its use is almost never associated with any pain, making it a good alternative for anyone who has a problem with alprostadil. Papaverine has a slightly greater tendency to cause scarring at the injection site and is associated with a greater risk of priapism (prolonged erection) because it remains active in the body for a somewhat longer period of time. Regitine (phentolamine) is often used in combination with papaverine, or in conjunction with both alprostadil and papaverine, to heighten their effectiveness. Regitine is not active by itself and is therefore never used independently. Neither papaverine nor phentolamine has been approved by the FDA for the treatment of erectile dysfunction. And both must be prescribed at the correct dosage as they are not broken down chemically in the penis itself, and thus have a greater chance of causing a prolonged erection if not used appropriately.

IF THE ONLY FDA-APPROVED, SELF-INJECTION DRUG FOR THE MANAGEMENT OF ERECTILE DYSFUNCTION IS ALPROSTADIL, DOES THIS MEAN THAT THE OTHER TWO DRUGS ARE NOT SAFE?

Medications are approved by the FDA for specific functions. They may be used for other purposes at the discretion of the physician. The fact that a drug is not FDA-approved does not mean that it is not safe; it means simply that a drug company has not gone through the costly and time-consuming licensing and testing of the drug for a specific purpose. The three drugs that are currently being used in penile injections are all safe and effective when used properly.

WHAT SIDE EFFECTS ARE ASSOCIATED WITH THE USE OF THESE MEDICATIONS?

One possible side effect of these medications is *priapism* (prolonged erection). Priapism almost never occurs in individuals who adhere to the prescribed dose of medication and who are properly trained in the injection procedures. As rare as it is, priapism does occur with greater frequency with the injectable medications than with PDE-5 inhibitors.

A second potential side effect of penile injections is scarring at the injection site, experienced by approximately 7 to 10 percent of individuals. This problem seldom occurs in men who have been properly trained in the techniques of injection and compression of the injection site. When scarring does occur, it takes the form of a small nodule in the lining of the erection chambers of the penis. These nodules typically disappear once the injections are stopped. It is important to be medically monitored and treated so that the scarring does not progress, as it may lead to penile curvature and cause difficulty maintaining an erection. Any man who is self-injecting should be examined by a physician every 3 months for possible scarring.

WILL I BECOME DEPENDENT ON ORAL OR INJECTABLE MEDICATIONS THAT ARE USED FOR ERECTILE DYSFUNCTION?

Oral PDE-5 inhibitors, alprostadil, papaverine, and phentolamine are used only to potentiate the process of having an erection. No chemical dependency is associated with their use. Depending on the status of your MS symptoms, you may find that you need to use the oral or injectable medications at some times but not others. They can be a helpful adjunct when you are unable to achieve or maintain an adequate erection.

WHAT IS A PENILE PROSTHESIS, AND HOW DOES IT WORK?

A penile prosthesis is a mechanical device designed to give a man with erectile dysfunction the option of having an erection. There are two types of penile prostheses, semirigid and inflatable.

- With the semirigid type, a flexible rod is surgically implanted in each of the erection chambers (corpus cavernosa) of the penis. These rods can be bent upward when an erection is desired and bent downward at other times. Following insertion of the rods, the penis remains somewhat enlarged, with a permanent partial erection.
- With the inflatable type of prosthesis, a saline fluid is pumped from a reservoir behind the abdominal wall into expandable cylinders inserted into the erection chambers of the penis. The fluid causes the balloons to inflate, resulting in an erection. The man pumps the fluid into the chambers when he desires an erection and transfers the fluid back into the reservoir when he no longer wants the erection. The reservoir is surgically implanted behind the abdominal wall and the pump is implanted in the scrotum. Silicon tubing is used to connect the reservoir, pump, and balloons. Since the entire device is inserted through a single, relatively invisible incision in the scrotum, this type of prosthesis is barely noticeable. However, operating the pump through the scrotum wall can be difficult for individuals with reduced hand sensation or strength.

A spouse or long-term sexual partner should be included in the decision to get an implant, as well as in the selection of the type of prosthesis to be used. Extensive presurgery consultation with a urologist or physician familiar with MS will help to ensure that the man and his partner have realistic expectations after the surgery. Approximately 80 percent of men using these types of prostheses find them quite satisfactory. Many experience normal erectile sensations and normal orgasm. In addition, they are able to have an erection for as long as they choose to do so.

WHAT COMPLICATIONS ARE ASSOCIATED WITH PENILE PROSTHESES?

As with any surgery, there are possible complications related to anesthesia and bleeding. Infection occurs in approximately 3 percent of men receiving prostheses and can be quite serious. The entire device must be removed if an infection occurs.

Replacement of the implant following treatment of the infection is usually feasible, but often more complicated.

HOW WOULD I KNOW IF I AM A SUITABLE CANDIDATE FOR A PENILE PROSTHESIS?
A penile prosthesis is only recommended when all other efforts to manage erectile dysfunction are not feasible or are unsuccessful. In other words, you would be considered a candidate for a prosthesis only if noninvasive measures were unsuccessful, oral and self-injection therapies were ineffective, or an effective dose level or combination of medications could not be found.

ARE THERE ANY NONMEDICAL SEXUAL AIDS AVAILABLE TO HELP WITH ERECTILE PROBLEMS?
A number of sexual aids are available by mail order that do not require a physician's prescription (see mail order catalogs listed). Some people prefer strap-on latex penises, some of which are hollow and can hold a flaccid or semi-erect penis. Strap-on, battery-operated vibrators in the shape of a penis are also available.

Choosing a sexual device to aid with erections is best done with the advice of a urologist or sex therapist familiar with MS. If you have a long-term sex partner, it is important to include this person in the discussion. This will decrease anxiety and uncertainty when the devices are used and enhance intimacy by allowing both sex partners to explore them together. Counseling with a mental health professional who is knowledgeable about MS can facilitate the process if you have problems communicating or feel inhibited about talking through these issues.

RECENTLY IT HAS STARTED TO BE PAINFUL FOR ME WHEN WE HAVE SEX. MY HUSBAND SAYS I FEEL TIGHT AND DRY. WHAT IS THE BEST WAY TO DEAL WITH THIS PROBLEM?
Similar to the erectile response in men, vaginal lubrication is controlled by two different pathways in the brain and spinal cord. *Psychogenic* lubrication typically originates in the brain and occurs through fantasy, reading erotic novels, or exposure to sexually related stimuli. *Reflexogenic* lubrication occurs through direct stimulation of the genitals or anus via a reflex response in the sacral (lower) part of the spinal cord. MS can affect nerve pathways that control either or both types of lubrication. In addition, some medications used to treat bladder symptoms in MS can reduce vaginal lubrication. Psychogenic lubrication can sometimes be enhanced by establishing a relaxing, romantic, and/or sexually stimulating setting for sexual activity, incorporating relaxing massage into foreplay activities, and prolonging foreplay before intercourse. Reflexogenic lubrication can sometimes be increased by manually or orally stimulating the genitals prior to attempting intercourse.

Vaginal dryness can also be dealt with by applying generous amounts of water-soluble lubricants such as Astroglide, Replens, or K-Y Jelly, which are available over-the-counter in most pharmacies and drugstores. If condoms are used for birth control or disease prevention purposes, it is recommended that you use those that are lubricated and apply additional lubricant to the vaginal area as needed. Water-soluble lubricants that are marketed for sexual activity purposes can also be purchased by mail order via the catalog services listed at the end of the chapter.

Health care professionals do not recommend the use of petroleum (oil)-based jellies (e.g., Vaseline) for vaginal lubrication since they are not water-soluble. Petroleum-based jellies can leave residues in and around the vaginal and urethral openings that could set the stage for bacterial infections to develop.

Women may have thinning of the vaginal lining and decreased lubrication from decreased estrogen levels. These can be supplemented either systemically or locally (in the vagina).

**SPASTICITY IN MY LEGS SOMETIMES MAKES SEXUAL ACTIVITY
VERY UNCOMFORTABLE. IS THERE ANYTHING I CAN DO ABOUT THIS PROBLEM?**
Spasticity can make straightening the legs or changing leg positions for sexual activity uncomfortable or even painful. Active symptomatic management of spasticity will minimize its impact on sexuality (see Chapter 4 and Appendix B). Range-of-motion and other physical therapy exercises are commonly employed, as well as antispasticity medications such as Lioresal (baclofen) or Zanaflex (tizanidine). Administering antispasticity medication prior to anticipated sexual activity can be helpful. Be sure, however, to discuss any medication changes with your physician.

Exploring alternative sexual positions for intercourse is sometimes helpful when spasticity is a problem. Women who have spasticity of the adductor muscles may find it difficult or painful to separate their legs. The impact of adductor spasms can be minimized by lying on your side, with your partner approaching you from behind. Placing a towel between your legs while lying in this position might help you feel more comfortable. You may find that lying on your back, perpendicular to the bed, with both legs (from the knees down) hanging off the edge of the bed, makes intercourse easier and more comfortable.

A man who has difficulty straightening his legs may find that sitting upright in an armless chair allows his partner to mount his erect penis in either a face-to-face or face-to-back position. However, everyone's body is different, and the key to finding alternative sexual positions is open exploration and communication between partners.

**MY WIFE'S MS MAKES HER SO TIRED THAT BY THE TIME WE GET THE
CHILDREN TO BED SHE'S TOO WORN OUT TO WANT TO HAVE SEX.
IS THERE ANYTHING WE CAN DO ABOUT ALL THIS FATIGUE?**
Energy conservation and fatigue management are important interventions to promote sexual activity and enjoyment. Fatigue is managed from physical therapy, occupational therapy, and pharmacologic perspectives. It can be helpful to have consultations at an MS center that offers comprehensive care or to obtain referrals to MS experts in these areas. If medications such as Symmetrel (amantadine) or Provigil (modafinil) are prescribed for fatigue management, administration prior to anticipated sexual activity may be helpful (see Chapter 4 and Appendix B).

Even with effective symptom management, you and your wife may still want to explore other strategies to enhance your sex life and reduce the impact of her fatigue. Couples frequently engage in sexual activity in the evening, when energy is at its lowest ebb. Talk over the possibility of having sex in the morning, when fatigue is at a minimum. Although making a "date" to awaken earlier for sexual activity may initially seem undesirable, this kind of adaptation may be necessary for retaining an enjoyable sex life. Some couples are fortunate to have the flexibility in their schedules to make a periodic "lunch date" for intimate play.

Some sexual positions require less energy than others, and alternative positions that minimize weight bearing or tiring movements can minimize fatigue. As you try to initiate some of these changes in your sexual life, be aware that they require open communication and the willingness to engage in some trial-and-error exploration. Counseling may be helpful if you and your wife find it difficult to communicate about alternatives.

I'VE BEEN HAVING A LOT OF DIFFICULTY CONTROLLING MY URINE LATELY. I'M SO WORRIED ABOUT HAVING AN ACCIDENT DURING SEX THAT I KEEP MAKING EXCUSES TO MY PARTNER. I WANT TO HAVE SEX BUT I'M AFRAID THAT IF I WET MYSELF—OR HIM—HE'LL NEVER WANT TO HAVE SEX AGAIN!

Fortunately, successful bladder management is attainable for most people (see Chapter 8). A critical first step in this process is careful bladder assessment, guided by your MS health care team or a urologist who is familiar with MS.

Try discussing your concerns about incontinence openly with your partner. Most are willing to "take the chance" once they are informed of the issues and assured that everything is being done to manage the bladder problems. Discussing your fears with him, and strategizing together with your health care team to minimize the risk of incontinence during sexual activity, will also give you more confidence. You may need to tailor your symptomatic management strategies a bit to allow for anticipated sexual activity.

- If, for example, you are taking ***anticholinergic*** medications, such as Ditropan (oxybutynin), Detrol (tolterodine), or Enablex (darifenacin) for bladder storage dysfunction, you might try taking the medication 30 minutes before anticipated sexual activity to minimize bothersome bladder contractions. These medicines increase vaginal dryness, so you may need to compensate by using water-soluble lubricants.
- You can also minimize incontinence by restricting fluid intake for an hour or two before sex and doing *intermittent catheterization* just before sexual activity.
- Wearing a condom during sex is advised for men who are concerned with small amounts of urinary leakage.
- Many couples will also put down a towel on the bed prior to engaging in relations, so that they are not as concerned about urinary leakage.
- A woman who has an ***indwelling catheter*** can manage by taping the catheter securely to the stomach, emptying the collecting bag before sexual activity, and putting additional tape around the top ring to minimize the chances of leaks. You can avoid putting pressure on the catheter or the collecting bag by lying in a "nestled spoons" position, with the woman in front and using rear-entry intercourse. An alternative position for a woman with a catheter is to lie on her back with her legs over the man's shoulders. He can support himself on his arms in order to reduce the weight on her. A variation of this position is for the man to sit on his knees, between the woman's legs, and position her legs over his shoulders. The latter position allows for less vigorous, gentler "rocking" movements and allows a woman with spasticity to keep her legs closer together.

These are examples of ways in which sexual activity can be modified in order to compensate for MS-related changes. Each couple will need to find the solutions that best meet their needs. Some couples will find these solutions through patient trial-and-error exploration. Others will find it useful to consult with an experienced sex therapist.

Trying new sexual positions that will compensate for MS symptoms and disabilities can be anxiety-provoking for many people. Taking the time to acquire information, explore, discuss, and obtain frequent feedback during sexual experimentation will help alleviate fears. Able-bodied partners may be fearful of causing pain, or they may feel insecure about knowing what to do and how to do it. Setting aside regular time to talk about sex gives it more importance in the relationship and sets the stage for the couple to air their fears and concerns and improve their communication.

MY WIFE HAS DIFFICULTY MOVING VERY MUCH DURING SEX SINCE SHE LOST SO MUCH STRENGTH IN HER ARMS AND LEGS. WILL I HURT HER IF WE TRY SOME DIFFERENT POSITIONS?

Weakness is a common MS symptom that frequently requires finding new positions for satisfactory sexual activities. Reclining positions do not place as much strain on muscles and are therefore less tiring. Pillows can be used to improve positioning and reduce muscle strain. Inflatable pillows, specifically designed to provide back support during sexual activity, can help minimize back strain. These wedge-shaped pillows have individually inflatable sections that allow for firmness adjustment and do not restrict movement. Oral sex requires less movement than intercourse, and using handheld or strap-on vibrators can help compensate for hand weakness while providing sexual stimulation.

Anxiety about hurting your sex partner is fairly common when significant changes in physical functioning have occurred. Open discussions with each other before attempting new positions or sexual activities will allow your wife to educate you about her MS symptoms and enable you both to air your concerns while planning for sexual encounters. Conducting a "positioning" exercise before sex will help you both determine if the new positions are comfortable without introducing anxiety during sexual activity. If your wife has a physical therapist who knows her body strengths and weaknesses well, he or she may be able to advise you both about positions for sexual activity that take into account your wife's vulnerabilities.

I FIND THAT I LOSE MY TRAIN OF THOUGHT WHEN I HAVE SEX. MY INTEREST AND DESIRE START OUT FINE, BUT THEN MY MIND DRIFTS AND I LOSE INTEREST. THIS IS VERY FRUSTRATING FOR ME, AND MY PARTNER FREQUENTLY FEELS LIKE HE'S NOT DOING SOMETHING RIGHT. IS THERE ANYTHING I CAN DO ABOUT THIS PROBLEM?

Changes in attention and concentration are common in MS and may derail the ability to sustain sexual interest and excitement. Partners sometimes misinterpret this symptom to mean that they are deficient or uninteresting as lovers. The person with MS sometimes feels guilty or inadequate. These negative feelings can increase the distractibility or lead the person to avoid sex altogether. Accepting distractibility as a valid MS symptom and discussing ways to help compensate for it are crucial steps to finding a solution.

Attention/concentration problems tend to be worse when a person is fatigued, so it is vitally important to evaluate fatigue level and compensate accordingly. In general, minimizing nonromantic or nonsexual stimuli and maximizing sensual and sexual stimulation during sex is the strategy for compensating. You can help minimize this problem by creating a romantic mood/environment, using multisensory stimulation (e.g., talking in sexy ways, engaging in sensual and erotic touching, and playing music that has strong romantic associations). Developing an atmosphere of acceptance and permission for the person to "reenter the sexual experience" after losing focus can help. Sometimes, switching briefly from erotic to sensual (but nongenital) touching can facilitate interest when attention wanders. Refer to Chapter 14 for suggestions on the general management of attention/concentration problems.

MY HUSBAND HAS CHANGED A LOT SINCE HE GOT MS. HE GRABS ME A LOT, EVEN IN FRONT OF OTHER PEOPLE, AND SEEMS TO WANT TO HAVE SEX ALL THE TIME. WE ALWAYS HAD A COMFORTABLE SEX LIFE, BUT NOW IT ALMOST FEELS LIKE HE'S A STRANGER IN SOME WAYS, AND I'M NOT COMFORTABLE ANYMORE.
"Behavioral disinhibition," or acting on one's sexual impulses in an uncontrolled way, is occasionally (but rarely) reported in MS. It may be associated with MS-related **cognitive impairments** (see Chapter 14) or a separate and distinct type of depression that has both manic (hyperactive) and depressive features called *bipolar disorder* (formerly called manic depression). In general, referral to a psychiatrist who is familiar with MS is important so that an accurate understanding of the symptom can be reached. Medications can sometimes manage this symptom if the impulsive hypersexuality is part of the manic phase of bipolar disorder. Regardless of the origin of the disinhibition, counseling is important to help the person with MS and the sexual partner cope with the impulsivity. If the symptom is associated with cognitive changes or other changes in judgment, the appropriateness of cognitive rehabilitation could be explored.

I'VE BECOME SO DISCOURAGED LATELY. NOTHING SEEMS WORTH THE EFFORT. MY WIFE WANTS TO HAVE SEX WITH ME, AND IT'S THE FURTHEST THING FROM MY MIND. I'M TOO ANGRY AND SAD ALL THE TIME TO EVEN THINK ABOUT SEX. I KNOW IT'S NOT FAIR TO HER BUT I CAN'T SEEM TO SHAKE THIS MOOD.
MS is frequently associated with emotional challenges that include grief, demoralization, changes in self-esteem and body image, and clinical depression (see Chapter 16). These emotional states can temporarily dampen interest in sex or the ability to give and receive sexual pleasure. Addressing these emotional challenges in an effort to enhance sexuality has several aspects: education, assessment, professional treatment, and coping interventions.

Education about the emotional challenges in MS is available through the National Multiple Sclerosis Society. In addition, groups in which people with MS and their partners can share information about MS are widely available. These resources can help you and your wife to understand the feelings you are experiencing and recognize the ways these feelings can affect your sexual relationship.

Assessment of a person's emotional responses to the stresses imposed by MS can be done by a mental health professional who is familiar with the disease. Correctly identifying the type of emotional distress a person is experiencing is a prerequisite to providing the appropriate treatment. In other words, it is necessary to find out what is causing your distress in order for you to be able to "shake this mood." A normal grief reaction to the stresses and losses imposed by the illness might be dealt with very effectively in a support group or short-term, individual psychotherapy. A more acute clinical depression, however, might best be treated with some combination of psychotherapy and antidepressant medication.

Sometimes antidepressant medications can cause sexual problems, such as delayed orgasm or loss of libido. Talking with your doctor about possible sexual side effects, if they occur, can set the stage for managing them effectively. The SSRIs, such as fluoxetine, citalopram, escitalopram, sertraline, and so on, all have documented sexual side effects, including diminished libido, erectile dysfunction, and diminished orgasm. They stimulate certain brain receptors (postsynaptic 5-HT1 and 5-HT2), which decreases the release of dopamine and norepinephrine from brain structures. It is thought that the decrease in dopamine pathway stimulation is largely responsible for the sexual side effects, since some of these pathways are critical to libido, sexual arousal, and orgasm. There are a number of antidepressants on the market that do not typically have sexual side effects, and some may help to enhance sexual response by indirectly stimulating dopamine pathways. These antidepressants include buproprion (norepinephrine and dopamine reuptake inhibitor), mirtazapine (affects noradrenergic and specific serotonergic receptors), and trazodone (serotonin antagonist and reuptake inhibitor). Other medicines on the market that tend to directly or indirectly affect dopamine pathways and have been prescribed off-label to help with sexual dysfunction include buspirone (an antianxiety agent), methylphenidate (a stimulant commonly used to treat attention deficit hyperactivity disorder in children and adults), and pramipexole (a dopamine agonist used to treat Parkinson's disease and restless leg syndrome). However, all of these medicines have side effects that may make them unsuitable for specific individuals, and the determination of which medicine, if any, to try has to take into consideration your health, medical history, and current symptoms/problems. Talking with your doctor is essential. Sometimes coadministering one of these medications with an SSRI, or altering the timing of taking antidepressants can alleviate sexual side effects.

As you begin to experience some relief from these distressing feelings, you and your wife may find it easier to talk about the ways in which MS and your feelings about the disease have affected your sexual relationship. One of the most important coping strategies for dealing with emotional and body image changes is ongoing, intimate communication with your long-term sexual partner. It may be particularly difficult to explore new options, discuss disappointments, and express what both of you feel and want in the face of coping with all the other changes associated with MS. MS peer support groups, couples groups, and/or individual or couples counseling can facilitate this process.

MY HUSBAND HAS BECOME QUITE DISABLED, AND I AM HIS PRIMARY CAREGIVER. IT'S HARD FOR ME TO THINK OF HIM AS MY HUSBAND AND MY LOVER WHEN I ALSO DRESS, BATHE, AND CLEAN HIM. I KNOW HE WANTS ME TO HAVE SEX WITH HIM BUT I JUST DON'T FEEL LIKE IT ANYMORE.

Changes in former sexual patterns and roles represent significant challenges to intimacy and sexuality. Perceptions of being ill or disabled may be incompatible with an image of being sexually active and vigorous. Role changes that involve the "well" partner assuming many caregiving functions may challenge that person's ability to view his or her partner as a source of sexual excitement. When caregiving becomes a prominent part of a relationship, it is difficult to relax and have sexual fun. If possible, nursing activities should be done by someone other than the sexual partner so that the person with MS does not assume the role of "patient" in the intimate relationship. To the extent possible, the bedroom should be preserved as a private place for closeness and intimacy; medical equipment and other illness-related paraphernalia should be kept to one side or in another room. Ideally, time for intimate talk, cuddling, or sexual activity should be set aside, separate from the times for caregiving.

Obviously, these suggestions are not always viable. Finding "substitute" caregivers to provide nursing care is not always possible. Families do not always have the luxury of keeping medical equipment in a separate space. In addition, some couples are unwilling to give up the caregiving and care-receiving roles since much of the closeness that remains in the relationship may be in the context of these caregiving activities.

For someone who is attempting to juggle the dual roles of nurse/caregiver and sexual partner, it is very important to be able to discuss this challenge to intimacy. You may be hesitant to discuss your feelings with your husband because you do not want to upset him. In turn, he may find it difficult to express his frustration and resentment over the change in the sexual relationship because he does not want to risk hurting or angering you—his primary caregiver. Yet this reluctance to share these difficult and painful feelings represents a further loss of intimacy. You and your husband may find it helpful to talk over these issues with a family therapist experienced in chronic illness and sexuality.

SINCE MY WIFE WAS DIAGNOSED WITH MS, IT FEELS AS THOUGH WE ARE DRIFTING APART. INITIALLY, WE WORKED TOGETHER TO COPE WITH THE UNCERTAINTIES OF THE DIAGNOSIS AND THE AFTERMATH OF HER FIRST FEW EXACERBATIONS. YET WE SEEM TO BE FEELING LESS AND LESS CLOSE OVER TIME, EVEN THOUGH SHE IS NOT THAT PHYSICALLY DISABLED. IT'S HARDER FOR US TO BE SEXUAL WITH EACH OTHER AND TO FEEL CLOSE.

There is a heavy emphasis in present-day Western culture on youth, beauty, health, and physical vigor. Men and women in our culture often feel burdened by the pressure to be eternally young and vigorously sexual. The experience of MS, with its associated changes in body functions, can trigger a dramatic sense of sexual or sensual inadequacy in the face of these cultural pressures. It is difficult to feel sexual with another person when one's sexual feelings and performance are being threatened. Men and women with MS may have difficulty enjoying and expressing their sensual/sexual nature because of the widening gap between culturally based ideals and their own illness experience.

Pressures also exist for the sexual partner of someone with MS. The partner may begin to think of the person with MS as too fragile to engage in sexual activity or as a "patient" who is too ill to be sexually expressive. The physical, cognitive, and emotional changes sometimes associated with MS can also strain the intimacy between two people; a partner can begin to feel as though he or she is trying to relate to a person who is somehow different or unfamiliar. Similarly, the role changes that are sometimes required in the face of MS, such as one partner becoming the other's caregiver, can drastically alter the mutual feelings and expectations within a relationship.

All these changes can lead to an increasing sense of personal isolation within a relationship. Each partner may feel less and less able to understand the other's experience, feelings, and needs. In turn, a diminishing capacity to understand and work through these differences can create greater isolation and misunderstanding. Mutual resentment can begin to fester and grow.

Throughout this chapter, we have emphasized effective communication between partners (and between partners and health care providers) as a necessary step toward restoring sexual enjoyment and intimacy. However, there are many barriers to effective communication. Images of sexuality and sensuality are rampant in Western society, yet they are not depicted in a way that provides an open and acceptable means of discussion and problem solving. Most sexual language is either too "medicalized" or technical, or considered "dirty" or unacceptable to allow for easy conversation between lovers. Part of the solution to these barriers involves developing a more comfortable vocabulary about sexuality and intimacy. Education about MS symptoms and the anatomy and physiology of sexuality can help to provide a basis for mutual understanding and problem solving. The organizations listed at the end of this chapter can add to the information provided here. There also are many self-help books available at most bookstores that are designed to enhance communication, sexuality, and intimacy. Reading these materials together can help you become comfortable with the vocabulary you need to be able to discuss personal and intimate subjects. Talk to each other about what you are reading and how it might be applied to your relationship.

Another approach involves setting aside time each week to devote exclusively to restoring intimacy and talking about sexuality. This can set the stage for a couple to begin talking more easily about their intimate needs, wants, and differences. A helpful but more challenging adjunct to this process is to make regular "dates" when you are free from caregiving, child rearing, or household tasks. This kind of opportunity to focus exclusively on one another recalls the early romantic phase of most long-term intimate relationships, which has all too often been sacrificed to the pressures of careers, parenting, and coping with MS-related tasks. Partners need to rediscover each other as their roles and expectations are updated or reconciled with the changing MS situation. Many couples, however, become anxious or frustrated with their efforts to reconnect with one another. If you and your wife find the process to be too difficult on your own, you may find that couple's counseling can provide a safe atmosphere in which to begin exploring these aspects of your relationship.

I AM GAY AND HAVE MS, AND FIND IT DIFFICULT TO TALK TO MY DOCTOR ABOUT MY SEXUAL CONCERNS. WHAT RESOURCES ARE AVAILABLE FOR GAY AND LESBIAN PEOPLE WITH MS?

The experience of having MS frequently causes one to become "marginalized" in society. For example, social circles may become narrower, and/or job opportunities may become more constricted. MS societies and other MS organizations around the world combat this disabling tendency toward isolation by providing a variety of outreach services, education, training, and research funding. This marginalization is compounded greatly if one is gay or lesbian and has MS. Many people with MS who are not gay or lesbian have found that it is very difficult to discuss intimacy and/or sexuality issues with their health care team because of fears that they will be misunderstood, rejected, or judged negatively. If one is gay or lesbian with MS, the fear of receiving rejection or disapproval in the context of reaching out for help is even greater.

An important ingredient in combating the social isolation and lack of professional support entails networking and reaching out to other gay and lesbian people with MS to receive support and validation. Although the very nature of marginalization makes this difficult to accomplish, the Internet has been quite helpful for some in this regard. The Multiple Sclerosis Society of Great Britain and Northern Ireland, based in London, England (see Recommended Resources at end of chapter) can provide information for people with MS regarding gay or lesbian issues and Internet information.

GETTING THROUGH EACH DAY HAS GOTTEN VERY HARD FOR ME. NOTHING IS EASY ANYMORE, AND NOTHING CAN EVER BE SPONTANEOUS. WE USED TO HAVE SEX WHENEVER WE WANTED TO—JUST BECAUSE WE FELT LIKE IT. NOW WE HAVE TO PLAN IT ALL SO I'LL BE COMFORTABLE AND NOT TOO TIRED.

One of our common Western cultural expectations is that sex should be spontaneous and passionate, with the lovers becoming "swept away" in a torrent of romantic and intimate urges. Couples may feel disappointed if this or other internalized visions of what sex "should be" are not met—so disappointed, in fact, that they may fail to explore other sexual possibilities or even stop having sex altogether.

In addition, the changes imposed by MS frequently make it necessary for there to be some preparation for sexual encounters, possibly including changing the timing of certain medications, altering the time of day for sexual activity, and learning new sexual activities that compensate for disabilities. In the face of these adjustments, some couples may decide that sex—that day, that week, or even that month—is just not worth all the trouble. When a major symptom flare-up or any other life situation occurs that interferes with sexual expression, it is important to communicate with your partner about the changes and feelings you are experiencing. This will allow you to retain a sense of closeness and intimacy even in the absence of sexual activity. You can use this period of time to focus on other pleasurable aspects of the relationship, such as the sensual or "special person" aspects discussed earlier.

Failing to communicate, either verbally or nonverbally, about those times when sex "isn't worth all the effort" will put you at risk for withdrawing from each other even further. Joining together in the decision "not to have sex right now" will also enable you to ask each other "what do we want right now?" and "how can we go about achieving it for ourselves?"

REFERENCES

Christopherson JM, Moore K, Foley FW, Warren KG. A comparison of written materials vs. materials and counseling for women with sexual dysfunction and multiple sclerosis. *Journal of Clinical Nursing.* 2006;15:742–750.

Foley FW, LaRocca NG, Sorgen A, Zemon V. Rehabilitation of intimacy and sexual dysfunction in couples with multiple sclerosis. *Multiple Sclerosis: Clinical and Laboratory Research.* 2001;7(6):417–421.

Foley, FW, Zemon, V, Campagnolo, D, Devitt, M, Tyry, T, Marrie, R, Cutter, G, Sipski, ML, Vollmer, T. (2007, June). The epidemiology of sexual dysfunction in the United States. Platform presentation at the 21st Annual Meeting of the Consortium of Multiple Sclerosis Centers, Washington, D.C.

Sanders AS, Foley FW, LaRocca NG, Zemon V. The Multiple Sclerosis Intimacy And Sexuality Questionnaire-19 [MSISQ-191]. *Sexuality and Disability.* 2000;18(1): 3–26.

RECOMMENDED READING

Foley FW. Sexuality and intimacy in multiple sclerosis. In: Kalb R, ed., *Multiple Sclerosis: A Guide for Families.* 3rd ed. New York: Demos Medical Publishing, 2006.

Foley FW, Sanders A. Sexuality and multiple sclerosis. In: Halper J, Holland N, eds, *The Multiple Sclerosis Self-Care Guide.* 2nd ed. New York: Demos Medical Publishing. In Press.

Foley FW, Symonds S. *The Impact of MS on Sexuality and Loving.* London, England: Burnett Publications, 1999. (Booklet available from the Multiple Sclerosis Society of Great Britain and Northern Ireland, 25 Effie Road, Fulham, London, SW61EE, England.)

Joannides P. *Guide to Getting it On!* Oregon: Goofy Foot Press, 2004.

Kaplan HS. *The Illustrated Manual of Sex Therapy.* 2nd ed. New York: Brunner Mazel Publishers, 1987.

Kroll K, Klein EL. *Enabling Romance: A Guide to Love, Sex, and Relationships for the Disabled.* New York: Harmony Books, 1992.

Mooney TO, Cole TM, Chilgren RA. *Sexual Options for Paraplegics and Quadriplegics.* Boston: Little Brown, 1975.

Neistadt ME, Freda M. *Choices: A Guide to Sex Counseling with Physically Disabled Adults.* Malabar, FL: Robert E. Krieger Publishing, 1987.

Yaffe M, Fenwick E, Rosen R, Kellett J. *Sexual Happiness for Men: A Practical Approach.* New York: Henry Holt, 1992.

Yaffe M, Fenwick E, Rosen R, Kellett J. *Sexual Happiness for Women: A Practical Approach.* New York: Henry Holt, 1992.

Selected pamphlets from the National Multiple Sclerosis Society (1-800-FIGHT MS; 800-344-4867) or online at http://www.nationalmssociety.org/Brochures:

- *MS and Intimacy*
- *Fatigue: What You Should Know*
- *Sexuality and Multiple Sclerosis (3rd ed.)*—Michael Barrett, PhD (Available from Multiple Sclerosis Society of Canada, 250 Bloor St East, Ste 820, Toronto, Ontario M4W 3P9, Phone: 416-922-6065.)

RECOMMENDED RESOURCES

The Sexuality Information and Education Council of the United States (SIECUS): This organization, which has a Resource Center and Library, publishes an annotated bibliography on sexuality and disability, and runs database searches for more specific topics utilizing their own extensive reference library. SIECUS can be reached at www.siecus.org.

Sexuality and Disability: A quarterly journal that publishes scholarly articles on rehabilitation, disability, and sexuality. It also publishes guidelines for professional clinical practice, case studies, and information for consumers. The journal is available at: www.springer.com/psychology/community+psychology//journal/11195.

The American Association of Sex Educators, Counselors, and Therapists (AASECT): Certifies professional sex therapists who can document that they have met their criteria for minimum educational and clinical experience standards. AASECT-certified therapists also must agree to adhere to a code of ethics. Although many highly qualified sex therapists do not choose to join AASECT, you can obtain a list of AASECT-certified sex therapists by writing to them at www.aasect.org.

A number of discreet catalog services are available that sell sexually oriented materials. Most of these are not targeted toward people with disabilities, but they contain products that may be helpful to both disabled and nondisabled people. Some include the following:

- Eve's Garden International, Ltd., sells books, videos, and sexual aids/toys. Their catalog can be ordered from their offices at 119 W. 57th St, Ste 1201, New York, NY 10019-2383 (Phone: 800-848-3837; http://www.evesgarden.com).
- Good Vibrations, Inc., offers similar fare. Their catalog can be ordered from 938 Howard St, San Francisco, CA 94103 (Phone: 415-974-8990; 800-289-8423; http://www.goodvibes.com).
- Lawrence Research offers a catalog full of sexual novelties and aids, videos, and books, called the Xandria Collection catalogue (Phone: 800-242-2823; http://www.xandria.com).

Speech and Voice Problems: Assessment and Management

Pamela H. Miller, MA, CCC-SLP

Multiple sclerosis (MS) ***plaques*** (also called ***lesions***) in the brain can interfere with muscle control in the lips, tongue, soft palate (the soft muscle tissue extending back from the roof of the mouth), vocal cords, and diaphragm (the dome-like muscle under the lungs that plays an important role in breathing). These muscles control speech production and voice quality, as well as the process of swallowing. A person who develops problems with speech or swallowing is usually referred by his or her physician to a ***speech/language pathologist***, who specializes in the diagnosis and treatment of speech and swallowing disorders. The evaluation and treatment of problems with speech production and voice quality are discussed in this chapter, while MS-related swallowing difficulties are the subject of Chapter 13.

Many speech/language pathologists also evaluate and treat cognitive-communication symptoms, including problems with attention, memory, finding the words to express ideas while speaking or writing, and processing or remembering what is heard or read. Cognitive-communication disorders are discussed in Chapter 14.

Normal speech and voice production is complex, requiring the following five systems to work smoothly together:

- *Respiration*—using the diaphragm to fill the lungs fully, followed by slow, controlled exhalation for speech
- *Phonation*—using the vocal cords and airflow to produce voice sounds of different pitch (highness or lowness of tone), loudness, and quality
- *Resonance*—raising and lowering the soft palate to direct the voice to vibrate in either the mouth or nose, further affecting quality
- *Articulation*—making quick, precise movements of the lips, tongue, and soft palate for clarity of speech
- *Prosody*—combining all the above elements for a natural flow of speech, with adequate speaking rate, appropriate pauses, and variations in loudness and emphasis to enhance meaning

Approximately 41 to 51 percent of people with MS experience speech and voice disorders during the course of the disease. The disorders are caused by ***spasticity***, weakness, slowness, and incoordination of the muscles in the tongue, lips, soft palate, vocal cords, and diaphragm.

Dysarthria is the term used to describe motor speech disorders that result in the slurred or unclear articulation of words. Impairments in volume control, articulation, and emphasis have been reported as the three most common features of dysarthria.

- Impaired volume control refers to a voice that is too quiet, too loud, or tends to fluctuate because of poor breath support and control.
- Poor articulation results in speech that is slurred and sometimes difficult to understand in conversation.
- Problems with emphasis result in speech that is slowed or unnatural because of inappropriate pauses, placement of excess and equal stress on each word, or difficulty in varying pitch and loudness to emphasize important words.

The term *dysphonia* refers to disorders of voice quality. Dysphonia commonly involves the following features:

- *Harsh voice quality* resulting from spasticity or too much muscle tone in the vocal cords, which gives the voice a strained, brassy sound
- *Impaired pitch control* due to tremor or spasticity in the vocal cords, which results either in pitch breaks (similar to the "cracking" that is heard in an adolescent whose voice is changing), or in a monotone or flat voice (lacking the pitch variation that produces a natural line of melody while speaking)
- *Hypernasality* is a nasal speech quality caused by weakness, slowness, or incoordination of the soft palate that allows too much air to resonate in the nasal cavity
- *A pitch level that is higher or lower than usual* (caused by changes in muscle tone) or an uneven, gravelly voice quality (caused by trying to speak when there is very little air left in the lungs)
- *Breathiness* (caused by vocal cords that allow too much air to escape)
- *Hoarseness* (resulting from vocal cords that fluctuate between coming together too tightly and too loosely), which sounds similar to laryngitis

Problems with speech and voice can come and go. They sometimes worsen temporarily with MS *exacerbations* (also called relapses or attacks) or during bouts of severe fatigue, and then gradually improve. Depending on the course that the disease is following, these symptoms may also progressively worsen. Anyone who experiences problems with speech or voice that interfere with everyday communication, or limit participation in social or daily activities should request a physician's referral to a speech/language pathologist, who is trained to evaluate symptoms and design an individualized treatment program. Therapy can alleviate many types of speech and voice problems; the sooner that therapy is begun, the greater the improvement is likely to be.

WHAT WILL THE SPEECH/LANGUAGE PATHOLOGIST DO TO EVALUATE MY SPEECH AND VOICE?

The speech/language pathologist will first complete an *oral peripheral examination*. This examination includes:

- An assessment of the oral muscles necessary for speech (lips, tongue, and soft palate) in terms of strength, speed, range, accuracy, timing, and coordination. To evaluate the strength and control of your tongue muscles, for example, you may be asked to stick out your tongue, wag your tongue from side to side as quickly as you can, and lick your lips around in a circle and then change directions. To evaluate the functioning of your lips and soft palate, you may be asked to puff up your cheeks with your lips tightly closed, and resist pressure on your cheeks so that no air is permitted to escape. You may also be asked to show your teeth, pucker your lips, and alternate between a pucker and a smile. To determine how quickly you can coordinate the lip and tongue movements necessary for speech, you may be asked to say "pataka" as quickly and evenly as you can.

- An examination of your teeth and hard palate.

    A *motor speech evaluation* will be done to assess how well all systems work together: breath support and control, voice production, resonance, articulation, and flow of speech.

- The precision of your pronunciation (articulation) and the ease with which you are understood by others (intelligibility) are measured at the sound, word, sentence, and conversational levels.
- A baseline sample of your speech may be recorded and transcribed.
- Conversational speech may be analyzed for its natural flow (prosody): Are there appropriate pauses, or do they occur too often or at illogical places? Are important words emphasized with more loudness and higher pitch to enhance meaning, or are all words spoken with the same or no emphasis?
- The rate at which you speak may also be measured to determine if your speech is too fast or too slow when compared with the norm.

    The speech/language pathologist will also do a voice evaluation to assess the functioning of the vocal cords, respiratory muscles, and soft palate as they relate to pitch, loudness, resonance, and voice quality.

- To assess respiratory function for speech, you may be asked to fill your lungs deeply, say "ahhh" for as long as you can, repeat "ah" many times quickly, and count as high as you can in one breath.
- To determine how well you can control pitch and loudness, you may be asked to sing up the scale ("do, re, mi...") or count from one to ten while gradually increasing your volume from a whisper to a shout. Instrumental voice analysis using computerized speech lab software may also be performed.
- Referrals to an *otolaryngologist* (also known as an ear, nose, and throat [ENT] specialist) for examination of the vocal cords, or to a pulmonologist for a baseline pulmonary (lung) function test may also be indicated.

    The speech/language pathologist will also complete a communication profile and needs assessment to determine the adequacy of your speech and voice at home, at work, and in the community. For example, the communication requirements of a public speaker, teacher, or retired person living with a spouse of 25 years may be very different. The profile evaluates the complexity of your typical speaking situations (the familiarity and size of the audience, and the demand for speed and intelligibility). It also assesses the perceptions and responses of your primary communication partners. What is their attitude? How well do they understand you? What do they do to help the communication? The ultimate goal of speech and voice therapy is to improve the intelligibility, rate, and naturalness of your speech to enhance your communication with others, in whatever setting you find yourself. Information from the communication profile provides the overall framework within which treatment planning on specific speech and voice problems occurs.

A brief assessment of cognitive function may also be included in the speech/language evaluation. Information about any problems you may be having with attention, memory, verbal fluency, and problem solving will be useful to the speech/language pathologist in designing a treatment plan and determining appropriate treatment goals, since problems in any of these areas could impact your progress. The results of the brief cognitive assessment can guide the choice of learning and memory strategies to be used in the therapy, and may also help to predict how much improvement to expect.

An audiological assessment may be necessary to determine if there is a hearing loss or problem with auditory discrimination. It is important to rule out hearing problems since they may influence clarity of speech as well as the ability to self-monitor and self-correct errors. Your hearing may be screened by the speech/language pathologist, using pure tone audiometry, or you may be referred to an audiologist for a complete evaluation.

Determining the status of fatigue and visual-motor skills also has important implications for treatment planning.

■ Fatigue is a common MS symptom that can temporarily interfere with speech and voice production. You may be asked to describe the frequency and severity of your fatigue, the conditions or activities that seem to precipitate it, its impact on your speech, and the strategies you use to manage your fatigue.

■ Motor problems, such as spasticity and tremor, and visual problems such as *optic neuritis*, *nystagmus* (jiggly eye movements), *diplopia* (double vision), and visual scanning difficulties, can also occur with MS. Information about visual-motor abilities is helpful when planning the visual and written material to use in therapy, and when selecting the appropriate type of alternative communication device.

WHAT IS INVOLVED IN THE TREATMENT OF SPEECH AND VOICE PROBLEMS?
Therapy is recommended with a speech/language pathologist if speech or voice problems interfere with everyday communication needs and limit participation in social or daily activities. The type and amount of treatment will vary with each individual. A treatment plan can be devised based on the person's specific problem areas and communication needs. Therapy usually begins with learning about normal speech and voice production. Improving speech intelligibility and naturalness are the ultimate goals. It is important to learn to use the lips, tongue, soft palate, vocal cords, and diaphragm, with improved strength, range, and coordination while talking. Active self-monitoring is essential and can be enhanced with the use of a tape or digital recorder, speech analysis computer software, and *spirometer* (an instrument that measures how completely the lungs are filled).

The person may be taught new strategies and compensatory techniques for improving the clarity of speech, including slowing down, overarticulation (exaggerated enunciation), phrasing, strategic pauses, and syllable tapping (tapping as you say each syllable). Practicing these techniques in increasingly more difficult and less structured speaking situations—during individual and then group therapy sessions—can help a person generalize these new skills. Training family members in ways to provide useful cues can help promote treatment carryover outside the therapy sessions.

Home programs to enhance progress can be developed, incorporating, for example, the use of a mirror during speech exercises, and the use of a recorder while practicing and self-evaluating the new speaking strategies and compensatory techniques.

Training in the use of an augmentative or alternative communication (AAC) device can be provided for any person who is unable to speak loudly or clearly enough to be understood by others. For example, a simple voice amplifier (with headset microphone, loudness control, and speaker) can enhance one-to-one or even room-to-room communication for those who cannot speak loudly enough to be heard, or who become easily fatigued by the effort to do so. For those who are unable to articulate clearly enough to be understood, there are AAC devices ranging from a simple alphabet board to computer-assisted, electronic communication systems (see Recommended Resources list at the end of the chapter).

Referrals may also be made to other members of the medical team, based on individual needs, including a ***neurologist***, otolaryngologist (or ENT specialist), pulmonologist, respiratory therapist, or ***occupational therapist***.

ARE THERE MEDICINES THAT CAN HELP MY SPEECH AND VOICE PROBLEMS?

Speech and voice problems in MS result from underlying neuromuscular impairments, complicated by a variety of other MS symptoms. Therefore, a treatment plan that combines medical management of MS-related ***spasticity***, tremor, and/or fatigue with the learning of appropriate speech/voice techniques is often the best option (see Chapter 4 and Appendix C):

- Medications to treat spasticity (such as Lioresal [baclofen] or Zanaflex [tizanidine]) may be helpful to try, because spasticity can affect voice quality, loudness, and how clearly or quickly a person speaks. For example, spasticity, or too much muscle tone, may restrict full movement of the diaphragm, thus causing reduced breath support and loudness. Or, excess muscle tone in the vocal cords may result in a harsh, strained voice quality. Increased tone may also restrict movements of the lips, tongue, and soft palate, causing a slower speaking rate, imprecise articulation, and/or nasal voice.

- Various medications (such as Klonopin [clonazepam], Inderal [propranolol], Mysoline [primidone], and Doriden [glutethimide]) have been tried singly or in combination to reduce tremor. Unfortunately, MS-related tremor is one of the most difficult symptoms to treat, and an individual's response to the medicines is unpredictable. Tremor may cause involuntary, rhythmic movements of any muscle group, including the arms, legs, trunk, head, vocal cords, jaw, lips, and tongue. The result may be an uneven voice quality, irregular articulation breakdowns, and incoordination of breath support for speech. Tremor can also be very fatiguing.

- Medications to manage fatigue (such as Symmetrel [amantadine], Provigil [modafinil], and Nuvigil [armodafinil]) may be useful because many people notice that their speech is more slurred, and their voice is weaker when they are experiencing MS fatigue. This is understandable because normal speech and voice production require fast, coordinated, complex movements of the lips, tongue, soft palate, vocal cords, and diaphragm. When a person is fatigued, movements may be slower, weaker, and less coordinated.

A speech/language pathologist can provide objective monitoring of the effect of specific medication on speech and voice for the physician, to aid in treatment planning.

MY THOUGHTS STILL FLOW AS WELL AS THEY USED TO, BUT I CAN'T SPEAK AS QUICKLY AND CLEARLY NOW. IT SOUNDS AS THOUGH I HAVE A MOUTHFUL OF MARBLES. WHAT IS CAUSING MY SPEECH TO SOUND SO SLURRED?

Feeling "out of sync," as if your mouth is unable to keep up with your thoughts, is a common complaint. Clear speech requires precise, rapid, coordinated movements of your lips, tongue, and soft palate. MS can cause the mouth and throat muscles to become weaker and less coordinated, resulting in the neuromuscular speech disorder called dysarthria. Slurred speech or imprecise articulation is a common feature of dysarthria. It can occasionally become severe enough to interfere with the ability of others to understand what you are saying.

A speech/language pathologist can help you improve the clarity of your speech. First, it is important to become consistent in identifying when your speech sounds slurred. This may require you to improve your self-monitoring skills by evaluating your own recorded speech samples. Hearing the problem is the necessary first step to being able to make adjustments. The following techniques are helpful in improving speech intelligibility while also striving for naturalness:

- *Speak louder.* Recent studies have shown this to be beneficial in improving both speech intelligibility and naturalness. With increased loudness, speech tends to become more precise, with better, more natural intonation patterns.
- *Overarticulate.* Open your mouth a little more while talking and exaggerate the movements of your tongue, lips, and jaw.
- *Pause strategically.* Instead of trying to say too many words at once, it is better to utilize a strategy called "phrasing," by which you learn to pause at logical places in long sentences. This takes extra time and planning, but can promote clear speech.

TALKING SEEMS TO TAKE MUCH MORE EFFORT THAN IT USED TO. I CAN GET VERY TIRED AND NOT HAVE ENOUGH BREATH TO SAY COMPLETE SENTENCES LOUDLY ENOUGH FOR OTHERS TO UNDERSTAND ME. WHY IS THIS HAPPENING? WHAT CAN I DO ABOUT IT?

Talking is a complex activity that we take for granted until something like MS interferes. Clear, audible speech requires physical effort and precise timing by many muscle groups. Speaking for extended periods can thus be quite tiring, particularly for those individuals who also experience MS-related fatigue. A speech/language pathologist can help you become efficient at speaking loudly while simultaneously learning to pace yourself.

Adequate breath support and control are needed for loud speech. Air is the "gasoline" needed to drive the necessary muscles. You start by completely filling your lungs, using your diaphragm to inhale quickly and deeply. Then slowly extend your exhalation to produce words. It is important to identify how many words are loud enough before you run out of air and lose necessary volume. Then you can begin to modify your speech and breathing patterns to raise your volume and improve audibility. Use a technique called *phrasing* to plan pauses for breathing rather than saying too many words in one breath. For example, you may find that breaking sentences into five-word breath units helps you to maintain adequate loudness.

Besides teaching diaphragmatic breathing and phrasing techniques, the speech/language pathologist can provide other options, as needed. For example, the *push technique* requires you to push down with your elbows on the armrests of your chair while talking. This can help your vocal cords come together more strongly to help create a louder voice. Using a spirometer can assist you in observing and measuring how fully you are filling your lungs. A recorder and speech analysis software can give you feedback on how loud you sound and if you are reaching the goals set in therapy. Voice amplifiers with headset, collar, or neck loop microphones are sometimes recommended when loudness cannot be improved to a functionally adequate level. However, a speech/language pathologist should first evaluate the problem, recommend the most appropriate equipment, and then train you in its use.

MY WIFE SPEAKS SO SOFTLY I CANNOT HEAR HER. SHOULD WE CONSIDER PURCHASING A VOICE AMPLIFIER? HOW EFFECTIVE ARE THEY?
A variety of portable, battery-operated voice amplifiers are available. They are worn using a headset with attached microphone, and a small receiver with amplifier and volume control that is clipped onto the body. For some people with MS, whose speech is otherwise too soft to hear, this simple device can open their world and make one-to-one communication possible. For others with various physical, behavioral, and/or cognitive challenges, it tends to be less effective. To evaluate candidacy for the effective use of a voice amplifier, the following are just a few of the questions that a speech/language pathologist must answer during individual evaluation:

● How aware and motivated is the person with MS to learn its use?
● What is the person's cognitive status for learning and recalling this new procedure?
● Is breath support/control adequate to drive the microphone?
● Can the person produce some voice, or is it just a whisper?
● How well can the person control the lips and tongue to accurately shape the speech sounds that need to be amplified?
● Is there a supportive communication partner who can be easily trained?
● What are the typical speaking situations and communication needs?
● How realistic are the person's expectations?
● Will MS fatigue play a significant role in effective, consistent usage?

WHY DOESN'T MY VOICE SOUND THE WAY IT USED TO? SOMETIMES IT SEEMS HOARSE, AS IF I HAVE LARYNGITIS. OTHER TIMES IT SOUNDS STRAINED OR HARSH.
Your voice quality is largely determined by how your vocal cords function. MS can cause spasticity, weakness, slowness, and incoordination of any muscle group. Your

vocal cords are muscles, too, and can therefore undergo these changes. This can occur temporarily during MS exacerbations or more continuously as a result of disease progression. The types of voice problems or dysphonia that are characteristic of MS include harshness, hoarseness, breathiness, and hypernasality.

A harsh, strained voice quality occurs when there is too much muscle tone or tightness in the vocal cords due to MS-related spasticity. Lioresal (baclofen), a medication to relieve spasticity (see Chapter 4 and Appendix C), may be helpful. A speech/language pathologist can help you and the prescribing physician monitor the effectiveness of the antispasticity medication on your voice and speech quality. Voice therapy can help to reduce harshness by emphasizing relaxation techniques for your throat and vocal cords, improving breath support, promoting "easy onset" of your voicing, and a breathier speech quality. The "yawn-sigh" approach, in which the vocal cords are automatically relaxed during a yawn to promote a softer voice quality during the exhaled sigh, may also help with this problem.

A hoarse voice quality results when something interferes with the way your vocal cords come together during speaking. Hoarseness is a combination of harsh and breathy voice qualities. Your vocal cords may fluctuate between coming together too tightly (harsh) and too loosely (breathy), resulting in hoarseness. When hoarseness lasts more than 7 to 10 days, it is important to have an otolaryngologist or ENT specialist evaluate medical causes that can be treated, such as colds, allergies, abnormal growths, and paralysis. After these are ruled out, voice therapy that emphasizes increasing breath support and loudness, lowering your usual pitch, and self-monitoring for a "clear" target voice quality may reduce the problem.

WHAT CAUSES MY VOICE TO FLUCTUATE SO MUCH? IT DOESN'T SEEM TO BE WITHIN MY CONTROL. SOMETIMES I HAVE BURSTS OF LOUDNESS. OTHER TIMES, MY PITCH CHANGES OR MY VOICE TURNS OFF MID-SENTENCE.
Such wide variations in pitch, loudness, and voice control are probably due to MS lesions in the *cerebellum*, the part of the brain responsible for regulating and coordinating complex voluntary movements. Either fine tremor or wide, jerking, shaking movements, also called cerebellar tremor or **ataxia**, may be seen in MS. Tremor can be one of the most disabling symptoms of MS. It may affect a variety of muscle groups (including the arms, legs, trunk, head, vocal cords, jaw, lips, and tongue) and interfere significantly with the daily activities of walking, self-care, sitting balance, head control, writing, swallowing, speech, and voice.

Cerebellar lesions can interfere with the vocal cord action required to produce vocalizations. You may experience sudden changes in pitch because of uncontrolled fluctuations between vocal cord elongation (high pitch) and contraction (low pitch). Bursts of loudness may result from abrupt vocal cord tension and diaphragm contraction. Intermittent aphonia (the loss of voice in mid-sentence) may occur because of unexpected parting of the vocal folds, when they should be vibrating together to produce a voice. Continuous vocal cord tremors may interrupt the smoothness of your voice quality.

Problems with cerebellar tremor or ataxia are very difficult to treat (see Chapter 4). No medication has been developed specifically for tremor control. However, some medications designed to treat other conditions have been found to have secondary anti-tremor properties. Muscle relaxants, seizure medications, and certain beta-blockers have been tried on individuals with MS. A speech/language pathologist can help evaluate the effectiveness of a medication on your speech and voice. Other treatment approaches for reducing the impact of cerebellar tremor on speech and voice include improving sitting posture, trunk stabilization and head control, learning relaxation techniques and EMG/biofeedback to enhance muscle control for smoother respiration and voicing, and using a tape or digital recorder and/or speech analysis software to monitor pitch, loudness, and voice quality. Therapy that emphasizes active self-monitoring, practicing the new vocal skills while reading aloud and conversing, and reducing physical effort during speech, may also be beneficial.

HOW OFTEN AND FOR HOW LONG WILL I NEED TO SEE THE THERAPIST?
The frequency and duration of your therapy depends on the type and severity of your problems and your communication needs. Individualized treatment planning may also be impacted by insurance coverage. However, a lot can generally be accomplished in twice-weekly outpatient therapy, with a re-evaluation and update of goals after 2 or 3 months. Involving the primary communication partner in treatment sessions and diligently following the home program are essential for successful carryover of techniques.

DO SPEECH AND VOICE PROBLEMS CAUSED BY MS EVER REMIT LIKE OTHER MS SYMPTOMS?
If you experience slurred speech only during times of fatigue, you have probably noticed that the problem disappears once you are rested. If you experience the kind of MS-related fatigue that persists in spite of adequate sleep or rest, an occupational therapist can teach you energy efficiency strategies to help manage your fatigue. A physician may also prescribe medication (e.g., Symmetrel [amantadine], Provigil [modafinil], and Nuvigil [armodafinil]) to help control the fatigue (see Chapter 4 and Appendix C). Speech and voice problems that occur during an MS exacerbation may improve or resolve following treatment with high-dose *steroids*. Thus, managing fatigue and treating exacerbations can at times help speech and voice symptoms to remit. However, referral to a speech/language pathologist is recommended if symptoms persist even when you are rested, or one month after medical treatment is received for an MS exacerbation.

SOMETIMES I AVOID TALKING TO OTHERS BECAUSE IT FEELS BAD NOT TO BE UNDERSTOOD. PEOPLE SEEM TO LOSE INTEREST BECAUSE IT TAKES MORE TIME TO LISTEN TO ME. SOMETIMES THEY EVEN NOD WHEN I KNOW THEY DO NOT UNDERSTAND WHAT I'M SAYING. WHAT SHOULD I DO?
You are not alone in your frustration. People with MS who have moderate to severe dysarthria often experience similar feelings. Some also express resentment that their impaired speech causes others to "talk down" to them in the mistaken belief that they are not capable or intelligent. A useful strategy is to let people know about your speech difficulty and explain what assistance you need from them. It takes time and practice to feel comfortable asserting yourself in these ways. You might try out the following explanation: "The reason my speech is slow and hard to understand is

because of my MS. My brain works fine, but my lips and tongue don't always coop-erate." You can then give your listener guidance in how to respond to you by saying, "I am trying to speak clearly, but please tell me when you don't understand." These simple statements will help you and your listeners to feel more comfortable because they give your listeners permission to talk about any difficulty they might have in understanding what you are saying.

We live in a fast-paced world. Assess the situation and watch the body language of your listeners. This will enable you to judge which people and situations can allow the extra time that you need. Estimate the time needed and ask first: "Do you have...minutes to talk about...?" It is important that you do not avoid talking to others. It can be a challenge, but you have a right as a speaker to be understood and a responsibility to let listeners know what you need from them. A speech/language pathologist can help you become comfortable and proficient in this process. It is best to build your comfort level gradually with this new approach, first with a therapist and then family and close friends, before trying it with strangers.

IF MY SPEECH GETS ANY WORSE, EVEN MY FAMILY WILL NOT UNDERSTAND WHAT I AM SAYING. ARE THERE OTHER WAYS OF COMMUNICATING THAT I CAN LEARN?

The speech problems typical of MS can usually be improved with therapy. Although your speech may not be as loud, precise, fast, or flowing as it was, learning the appropriate techniques will usually allow you to be adequately understood by others. However, alternative modes of communication are necessary in certain situations. Many options are available, ranging from the simple to the "high tech." The selection depends on your specific needs, abilities, and financial resources. Some of the simpler communication aids include light and buzzer switches to get the attention of others; yes/no signals, eye blink systems, alphabet charts to spell out messages with finger or eye movements, and picture/word communication charts.

Many electronic and computer-assisted forms of communication are also available. They vary in size, portability, complexity, function, input, output, and cost. Some are laptop size for you to type in the message and have it printed out. Others can be programmed so that one keystroke produces a frequently used complete sentence. Some computers actually speak the messages you program in or type. Because of the variety and complexity of the available technology, you should be evaluated by a speech/language pathology and occupational therapy team that has expertise in this area. This specialty team can help you identify the type of equipment best suited to your needs by taking into account whatever physical limitations you may have, as well as your visual-motor, cognitive, and communication skills. You can then pur-chase or construct the appropriate communication aid and be properly trained in its use (see Recommended Resources list).

ARE THERE ANY NEW TRENDS IN SPEECH THERAPY IN MS?

In recent years, three significant trends have appeared in the literature: (1) more objective measurement of the specific acoustic differences of dysarthric speech in MS, (2) identification of evidence-based treatments that are more beneficial, and (3) more attention to quality-of-life issues in goal setting.

- Physiologic instrumentation using such equipment as a sound lab, specialized computer software, and spectrographic displays has been used to objectively measure variations in sound/syllable duration, rate of articulation, vocal intensity, and size of working space for vowel and consonant production. Lip and tongue transducers have been used to objectively measure range, force, and *diadochokinesis* (or rapid alternating movements) of their function. For example, results of a recent study by Hartelius and Lillvik using this technique found that tongue function is more severely affected than lip function in MS, and that tongue dysfunction can even be detected in people with MS who do not have dysarthria.

- A series of four practice guideline reports have been published regarding dysarthria management in the *Journal of Medical Speech/Language Pathology* (2001–2004) and are available at www.ancds.org. Guidelines for improving speech intelligibility and naturalness are forthcoming.

- The World Health Organization's international classification of function, disability, and health has had a significant impact in rehabilitation since 2002. Addressing body function and structure, within the context of activity limitations, participation restrictions, and environmental factors has influenced assessment protocols and treatment planning. In dysarthria therapy, the trend is to shift away from focusing on the impairment (i.e., oral exercises to normalize movement patterns, which actually have been found to be ineffective), toward the acquisition of specific communication skills to aid participation in functional real-world activities (i.e., speaking with adequate loudness and intelligibility for necessary telephone skills at work or home). Improved speech intelligibility, naturalness of speech, and quality of life are the ultimate goals.

RECOMMENDED READINGS

Darley F, Brown J, Goldstein N. Dysarthria in multiple sclerosis. *Journal of Speech & Hearing Research*. 1972;15:229–245.

Interactive Therapeutics. *A Guide for the Patient and Family* (Interactive Therapeutics, Inc., P.O. Box 1805, Stow, OH 44224 0805 Tel: 800-253-5111).

Murdoch BE, Theodoros DG (eds.). *Speech and Language Disorders in Multiple Sclerosis*. London: Whurr, 2000.

Robertson SJ, Tanner B, Young F. *Dysarthria Sourcebook: Exercises to Photocopy*. Bicester, Oxon: Winslow Press, 1986.

Sorensen P. *Dysarthria in Multiple Sclerosis: Diagnosis, Medical Management, and Rehabilitation*. Burks J, Johnson K (eds.). New York: Demos Medical Publishing, 2000.

Sorensen P, Brown S, Logemann J, Wilson K, Herndon R. Communication disorders and dysphagia. *Journal of Neurologic Rehabilitation*. 1994;8:137–143.

Yorkston KM, Beukelman DR. Decision-making in AAC intervention. In: Beukelman DR, Yorkston KM, Reichle J (eds.). *Augmentative and Alternative Communication for Adults with Acquired Neurologic Disorders*. Baltimore: Paul H. Brookes, 2000.

Selected materials available from the National Multiple Sclerosis Society, available by calling 800-344-3867:

- *Speech and Swallowing: The Basic Facts (also available online at www. nationalmssociety. org/Brochures)*
- *Dysarthria in Multiple Sclerosis (also available online at www. nationalmssociety. org/ ClinicalBulletins)*

RECOMMENDED RESOURCES

For information about Medicare funding and AAC device coverage criteria.
www.aac-rerc.com

For information about AAC devices, vendors, materials, and tutorials.
www.aac.unl.edu

For information about dysarthria symptoms, evaluation, and treatment, as well as practical communication tips for both the person with dysarthria and the listener.
www.asha.org/public/speech/disorders/dysarthria

To locate a speech pathologist in your area.
www.asha.org/findpro

For information about speech-language pathology services, coverage, and resources.
www.asha.org/public/coverage/slpfundingresources

For information about augmentative and alternative communication (AAC) systems, and how to connect with trained professionals and related organizations.
www.asha.org/public/speech/disorders/AAC

For information specific to alternative and augmentative communication products.
www.freedomofspeech.com

For information about Speech-to-Speech (STS), a telephone relay service that provides trained communication assistants (CAs) for people with difficulty being understood by the public on the telephone. CAs, who are familiar with many different speech patterns and language recognition skills, make the call and then repeat the words exactly. This service is available for business, medical, and personal communication.
www.speechtospeech.org

For toll-free phone numbers to access the service called STS in your state.
www.fcc.gov/cib/dro/sts.html

Swallowing Problems: Assessment and Management

Jeri A. Logemann, PhD

In addition to the problems with speech and language discussed in the previous chapter, the ***speech/language pathologist*** is also trained to diagnose and treat symptoms related to the swallowing mechanism. Normal swallowing is a rapid, safe, and efficient process that occurs in four stages.

STAGE ONE—ORAL PREPARATION

When food is placed in the mouth, chewing reduces it to a consistency appropriate for swallowing. Chewing requires the coordinated action of lips, tongue, and jaw muscles to move the food onto the teeth, pick up the food as it falls from the teeth, mix it with saliva, and replace it onto the teeth. The saliva that is mixed into the food during chewing helps with the digestive process and acts as a natural acid neutralizer. Chewing takes a variable amount of time, depending on the amount and thickness of food put in the mouth. When chewing has reduced the food to a consistency appropriate for swallowing, the tongue subdivides it and forms a ball, or *bolus*, of the right size to be swallowed. The thicker or more viscous the food, the less a person can swallow at one time. Trying to swallow too much food at one time is uncomfortable and may result in gagging.

STAGE TWO—ORAL STAGE

The tongue pushes the bolus of food up and backward through the mouth, applying pressure to the tail end of the bolus. As the tongue pushes the food up and backward, the movements of the tongue and bolus stimulate ***sensory*** nerve endings; these, in turn, signal the brain to trigger a series of muscle contractions in the *pharynx* (throat), called the *pharyngeal swallow*. Figure 13-1 illustrates the oral stage of swallow.

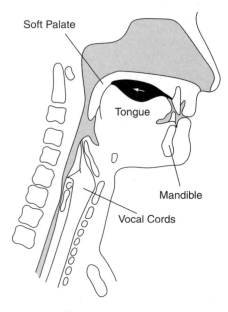

FIGURE 13-1. This side view of the mouth and throat shows the mouth containing the bolus, with the tongue applying pressure to the food.

STAGE THREE—PHARYNGEAL STAGE

The triggering of the pharyngeal swallow sets in motion a series of neuromuscular actions. The *soft palate* (the soft portion at the back of the roof of the mouth) lifts and closes the back entrance to the nose, preventing food or liquid from entering the nasal passages. The *larynx* (voice box) is the entrance to the airway. It lifts up and closes to help prevent food or liquid from entering the *trachea*, or airway, thereby preventing accidental **aspiration** of food or liquid into the lungs. The base of the tongue and the walls of the throat move toward each other until they touch. This movement generates the pressure needed to push the food through the throat. The valve at the bottom of the throat relaxes and opens to allow the bolus to pass easily into the *esophagus* (muscular tube leading down to the stomach). Figure 13-2 shows the onset of the pharyngeal stage of swallow. Figure 13-3 illustrates the middle of the pharyngeal stage of swallow.

STAGE FOUR—ESOPHAGEAL STAGE

Sequential muscle contractions in the walls of the esophagus propel the bolus through the esophagus, and the valve at the bottom of the esophagus opens to let the food enter the stomach. In normal swallowing, it takes approximately 2 seconds for the food to move through the mouth and throat before entering the esophagus. Once in the esophagus, it takes anywhere from 8 to 20 seconds for the food to travel to the stomach. When the swallowing mechanism is working normally and efficiently, food particles and liquids seldom make their way into the airway or windpipe. This usually happens only when someone is doing two things at once, such as talking or laughing while trying to swallow. A person who tries to talk while eating may begin to cough or choke because a particle of food has slipped into the

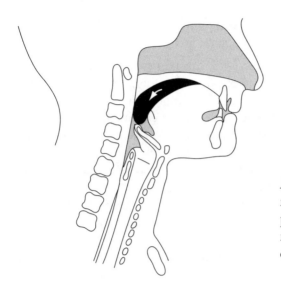

FIGURE 13-2. This side view of the mouth and pharynx shows the tongue pushing the food (bolus) out of the mouth. The entrance to the nose is closed and the airway is closing.

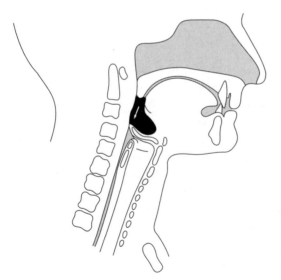

FIGURE 13-3. This side view of the mouth and pharynx shows the food at the base of the tongue. The entrance to the nose is still closed. The airway is closed. The junction into the esophagus is almost open.

airway. Once a normal swallow is completed, very little food is left in the mouth, throat, or esophagus.

WHAT IS DYSPHAGIA?

Dysphagia means difficulty swallowing. Approximately 30 muscles in the mouth and throat and eight cranial nerves are involved in the swallowing process. *Plaques* (lesions) in various parts of the brain, including the *brainstem* and/or the *cranial nerves*, can cause problems at any point in the swallowing process, from the time the food enters the mouth until it reaches the stomach.

- A slowing of the nerve impulses that control the mechanisms of swallowing can interfere with the voluntary movements involved in chewing, with the initiation of the pharyngeal swallow, or with the strength or range of movements that are required to push the food through the mouth, throat, or esophagus.
- Reduced muscle strength or coordination can allow food particles to remain in the mouth, throat, or esophagus after the swallow is completed.
- Food particles remaining in the mouth and throat may be accidentally aspirated into the lungs after the swallow when breathing resumes.
- If a delay occurs in triggering the pharyngeal swallow, the airway to the lungs remains open and the food can fall into the airway before the pharyngeal swallow triggers.
- Food or liquid can also escape into the nose or down into the windpipe during the pharyngeal swallow if a malfunction occurs in the valves in the throat.

The type of dysphagia a person develops will depend on the particular neuromuscular actions that are impaired. The swallowing problems most commonly seen in multiple sclerosis (MS) are a delay in the initiation of the pharyngeal swallow and a slowing of the passage of food through the pharynx.

WHAT ARE THE CHANCES THAT I WILL DEVELOP A SWALLOWING PROBLEM?

Most people with MS never experience this type of symptom over the course of the illness. Whether or not you develop a swallowing problem will depend entirely on the location of *demyelinating lesions*. Dysphagia can result if muscles of the mouth, throat, or esophagus are affected by the neurologic disease process. It has been estimated that 30 to 35 percent of people with MS develop a swallowing problem. We do not know if there are any specific characteristics that will predict whether someone will develop a swallowing problem. You should talk with your doctor about seeing a speech/language pathologist for a swallowing evaluation if you are finding it more difficult to chew or swallow your food, or seem to be coughing or choking during or after meals.

I HAVE BEEN REFERRED FOR A SWALLOWING EVALUATION. HOW IS THE EVALUATION DONE, AND WHAT WILL THE TEST BE ABLE TO TELL ME ABOUT MY SWALLOWING PROBLEM?

A speech/language pathologist usually conducts the swallowing evaluation. The speech/language pathologist will take a complete clinical history and evaluate your ability to control the muscles of your mouth and throat. During this examination, you will be asked to move your lips, tongue, and soft palate in various ways and to produce speech samples that require different types of muscle control. You will also be asked questions about your diet, the kinds of foods that are difficult for you to eat, and the problems you have noticed in eating or swallowing. You may be asked, for example, about:

- Episodes of coughing or choking during or after a meal
- How long it usually takes you to eat a meal

- Whether your voice becomes hoarse or gurgly during or after eating
- The frequency with which you get respiratory infections
- Whether you experience frequent heartburn or indigestion

Typically, the swallowing assessment also involves a radiographic study called *videofluoroscopy* (modified barium swallow). The barium you are given to swallow makes the structures of your mouth, throat, and esophagus visible on x-ray. The movements of these structures as you swallow different types of foods are recorded on film. During this examination, you will be asked to swallow varying amounts of liquids and solid foods with different consistencies. You may also be asked to chew and swallow a cookie with a small amount of barium on top.

The modified barium swallow is designed to help you, the speech/language pathologist, and your physician understand the specific nature of your swallowing problem. Depending on the results of the test, the speech/language pathologist may ask you to do various swallowing exercises in an attempt to improve or strengthen your swallow. You may also be given instructions on the safest ways to eat (e.g., optimal positioning of your head and neck, the size and frequency of meals, the correct way to chew) as well as the safest kinds of foods to eat (e.g., blenderized food, thickened liquids). The goal of this intervention is to identify ways to make it easier for you to continue to eat safely and comfortably.

WHAT OTHER SPECIALIZED TESTS ARE AVAILABLE IN ADDITION TO THE MODIFIED BARIUM SWALLOW, AND WHY MIGHT THEY BE USED?

The modified barium swallow is the best assessment of the overall function of the mouth and pharynx when swallowing difficulties are thought to be present. If there might also be esophageal problems, the doctor may order a barium swallow, an x-ray test designed to examine the functioning of the esophagus. Larger amounts of liquid are swallowed during the barium swallow than during the modified barium swallow. Another possible test is the endoscopic examination of swallowing, which involves the placement of a small fiberoptic tube through your nose and over the soft palate into the pharynx. This study does not involve x-ray but looks only at the pharynx, or throat, before and after the swallow. Because MS can cause oral problems, pharyngeal problems, or the two in combination, and because the relationship between the movements in the mouth and in the pharynx is so important, the endoscopic examination is usually not the swallowing examination of choice. However, the equipment is portable and can be taken to the person's bedside more easily than the modified barium swallow test that requires x-ray equipment. So, if a person is in a hospital or skilled nursing facility and needs an assessment of swallow, a fiberoptic endoscopic examination may be used.

If you are having difficulty with food coming back up from the stomach after it is swallowed, a gastroenterologist (a doctor specializing in the esophagus, stomach, and the rest of the GI tract) may examine you with a test called *reflux monitoring*. Reflux monitoring involves a tube placed through the nose down into the throat and esophagus. The purpose of the test is to identify how many events of reflux (food coming from the stomach back into the esophagus or throat) occur during a day, and whether or not the food comes all the way up into the throat. Many medications can be helpful for this problem.

WHEN SHOULD I ASK THE DOCTOR FOR A SWALLOWING EVALUATION?
If you are experiencing slowness of eating, difficulty in swallowing particular foods, or coughing associated with swallowing either during a meal or after a meal, you should discuss these symptoms with your doctor and ask about a swallowing assessment. Similarly, if you find that food sticks in your throat or in your chest, you should ask your doctor for a swallowing assessment. Slow eating, the feeling of food catching, coughing, choking, or throat clearing frequently during a meal can all be indications of a swallowing problem.

I HAVE HEARD THAT SOME MEDICAL FACILITIES HAVE A DYSPHAGIA TEAM. WHO MAKES UP THE DYSPHAGIA TEAM, AND WHAT DOES EACH MEMBER OF THE TEAM OFFER?
The dysphagia team will differ somewhat from one facility to another, but usually includes the patient's physician, a speech/language pathologist as the team coordinator, an *occupational therapist*, a *physical therapist*, a dietitian, and sometimes a dentist. Each professional offers different information and types of care. Generally, the physician oversees the information coming from all the team members and makes the final decisions with the patient about what types of management should be used. The speech/language pathologist typically does the swallowing assessments and treatments, and coordinates the team interventions. The occupational therapist usually recommends any adaptive eating utensils that may be needed for the person to be able to eat comfortably and independently. The physical therapist typically assists the person in optimal positioning and postural readiness for eating. The dietitian is very important in assessing the person's nutritional requirements and in determining the type of diet that best meets the person's nutritional needs and eating abilities.

IF THE SPEECH/LANGUAGE PATHOLOGIST RECOMMENDS SWALLOWING THERAPY, WHAT DOES THIS TREATMENT INVOLVE, AND FOR HOW LONG AM I LIKELY TO NEED IT?
Swallowing therapy usually involves exercises to strengthen the muscles used in swallowing and to improve the coordination of muscles during swallowing. Therapy often involves practicing muscle movements and learning safe swallowing strategies. Each person is different, so the exercises and techniques you are given may differ from those prescribed for someone else. The length of time swallowing therapy must be continued will also vary from one individual to another. Generally, however, a month or so of twice-weekly therapy sessions will provide you with enough training to proceed independently with your swallowing practice. Some people need to continue to exercise daily to keep their muscles operating at maximum strength and efficiency.

WHAT ARE SOME OF THE EXERCISES AND SWALLOWING STRATEGIES THAT A SPEECH/ LANGUAGE PATHOLOGIST MAY TEACH ME?
A speech/language pathologist may teach you how to coordinate your breathing and swallowing and/or protect your windpipe during swallowing so that no food or liquid goes into your lungs. You may also be given specific exercises to strengthen your tongue and lip function and/or make the swallow come faster.

WHY CAN'T THIS BOOK TELL ME HOW I SHOULD SWALLOW?
MS can affect swallowing in many different ways. What works to improve swallowing in one individual may actually make swallowing worse for another. Therefore, the safest, most effective strategy is to see a speech/language pathologist for a thorough swallowing assessment and development of a personalized treatment plan.

IF I START HAVING TROUBLE WITH MY SWALLOWING,
HOW OFTEN WILL THE DOCTOR WANT A SWALLOWING EVALUATION?
There is no set schedule for swallowing evaluations. Generally, the evaluation should be repeated if you have had a change in your symptoms. For example, you will need a re-evaluation if you begin to cough more frequently or have a gurgly voice during or after eating. You may also ask for a re-evaluation if you notice that swallowing is more difficult, or that it requires more energy and effort to swallow, or more time to eat a meal. Sometimes your doctor will want regular re-evaluations of swallowing to see if a particular medication has a positive effect on your swallowing ability.

WHY DO I SOMETIMES HAVE TROUBLE SWALLOWING LIQUIDS,
BUT HAVE NO TROUBLE AT ALL WITH SOLID FOODS?
Some people have more difficulty swallowing liquids, particularly if there is a delay between the end of the oral stage of swallowing (the movement of food through the mouth) and the beginning of the pharyngeal stage of swallowing (the movement of the food through the throat or pharynx). Since the airway remains open until the pharyngeal stage of swallowing has actually begun, the longer the delay, the greater the chance that liquid can slip into the airway and lungs. Because liquids have a thinner consistency than solids, they generally move faster and with less muscle effort than solids. Liquids are therefore likely to find their way into the open airway before solid foods do. Adding a thickening agent to the liquids you drink can often help to alleviate this problem.

WHY ARE SOME SOLID FOODS MORE DIFFICULT THAN OTHERS
FOR ME TO SWALLOW?
Because solid foods are thicker in texture than liquids, they require a great deal more pressure to push backward through the mouth and throat. Some solid foods are naturally thicker than others (peanut butter is the worst, of course). Generating more pressure requires greater muscle strength. If neurologic changes are impeding the muscle action in your mouth or throat, the resulting weakness may affect your ability to swallow solid foods. You will probably have more trouble swallowing the thickest foods and less trouble with thinner ones.

Weakness in the muscles used for chewing can also affect your ability to swallow. If chewing is difficult or tiring, you may be trying to swallow foods that are only half chewed. Half-chewed foods are much more difficult to swallow than foods that have been broken down to a softer consistency. If you are having trouble chewing, you may benefit from chewing exercises or from chopping or blenderizing the food before putting it on your plate. If you notice that your chewing gets weaker throughout a meal, you may want to eat five small meals rather than three large ones.

I SEEM TO HAVE A MOUTHFUL OF SALIVA MUCH MORE OFTEN THAN I USED TO, AND I SOMETIMES START TO CHOKE ON IT. IS THERE ANYTHING I CAN DO ABOUT THIS PROBLEM?

A mouthful of saliva that is not easily swallowed may result from a delay in triggering the pharyngeal swallow. You may benefit from swallowing therapy designed to improve the triggering mechanism and reduce the delay. You should talk with your speech/language pathologist about exercises for this problem. Excess saliva may also occur when you are not paying attention to the need to swallow or are unable to feel it. In that event, it may be helpful to train yourself to swallow more often and to receive cues from others. You may also want to keep a lozenge in your mouth to stimulate more saliva, which will, in turn, stimulate more swallows. A sour candy may naturally stimulate more swallows than a milder or less tasty lozenge.

A third possibility is that you are experiencing a symptom of gastroesophageal reflux disease, or GERD, that is unrelated to your MS. One symptom of GERD is called *water brash,* which means a sudden (less than one second) rush of saliva that acts as a natural neutralizer for the acid from the reflux. We do not know how often patients with MS experience GERD, and this is certainly not the most likely cause of your excess saliva. If, however, you have any other symptoms of reflux (heartburn, coughing or gagging after meals, waking at night coughing or gagging) you may wish to see your family physician or a gastroenterologist for an evaluation.

I USED TO SWALLOW AUTOMATICALLY, WITHOUT EVEN HAVING TO THINK ABOUT IT. NOW I'M HAVING A PROBLEM STARTING AND FINISHING THE SWALLOW. SOMETIMES I EVEN FEEL AS THOUGH I HAVEN'T SWALLOWED EVERYTHING THAT NEEDS TO GO DOWN. WHY IS THIS HAPPENING, AND CAN I DO ANYTHING ABOUT IT?

This problem probably indicates both a delay in the pharyngeal stage of swallowing and muscle weakness that allows food particles to remain in your mouth or throat following each swallow. These problems can sometimes be alleviated with swallowing therapy. Certain icing techniques can help trigger the pharyngeal stage of swallowing. Exercises may strengthen muscles used during swallowing. Sucking on a sour candy or taking a very small sip of sour lemonade between every few bites of food may help you to trigger these swallows more efficiently. A safe swallow strategy such as "hold your breath, swallow, clear your throat, and swallow again for each bite or sip" can help to clear out leftover food or liquid from the throat.

WHAT ADVICE CAN YOU GIVE MY CAREGIVER TO USE DURING MEALTIME?

Caregivers should observe their friend or family member during mealtime to determine whether coughing or choking at meals is increasing, or swallowing and eating are slowing down or becoming more difficult. If so, the caregiver should remind the person about those strategies that have been recommended by the speech/language pathologist. Sometimes, during the course of a meal, a person may forget the strategies he or she is supposed to be using. Head position, amount of food or liquid taken per swallow, time between swallows, and other variables can make a difference between a successful and unsuccessful swallow. Once the speech/language pathologist has recommended specific eating procedures, the caregiver can provide gentle reminders for the person to use these strategies.

**WHAT SPECIAL EQUIPMENT DO YOU RECOMMEND TO
HELP A PERSON EAT INDEPENDENTLY?**
Modified eating utensils may be needed to facilitate independent eating (see Chapter 10). An occupational therapist can recommend those devices that are most suited to your needs, and tell you where to get them.

**SOMETIMES MY HUSBAND CHOKES SO BADLY, I GET SCARED HE MIGHT CHOKE
TO DEATH. WHAT IS THE HEIMLICH MANEUVER, AND WHEN SHOULD I GIVE IT?**
The Heimlich maneuver is the best-known method of removing an object from the airway of a person who is choking. You can use it on yourself or someone else. If someone is choking, and cannot breathe because food is blocking his or her airway, the Heimlich maneuver can be used to dislodge the food. Caregivers and the person with MS should be familiar with this intervention. The Heimlich maneuver should not be performed if the person is coughing, speaking, or breathing. If the person cannot cough, speak, or breathe, proceed as follows:

1. Stand behind the choking person and wrap your arms around his or her waist. Bend the person slightly forward.
2. Make a fist with one hand and place it slightly above the person's navel.
3. Grasp your fist with the other hand and press hard into the abdomen with a quick, upward thrust. Repeat this procedure until the object is expelled from the airway.

If you must perform this maneuver on yourself, position your own fist slightly above your navel. Grasp your fist with your other hand and thrust upward into your abdomen until the object is expelled.

If a person with MS requires the Heimlich maneuver, he or she is in need of a swallowing evaluation.

CAN YOU GIVE ME SOME SIMPLE WAYS TO MAKE MY SWALLOWING BETTER?
Because MS varies so much from one person to another, swallowing problems caused by MS also vary greatly. There is no single way to improve the swallow for everyone. In fact, any universal suggestions could be dangerous for some individuals. Therefore, the best way to manage your swallowing problem is to have a detailed evaluation of your swallowing and let a speech/language pathologist devise a therapy program for your particular swallowing problems.

**I HAVE BEEN TOLD TO CUT MY FOOD INTO VERY SMALL PIECES (OR PUT IT
THROUGH A BLENDER) AND THICKEN ALL THE LIQUIDS I DRINK BECAUSE
I AM COUGHING AND CHOKING MORE OFTEN. THE PROBLEM STILL
SEEMS TO BE GETTING WORSE. WHAT WILL HAPPEN IF I CAN'T SOLVE THE
CHOKING PROBLEM?**
If you cannot solve the choking problem with therapy, modified swallowing techniques, or changes in the consistency of your food, your doctor may recommend that you begin non-oral (not by mouth) feedings. Frequent coughing or choking is an indication that you may be aspirating food or liquids into your lungs, which can, in turn, increase your risk of getting ***aspiration pneumonia***. In addition to the increased risk of aspiration and pneumonia, severe swallowing problems may deprive you of

adequate nutrition and fluids. People who find it too tiring to eat properly, or whose eating is frequently interrupted by bouts of coughing or choking, may not be able to eat or drink sufficient amounts to maintain their weight. Your doctor may recommend non-oral feedings to ensure that you get adequate nutrition and liquids.

There are two basic types of non-oral feeding that allow food and liquids to be taken into the body without being swallowed. A *nasogastric tube* (that goes through the nose and throat and into the esophagus and stomach) is typically used on a very temporary basis (following surgery, for example) when the person is expected to be able to resume eating by mouth within a few days or weeks. The nasogastric tube can be irritating to the nose and throat if left in for a prolonged period. A percutaneous endoscopic gastrostomy (PEG) is used if non-oral feedings are likely to be needed for a longer time. The PEG involves the insertion of a feeding tube through the abdominal wall directly into the stomach. In this relatively simple procedure, an endoscope (a special instrument designed to illuminate the inside of an internal organ) guides the placement of the tube through a tiny incision in the stomach wall. The tube remains in place as long as non-oral feeding is necessary, and a special dietary formula is pumped into the tube on a scheduled basis.

Both types of non-oral feeding tubes can be removed when and if your swallowing improves. Therefore, if your doctor recommends that you begin non-oral feedings, you do not have to feel that you are making a permanent decision. You can choose to have the feeding tube removed at any time. Keep in mind that being well-nourished and getting adequate liquids are important for maintaining your strength. Losing weight and getting weaker can, by themselves, cause swallowing problems, and your chances of regaining your swallowing abilities are better when you are strong and well-nourished. So, while it can be a big decision to take some or all nutrition and fluids by tube, that decision may help you to recover improved swallowing later. Do not put off taking good nutrition and liquids by non-oral means if your physician recommends them.

IF I DO START NON-ORAL FEEDING, DOES THAT MEAN THAT I CAN NEVER EAT ANY FOOD BY MOUTH?
No. Even with non-oral feeding, you may be able to take certain kinds of foods by mouth. This will generally depend on the nature of your swallowing problem and the thickness of the foods you want to eat. Many individuals take non-oral tube feeding for part of their nutritional needs and eat certain foods orally. Sometimes people can safely and efficiently swallow some types of food but not others. If you are safely able to chew and swallow foods of a certain thickness or consistency, you will be given a list of foods that are safe for you to eat by mouth and the kinds of foods you should be sure to avoid. Generally, if you are able to manage one or two consistencies of food, your speech/language pathologist or physician will try to keep you eating those types of food by mouth. However, you may need total non-oral feeding if you are having difficulty swallowing all types of foods and liquids.

IF I NEED TO HAVE A PEG NOW, DOES THAT MEAN I WILL ALWAYS HAVE TO HAVE ONE?
No. You may only need a PEG for a few months. If your swallowing improves due to swallowing therapy or a *remission* in the disease, your physician will probably

recommend that you resume eating by mouth at least some of the time. If you have no further difficulties with swallowing, the PEG can be removed. It is important that you pay attention to your swallowing ability and report changes or improvements to your physician and speech/language pathologist. A re-evaluation of your swallowing, probably including a repeat videofluoroscopy, will indicate whether or not it is safe for the PEG to be removed.

IS THERE ANY CURE FOR MY SWALLOWING PROBLEMS, OR WILL THEY JUST KEEP GETTING WORSE?

Some people with MS experience swallowing problems that gradually worsen over time. Others have a temporary problem with swallowing that gradually improves to the point where they can eat efficiently and safely by mouth. Once improved, the swallowing problems may or may not return. Your best strategy is to see your physician and speech/language pathologist any time you feel that your swallowing has changed, so that they can provide you with the best kinds of exercises and management techniques—and keep exercising!

RECOMMENDED READINGS

Bergamaschi R, Crivelli P, Rezzani C, et al. The DYMUS questionnaire for the assessment of dysphagia in multiple sclerosis. *Journal of Neurological Science.* 2008;269(1-2):49–53.

Groher ME. *Dysphagia: Diagnosis and Management.* Boston: Butterworth Publishers, 1984.

Jones GW, Feldmann MC, Ireland JV, Reinhart R, Yozwiak A. *Dysphagia: A Manual for Use by Families.* Austin, TX: Pro-Ed, 1994.

Logemann JA. *Evaluation and Treatment of Swallowing Disorders* (2nd ed.). Austin, TX: Pro-Ed, 1998.

Poorjavad M, Derakhshandeh F, Etemadifar M, et al. Oropharyngeal dysphagia in multiple sclerosis. *Multiple Sclerosis.* 2010;16(3):362–365.

Schapiro RT. *Symptom Management in Multiple Sclerosis* (4th ed.). New York: Demos Medical Publishing, 2003.

Selected materials available from the National Multiple Sclerosis Society, 800-FIGHT-MS (800-344-3867) or online at www.nationalmssociety.org/Brochures:
- *Speech and Swallowing: The Basic Facts*

RECOMMENDED RESOURCES

Mayo Foundation for Health Education and Research—First Aid: The Heimlich Maneuver
http://www.mayoclinic.com/health/first-aid-choking/FA00025

American Dysphagia Network: A network for the prevention, diagnosis & treatment of swallowing disorders.
http://americandysphagianetwork.org/

Cognitive Challenges:
Assessment and Management

Nicholas G. LaRocca, PhD, and
Pamela H. Miller, MA, CCC-SLP

*C*ognition refers to a variety of high-level functions carried out by the human brain. These include our ability to:

- Understand and use language.
- Accurately recognize objects (visual perception) and use these perceptions to draw, assemble things, and find our way around (visual construction).
- Perform calculations.
- Focus, maintain, and shift our attention as needed, even when information is coming at us very rapidly (information processing).
- Learn and remember information (memory).
- Perform complex tasks such as planning and carrying out activities in the proper order, solving problems, and monitoring our own behavior (executive functions).

It was believed for many years, even by multiple sclerosis (MS) specialists, that the disease rarely caused changes in cognitive functioning. Such changes, if at all, were thought to occur only in the late stages of MS. Based on a number of research studies published since the early 1980s, however, it is clear that *cognitive impairment* is quite common in MS. The results of several large-scale, *controlled studies* suggest that at least half of all people with MS experience changes in their cognitive functioning. Not surprisingly, cognitive impairment can have a profound effect on a person's ability to perform important daily activities related to work, household chores, social interactions, driving, and managing MS and its symptoms.

TYPES OF COGNITIVE CHANGES THAT CAN OCCUR IN MS
Just as MS varies in terms of how it affects a person physically, considerable variability occurs in the cognitive symptoms of MS. Typically, MS affects only some cognitive functions, while others remain relatively intact.

- Both research and clinical experience suggest that memory *impairment* is the most common cognitive symptom in MS. However, changes in speed of information processing and executive functions occur often.

- Visuospatial deficits (i.e., impairments in visual perception and constructional abilities) are seen less frequently.
- Changes in calculation ability are relatively uncommon in MS, but a person may have difficulty doing activities involving calculation (such as balancing a checkbook) due to deficits in information processing, problem solving, or organization.
- Cognitive-based communication problems may also be seen in MS. Changes in the ability to comprehend or use high-level language skills can result from problems with attention, speed of information processing, planning, reasoning, and self-monitoring. A person with MS may have difficulty comprehending information (either heard or read) that is too complex or presented too rapidly. Distractions in the environment can also interfere with the comprehension of incoming information. A person may experience difficulty formulating thoughts and retrieving specific words to express ideas either verbally or in writing. While these problems are typically mild and tend to go unnoticed by most, they can at times interfere with communication at home, at work, or in the community.

RELATIONSHIP TO DISEASE DURATION AND SEVERITY
Cognitive impairment is only weakly related to disease course and duration of MS. In other words, a person can experience cognitive changes at any point over the course of the disease, regardless of the severity of his or her physical symptoms. Some people experience cognitive changes as one of their earliest MS symptoms, while others who have had MS for many years may have no cognitive deficits at all.

CAUSES OF MS-RELATED COGNITIVE CHANGES
- In general, the greater the number and the more extensive the plaques (lesions) that can be seen on a person's brain using magnetic resonance imaging (MRI), the greater the likelihood of changes in his or her cognitive functioning. However, this "rule of thumb" is imperfect. Cognitive impairment can be present even if few or no lesions are visible on MRI; conversely, some people whose MRIs show many MS lesions have few measurable cognitive deficits.

  The location of lesions is also an important predictor of their effects on a person's functioning. Most MS lesions tend to cluster in the *white matter* around the fluid-filled ventricles in the brain (the *periventricular region*) and the bundle of fibers connecting the two cerebral hemispheres, the *corpus callosum*. This area of the brain is involved in those cognitive functions that are most susceptible to impairment in MS, including memory, information processing, and executive functions. However, isolated lesions can appear anywhere in the white matter, at the junction of the white and gray matter, or in the gray matter itself.
- Several studies have confirmed that MS *demyelinating* lesions can be accompanied by axonal loss and brain *atrophy* even early in the course of the disease. This tissue loss is also a major factor in cognitive status: the greater the loss in tissue volume in the brain, the more severe the cognitive changes are likely to be.

● MS-related cognitive impairment has also been shown to be related to biochemical changes in the brain that are not visible on standard MRI scans.

In addition, cognitive deficits have been shown on functional MRI to result in striking changes in the specific areas of the brain that are activated during the performance of tasks involving memory, calculations, and other functions. All of these research findings have confirmed that deficits in cognitive abilities can occur at any time during the course of the disease, even if the MRI does not appear to be highly abnormal.

COGNITIVE ASSESSMENT

A person's MRI scan provides important—but not sufficient—information about cognitive functioning. Lesions can occur in so-called "silent regions" of the brain that have relatively little impact on cognitive functions. They can also occur in areas that are critical to cognition. This means that a single lesion in a critical area may have a devastating impact on a person's abilities, while multiple lesions in a "silent" area may produce no cognitive changes. Consequently, the only reliable way of determining whether a person has experienced cognitive changes due to MS is through the objective assessment of cognitive functioning using standardized cognitive tests. An objective assessment of the type and severity of cognitive involvement can then be used to guide treatment recommendations.

Cognitive function can be assessed using an extensive "battery" of tests. This type of assessment is typically carried out by a *neuropsychologist*, a *speech/language pathologist*, or an *occupational therapist*. While these specialists have somewhat different approaches to the assessment of cognitive impairment and utilize different types of tests, their common goal is to identify changes in cognitive functioning that interfere with everyday life. Most major medical centers and many *rehabilitation* facilities have qualified specialists in these areas. Evaluations of cognitive functioning typically involve an interview and several hours of testing because the functions being tested are quite complex.

To determine whether a person's cognitive functioning has changed as a result of MS, the examiner compares the individual's test performance with that of healthy adults who are similar in terms of age, education, and other factors that can affect test performance. If no changes have occurred, the individual's test performance should be comparable to that of this reference, or *normative,* group. In general, the lower the test performance relative to these norms, the more severe the impairment in that particular cognitive function. Unless other factors could reasonably explain identified deficits, it is assumed that they are attributable to MS.

TREATMENT

Cognitive rehabilitation refers to techniques designed to improve the functioning of people who have cognitive impairment due to MS and other central nervous system (CNS) disorders. Most of these techniques were developed for patients with acute changes in their cognitive functioning due to traumatic brain injury or stroke, but many are applicable to MS. Cognitive rehabilitation may be offered by different types of health care professionals, including neuropsychologists, speech/language pathologists, and occupational therapists.

There are two primary types of cognitive rehabilitation strategies, one aimed at restoring a function, the other focusing on strategies to compensate for a deficit.

- Restorative strategies are designed to improve the impaired function directly through repetitive drills and practice. Examples of this include memory retraining strategies based on repetitive list-learning, or attention retraining strategies based on practice and mastery of progressively more challenging exercises.
- Compensatory strategies assume that the impaired function will not improve. Consequently, the person is taught to compensate for identified deficits through the use of such strategies as visual imagery, techniques for minimizing distractions, or the use of various organizational strategies.

The ultimate aim of any cognitive rehabilitation technique is to improve a person's ability to function as independently and safely in his or her daily activities as possible, in spite of cognitive impairment.

ASSESSMENT

MY WIFE AND CHILDREN KEEP TELLING ME THAT I'M BECOMING FORGETFUL. HOW CAN I TELL IF MS HAS AFFECTED MY MEMORY?
Unfortunately, people are often inaccurate in judging their own cognitive functioning. Those who are extremely distressed (depressed or anxious) are more likely to believe that their memory is worse than it actually is or to believe that they are having problems with many cognitive functions when they may only have deficits in one or two areas. Conversely, others may be unable to acknowledge their cognitive deficits because it is too emotionally painful for them to accept that MS can affect cognitive as well as physical functioning. Finally, individuals with extensive cognitive impairment may have only limited awareness of their deficits because they have lost the ability to monitor their behavior and performance.

The perceptions of family members and close friends can also be inaccurate. To be fair, subtle cognitive deficits are often hard to detect in the course of normal social interactions, even for experts. However, relatives and friends sometimes observe cognitive symptoms and misinterpret them as indications of "depression," "disinterest," or "laziness." Family members may be aware of cognitive deficits, but feel reluctant to acknowledge them for fear that these deficits would require changes on their part (for example, in the distribution of household responsibilities). Conversely, some relatives and friends may become overly vigilant, interpreting even the most infrequent memory lapse as something abnormal, and therefore caused by MS.

An objective assessment can help determine whether cognitive impairment is present and, if so, its nature and severity. It often includes tests that measure specific areas typically affected by MS, such as attention, new learning, memory, information processing, word retrieval, verbal fluency, reasoning, and executive functions. Complex reading, writing, and other communication skills may also be examined. A psychological assessment of patient and family interactions can also yield helpful information. Such an in-depth assessment can lead to recommendations regarding treatments for underlying or related problems, be they cognitive, emotional, inter-personal, or some combination of these.

CAN I BE TESTED FOR COGNITIVE PROBLEMS WHILE I'M TAKING MEDICATIONS?
CAN MEDICATIONS AFFECT THE WAY MY MEMORY WORKS,
AND THEREFORE ALTER THE TEST RESULTS?
The interpretation of test results is simpler if a person is not taking medications because medication effects can *confound* or confuse the results. While you do not need to stop taking most medications to be evaluated, it is important to tell the examiner what drugs you are on and their dosages. This knowledge will enhance the examiner's ability to interpret the test results.

Many medications, such as antibiotics, have no known effects on the CNS and therefore do not affect a person's cognitive functioning. Other medications, such as some of the most commonly used medications to treat bladder dysfunction, hyper-tension and depression, may have significant effects on cognition and the perform-ance of certain neuropsychological tests.

Medications that pose the greatest problems for test interpretation are those that have known CNS effects. These include medications with sedative properties, such as tranquilizers and certain pain medications, some treatments for MS *exacerbations,* such as Solu-Medrol (methylprednisolone), and some bladder medications, such as Ditropan (oxybutynin). If at all possible, a person should be tapered off these medications prior to cognitive assessment so that they do not confound the test interpretation.

SOMETIMES MY MEMORY AND THINKING SEEM MUCH BETTER THAN AT
OTHER TIMES. WHEN I'M TIRED, MY MEMORY SEEMS EVEN WORSE THAN USUAL.
CAN FATIGUE AFFECT COGNITIVE FUNCTIONING?
Many people with MS report that memory and other cognitive functions seem to fluctuate, getting worse during periods of increased sleepiness, fatigue, or stress. This is true of everyone, whether or not they have MS. However, this is a bigger issue for people with MS since they are at greater risk for disabling fatigue. The research published to date indicates that physical fatigue has relatively little effect on cogni-tive performance. However, investigators have been able to identify the presence of cognitive or mental fatigue among persons with MS. *Cognitive fatigue* refers to a phe-nomenon in which cognitive performance declines following a period in which the person has been engaged in cognitively challenging tasks. If you were an accountant, for example, you might find that your memory, thinking, and ability to concentrate might decline following a couple of hours of work on a complicated job. Although feeling "fatigued" after a mentally challenging task is not unique to persons with MS, research has shown that the fatiguing effect of such tasks is significantly greater among persons with the disease than among healthy controls. Cognitive fatigue can occur even if an individual does not feel physically fatigued.

If you find that fatigue adversely affects your memory or other cognitive func-tions, try to plan your activities in such a way that you use the times you are least fatigued to do your most demanding work. Pace your activities, so that you can rest and refresh yourself following periods of intense mental effort. Try to place fewer demands on your memory at times when you are most likely to be fatigued. It is also important to keep in mind that the adverse effects of fatigue, including cognitive fatigue, are temporary and will reverse once you feel more rested—which for most people is within a few hours. You should also become familiar with the options available for managing your fatigue, such as regular aerobic exercise (see Chapter 9), energy conservation and work simplification techniques (see Chapter 10), and medications such as Symmetrel (amantadine) and Provigil (modafinil) (see Chapter 4).

DOES HEAT AFFECT COGNITIVE SYMPTOMS?

Many people with MS report that heat can adversely affect their symptoms, including cognitive functioning. This may be due in part to the fatigue that can result from prolonged exposure to high temperatures. Recent research has confirmed that heat can adversely affect cognitive functioning in people with MS. This research suggests that cooling suits, vests, or cold baths may enhance certain physical abilities in persons with MS, at least for a few hours; however, these benefits have not as yet been clearly documented for cognitive abilities. Whatever the effects of heat and cooling on cognitive functions, these effects are transient and will pass in a few hours. You may find that you feel better in general and as a result think more clearly, if you keep yourself comfortably cool.

I KNOW THAT THERE CAN BE EXACERBATIONS AND REMISSIONS OF PHYSICAL SYMPTOMS IN MS. ARE THERE EXACERBATIONS AND REMISSIONS OF COGNITIVE SYMPTOMS?

Although there has been no formal research on cognitive exacerbations and *remissions*, it has been observed clinically that cognitive function may get worse during an exacerbation and improve during remission. In rare cases, cognitive functioning can become dramatically worse in a very short period and then gradually improve. These dramatic changes are most likely the result of an *acute* inflammatory process. When MS is active, swelling occurs in the CNS as the *immune system* attacks myelin and a person's symptoms are at their worst. As this acute stage nears its end, people often notice improvement in their symptoms. This process generally runs its course in a matter of weeks. If cognitive impairment has developed gradually and been present for months or years, it is unlikely to improve substantially on its own.

RECENT TESTS BY A NEUROPSYCHOLOGIST INDICATED SOME PROBLEMS WITH MY MEMORY AND CONCENTRATION. WILL MY COGNITIVE PROBLEMS GET WORSE?

Unfortunately, very little is known about the course of cognitive impairment in MS. Some recent longitudinal studies suggest that MS-related cognitive impairment may be more stable over time than physical disability, or at least may progress at a slower rate. Although cognitive problems are unlikely to remit, rapid deterioration is also rare. This is one reason why there is increasing interest in the use of rehabilitative strategies for improving or compensating for cognitive deficits in people with MS. If, over the course of the next year or two, you notice that you are having more problems with your memory or concentration, or new cognitive problems appear, you may find it worthwhile to have another cognitive assessment to determine if there have been any objective changes in your cognitive function.

**DO COGNITIVE SYMPTOMS EVER OCCUR BEFORE PHYSICAL SYMPTOMS
IN A PERSON WITH MS?**

Although physical symptoms are usually the first clue that a person has MS, there have been instances in which a change in cognitive functioning was the first observable MS symptom. Likewise, after a person has been diagnosed with MS, cognitive changes may signal disease activity before new physical symptoms develop. To the surprise of many MS experts, only a weak relationship exists between cognitive impairment and physical disability. A person with very little physical disability may have striking cognitive deficits, while one with severe physical disability may be intact cognitively. Although some evidence suggests that cognitive impairment may be more common in those whose MS is following a progressive course, there are many exceptions to this rule. In short, knowing the extent of someone's physical disability tells you very little about that person's cognitive status.

**WHY AM I ABLE TO REMEMBER THINGS THAT I KNEW A LONG TIME AGO
BETTER THAN THINGS THAT JUST HAPPENED RECENTLY?**

People use the term *memory* to refer to a number of cognitive processes that are actually quite different. MS is much more likely to interfere with a person's ability to lay down new memories than with the ability to summon up old ones from the distant past. This is because the processing of new information is often slowed in MS, making it more difficult to consolidate the new information in a meaningful way. Thus, you may be able to recall your high school years or your first job (drawing on your *remote memory*) much more readily than what occurred in a meeting you attended yesterday (*recent memory*) or at breakfast when you agreed to stop at the grocery store on the way home from work (*prospective memory*). This can be particularly puzzling to friends and family members, who may misinterpret this as a sign that you do not care enough to remember details of shared conversations or activities. However, once these memory problems are understood as a symptom of MS, a number of strategies can be used to help manage or compensate for them.

**HOW ARE MS-RELATED COGNITIVE PROBLEMS DIFFERENT FROM
THOSE IN ALZHEIMER'S DISEASE?**

MS-related cognitive problems differ from those in Alzheimer's disease in several important respects. Cognitive impairment is the primary symptom in Alzheimer's disease, whereas not everyone with MS experiences changes in cognitive function. This difference results from the fact that Alzheimer's is a disease of the brain characterized by dramatic changes in and loss of nerve cells (***neurons***) in the "gray matter" of the brain (***cortex***). Although MS is known to affect the gray matter, MS is a disease that primarily involves the ***white matter*** in the brain, optic nerve, and spinal cord (CNS). And while MS produces some loss of neurons and damage to the cortex, these effects are much less extensive than those observed in Alzheimer's disease. A diagnosis of Alzheimer's disease requires impairment of at least two cognitive functions, one of which must be memory, with progressive worsening of these functions over time. Even in its early stages, Alzheimer's disease typically involves severe impairment of memory (both recent and remote) and breakdown of language (primarily comprehension and word retrieval), as well as possible visuospatial deficits.

Ultimately, a person with Alzheimer's disease loses the ability to recognize family and friends and to perform even the most basic personal care. In contrast, MS exerts selective effects on cognitive functioning, typically involving recent memory, information processing, and/or executive functions. Furthermore, MS-related cognitive impairment appears to be relatively stable or slowly progressive over time, so that a person may be able to function quite effectively for many years, given appropriate cognitive rehabilitation.

CAN COGNITIVE IMPAIRMENT AFFECT MY DRIVING ABILITY?
Driving is a very complex task, requiring the integration of visual-motor and cognitive-perceptual skills. It involves understanding and following directions, planning and remembering a route, multi-tasking (i.e., doing more than one thing at a time), safe decision-making, and quick response time. Research has shown that MS-related cognitive impairment can affect functions that are critical for driving, such as selective attention and the ability to process visual information quickly. Often, a person who is aware of having these deficits voluntarily restricts his or her driving or stops driving entirely. However, because driving is a major source of personal independence, this is often a difficult decision to make. Unfortunately, the procedures used by state departments of motor vehicles are not designed to detect driving problems related to cognitive impairment, so a person's license may be renewed even if he or she is unsafe to drive. If you are concerned about your driving, the best approach would be to obtain an objective driver's evaluation (often done by an occupational therapist with specialized training) and a cognitive assessment so that you can find out the impacts of both the physical and cognitive symptoms of MS on your driving. Many major medical centers and rehabilitation facilities offer these services; your chapter of the National MS Society (800-344-4867) can help you locate the one closest to you.

I KNOW THAT I HAVE BEGUN EXPERIENCING SOME CHANGES IN MY THINKING AND MEMORY. WHAT IS THE BEST WAY TO EXPLAIN THESE CHANGES TO MY FAMILY AND FRIENDS? PEOPLE ALWAYS SEEM TO SAY "OH, THE SAME THING HAPPENS TO ME ALL THE TIME—I CAN'T REMEMBER A THING!"
Well-meaning family and friends often try to reassure a person by saying that they have a similar problem with memory or word-finding. This can be frustrating when you are trying to explain your MS symptoms and request their help. You can try explaining to them that, although you may have experienced some of these problems before you had MS, your cognitive problems are different now and more severe. Explain to them that these are a direct result of your MS, much like your physical symptoms. If you have had a cognitive assessment of some kind, you may want to share the results of that assessment with them so that they can begin to understand how MS-related memory problems are different from everyday forgetting. You may want to set up a family meeting with a psychologist, social worker, or speech/language pathologist who is knowledgeable about cognitive problems in MS and can explain them to your family and friends. You might also want to include family members in the problem-solving portion of your cognitive rehabilitation sessions. Then you can work together to develop strategies to help you function better. Such

strategies might include using a family calendar to keep track of appointments and social events, designating a specific place to store commonly used household objects, and speaking one at a time so that you can take in information more effectively.

HOW CAN I EXPLAIN MY COGNITIVE PROBLEMS TO MY CHILDREN?
Children vary in their need to know about your illness, depending on their ages and the seriousness of your MS. They are usually able to take cognitive changes in stride as long as they understand that these are symptoms of MS and the changes do not interfere too drastically with the flow of everyday life. Children will probably be more upset by your distress over these problems (especially if you are angry and irritable) than by the cognitive problems themselves. A matter-of-fact explanation is probably best, using words such as "MS has affected the way my brain works, just like it has affected my walking." Children may ask if this means that you are "stupid" or "crazy." The answer, of course, is that this is not the case.

Be open to questions, but avoid flooding your child with too much information. Younger children may need to be reassured that you are going to be okay and that what is happening is not their fault, while adolescents may need to be reminded that they should not take advantage of your memory problems (or any other symptom of your MS). If your cognitive problems are a major source of distress for your children or if you find it too difficult to discuss these problems with them, you may want to seek professional help from a psychologist, social worker, or cognitive rehabilitation specialist. One or two family meetings are often enough to ease the way for better family communication about these problems.

SHOULD I DISCUSS MY COGNITIVE PROBLEMS WITH MY SUPERVISOR AT WORK?
There is no easy answer to this question. Like the decision to disclose the diagnosis of MS (see Chapter 20), the decision to inform your supervisor that you have cognitive problems due to your MS is complex. One approach is to disclose the information on a "need-to-know" basis. There may be little reason to tell your supervisor if you have some mild memory problems for which you have effective compensatory strategies and that do not affect your job performance. On the other hand, if your work is beginning to suffer because of your cognitive changes, it may be to your advantage to set up a meeting to talk frankly with your supervisor. Otherwise, any problems with your performance could be misinterpreted as lack of motivation, sloppiness, or a host of other incorrect factors. People often fear that revealing the presence of cognitive symptoms may be a "kiss of death," stigmatizing them as impaired and incompetent. Such fears are generally unfounded, however it is important to take into account your unique situation and the atmosphere of your workplace.

Many people find it helpful to work with a cognitive rehabilitation specialist or *vocational rehabilitation* counselor familiar with the cognitive symptoms of MS. A formal evaluation, including an assessment of the cognitive and communication requirements of your job, can guide the rehabilitation process. Take the time to become familiar with the compliance guidelines of the Americans with Disabilities Act concerning cognitive and communication disorders (see Chapter 20). Then, the rehabilitation or vocational specialist can meet with you and your supervisor to identify ways in which your job tasks or your work environment can be modified to enhance your effectiveness on the job. During the meeting with your supervisor to discuss the cognitive changes caused by your MS, be sure to emphasize your track record and strengths. Try to engage your supervisor in problem-solving about how you and your work environment could adapt to accommodate these changes.

MY WIFE, WHO HAS MS, SEEMS TO BE FORGETTING A LOT LATELY.
WHAT IS THE BEST WAY TO TALK TO HER ABOUT THIS?
Family members are often reluctant to bring up concerns about memory or other cognitive problems with a person who has MS for fear that it will be upsetting. Often, however, it is a great relief to the person with MS when these concerns are raised because he or she can stop pretending that everything is okay. This can also open the door to a constructive discussion of ways that the person with MS and the family can adapt so that these problems do not "snowball" and cause major disruptions in family functioning.

You should plan to raise your concerns about your wife's memory at a time of day when you and she are well-rested, will not be interrupted, and will have plenty of time to talk things over. You may want to start out by asking her how MS has been affecting her recently to see whether she brings up concerns about her memory. If she does, you could offer your own observations and then talk about getting an objective memory assessment and recommendations about what can be done. If she does not mention memory problems on her own, you could offer some recent examples and then ask her whether she thinks MS could be affecting her memory. You might want to add your observations about how these memory lapses have affected her, as well as how they have affected you and other family members, and suggest that she undergoes cognitive assessment to sort things out.

If your wife becomes irritated or defensive when you bring this up the first time, it is probably best to drop it and try again at another time. If you get a similar response the next time, it may be wise to call and inform her physician of your concerns so that he or she can raise the issue and recommend appropriate assessment. Memory problems can have several different causes, many of them treatable or amenable to rehabilitation once they have been properly assessed.

I HAVE MS AND MEMORY PROBLEMS. I AM ALSO EXPERIENCING SYMPTOMS OF
MENOPAUSE. MY FRIENDS WHO ARE GOING THROUGH MENOPAUSE TELL ME THAT
THEY HAVE LOTS OF MEMORY PROBLEMS TOO. HOW CAN I TELL WHICH IS WHICH?
Approximately half the MS population is over 50, and the majority is women. The net result is that there are a lot of people with MS who are entering or in menopause. Because cognitive changes are known to accompany menopause, women with MS have a dual risk for memory problems. There is probably no way to determine whether the changes you are experiencing are due to menopause or MS or both—and the fact is, it really doesn't matter. If these changes are causing problems in your daily activities, you might want to consider getting a cognitive evaluation to pinpoint the problems and identify some compensatory strategies for you to use.

TREATMENT AND REHABILITATION

....

ARE THERE ANY MEDICATIONS TO TREAT COGNITIVE DEFICITS?

At present, no medications are generally known to improve cognitive functioning in MS. Physostigmine, a medication that was originally used experimentally in Alzheimer's disease, proved to be of some benefit in a pilot study with a small number of people with MS. However, the beneficial effects were seen on only a few memory measures and were not evident to family members who rated the person's everyday memory performance. A related medication, Aricept (donepezil HCl), has been approved by the FDA for the treatment of memory disorders in Alzheimer's disease. For some time, there have been positive anecdotal reports concerning Aricept as a treatment for memory problems in MS. A study of 69 MS patients with memory deficits showed that Aricept had modest benefits for verbal memory, the ability to remember a list of words. Unfortunately, a larger multi-center trial of Aricept found no benefit in people with MS.

One medication used to treat fatigue, Symmetrel (amantadine), was shown to have some beneficial effects on information processing in persons with MS suffering from fatigue. Provigil (modafinil) is a drug that has shown some benefit in the treatment of fatigue in MS. However, no studies have been published examining whether this drug may benefit cognitive functioning in MS. A substance called 4-aminopyridine (4-AP), which is thought to improve nerve conduction, has also been shown to have modest effects on some neuropsychological measures. However, 4-AP is short-acting, has some problematic side effects, and is not readily available (see Chapter 4). A time-release formulation, called Ampyra was approved by the FDA in 2009 for the treatment of walking difficulty in MS. Ampyra was shown to improve walking speed among people with MS. However, to date there are no published studies examining its potential effects on cognitive impairment. In the short term, rehabilitative strategies may be the most promising method for improving the daily functioning of a person with MS-related cognitive problems.

Anecdotal reports indicate that another class of drugs referred to as *psychic stimulants* is being used "off-label" by many physicians to treat cognitive dysfunction in MS. These drugs are used to treat attention deficit hyperactivity disorder and their rationale for use in MS appears to be that they can improve focus and concentration and thereby improve cognitive functioning. However, the published research on this issue has been mixed and the most recent studies failed to show any benefit of these agents on cognitive functioning in MS.

ARE THE DISEASE-MODIFYING DRUGS EFFECTIVE AGAINST COGNITIVE DEFICITS?

The studies completed thus far of the various disease-modifying agents (See Chapter 6) have not focused primarily on cognitive dysfunction. Cognitive functioning has only been examined by secondary outcome measures in such studies. Moreover, the people participating in these drug trials did not necessarily have any cognitive dysfunction; they were included based on the physical effects of their MS. As a result, the major clinical trials of disease-modifying agents have not been particularly sensitive tests of their effectiveness against cognitive dysfunction.

Nevertheless, an increasing number of these studies have indicated that some of the disease-modifying agents provide modest benefit compared to *placebo* in slowing the progression of cognitive dysfunction. The 2-year clinical trial of Avonex (interferon beta-1a) involving 166 patients showed positive results on measures of information processing, memory, visuospatial abilities, and problem-solving. The results of a small study of Betaseron (interferon beta-1b) in 30 patients with *relapsing-remitting MS* were mixed, showing significant improvement in visual-delayed recall (only one of the 13 measures tested). The Copaxone (glatiramer acetate) study of 248 relapsing-remitting patients showed no significant improvement on retesting, but also showed no significant decline in cognitive functioning over the 2-year period. A study published in 2010 comparing higher (44 mcg) vs. lower (22 mcg) doses of Rebif (interferon beta-1a) showed a positive effect on cognition for the higher dose compared to the lower dose.

There is some reason to believe that the disease-modifying drugs may be more helpful for cognition than these limited results suggest. Avonex, Betaseron, Copaxone, Extavia (interferon beta-1b), Gilenya (fingolimod), Novantrone, Rebif, and Tysabri (natalizumab) have all been shown to slow the development of new lesions on MRI. Since cognitive dysfunction is related to lesion number and volume, limiting new lesions should be beneficial for cognition over the long term. More recent clinical trials assessed cognitive changes using more sophisticated neuropsychological testing. As we learn more about the long-term effects of these medications with different populations, we hope to obtain a clearer answer to your question.

I READ ON THE INTERNET THAT GINKGO BILOBA CAN IMPROVE MEMORY. CAN IT HELP WITH MY MS MEMORY PROBLEMS?

Ginkgo biloba is a dry extract made from the leaves of the ginkgo tree. The tree is a native of China, Japan, and Korea but is cultivated for ornamental purposes in many American cities because of its hardiness. It appears to have a variety of effects including reduction in cerebral edema (swelling), enhancement of the brain's ability to utilize certain neurotransmitters, and thinning of the blood. It has been shown to improve concentration and memory in patients suffering from peripheral arterial occlusive disease. Arterial occlusive disease is a condition in which certain parts of the brain experience a reduced blood supply because of partial blockage of arteries. There is no evidence that arterial occlusion plays any role in MS. To date the largest study of ginkgo biloba in MS found no significant effects on cognition.

Ginkgo biloba and other "natural" remedies are readily available in health-food and vitamin stores. It is often difficult to determine how standardized the dose of the active ingredients is in such products and many have been found to have impurities. In addition, many natural preparations may have unintended side effects (see Chapter 7). Over-the-counter products should be approached with care; before taking any drug, dietary supplement, herbal treatment, or natural remedy, it is important to discuss your plan with you physician.

I HAVE HEARD A LOT ABOUT HOW EXERCISE HELPS MENTAL FITNESS IN THE ELDERLY. CAN EXERCISE IMPROVE COGNITIVE FUNCTIONING IN MS?

At one time people with MS were discouraged from exercising, however that has changed dramatically. Exercise has been shown to have a wide range of benefits for people with MS including cardiovascular fitness, strength, mood, and quality of life. A recent study found that people with MS who had higher levels of cardiovascular fitness showed more highly preserved gray matter volume and white matter integrity in the brain, as well as better speed of information processing. Studies are currently underway to more closely examine the potential benefits of exercise on cognition in people with MS. However, there is no need to wait for these studies to be completed. Since exercise has many other benefits, you can discuss with your doctor whether an exercise program might be right for you.

I WOULD LIKE TO SEE IF COGNITIVE REHABILITATION CAN HELP ME WITH MY MEMORY PROBLEMS. HOW CAN I FIND OUT WHERE TO GET THIS TYPE OF TREATMENT?

Cognitive rehabilitation by a neuropsychologist, speech/language pathologist, and/or occupational therapist may be offered at a comprehensive MS center, an outpatient rehabilitation facility, or by individual practitioners. It is preferable for the specialists to have experience in the evaluation and treatment of mild cognitive impairment due to MS or other similar neurological conditions such as brain injury. Your physician or the National MS Society can refer you to such a facility or to individual practitioners in your area who have expertise in MS.

Depending on the cognitive rehabilitation specialist's assessment of your particular needs, one of three general approaches might be recommended:

- A *general stimulation approach*, in which activities such as listening to stories and playing word games encourage cognitive processing at several levels.
- A *process-specific approach*, in which a specific cognitive function is targeted for intervention through a hierarchical series of successively more difficult exercises.
- A *functional adaptation approach*, in which rehabilitation is performed in your own home or work environment.

Some approaches to cognitive rehabilitation are very focused and specific, whereas others are part of a broader rehabilitative approach that may also include psychological or vocational counseling and other types of therapies. The cognitive rehabilitation specialist should give you the rationale for the approach that he or she recommends, as well as an estimate of what kind of results to expect and how many sessions this will take. Unfortunately, there are few published studies of cognitive rehabilitation in MS and these have found mixed results, so the clinical experience of the cognitive rehabilitation specialist is very important.

IF COGNITIVE REHABILITATION IS DONE BY NEUROPSYCHOLOGISTS, SPEECH/LANGUAGE PATHOLOGISTS, AND OCCUPATIONAL THERAPISTS, HOW DO I KNOW WHICH TYPE OF PROFESSIONAL I SHOULD SEE?

Neuropsychologists became involved in cognitive assessment and retraining because of their interest in brain-behavior relationships. Speech/language pathologists offer cognitive rehabilitation because of their expertise in language- and communication-related problems. Occupational therapists direct their rehabilitation efforts at reducing the impact of cognitive impairment on a person's ability to carry out daily activities at home, at work, and in the community. For example, preparing a meal is a more cognitively complex activity than many realize. While each of these professionals brings to the rehabilitation process a somewhat different set of assessment tools and treatment strategies, they share a common goal of enabling people with MS to function comfortably and successfully in everyday life.

The type of professional you see for cognitive rehabilitation will probably be determined by the availability of these service providers in your area, as well as your specific goals. Your physician will be able to refer you to the nearest agencies or individuals with expertise in cognitive rehabilitation in MS or other similar conditions such as brain injury. If you have the luxury of choice, you might want to discuss your situation with the available professionals and decide which individual(s) and which treatment approach(es) seem best suited to your particular needs and personality style. Ideally, an interdisciplinary team of professionals can work together toward your common goals, bringing different perspectives to the process.

HOW LONG WILL COGNITIVE REHABILITATION TAKE?

There is no standard time frame for cognitive rehabilitation; its duration will depend on the nature and severity of your cognitive problems. Cognitive rehabilitation techniques were originally developed in inpatient settings, where sessions occurred daily or even more than once a day. Many of these techniques have been adapted for use in outpatient settings, with sessions occurring at least once a week (but preferably more often, to improve carryover to daily life) for several months.

You and your cognitive rehabilitation specialist should periodically review your progress together, in order to revise or set new goals as needed. When you have achieved the goals you set, it is often a good idea to taper the frequency of cognitive rehabilitation sessions (i.e., gradually increase the length of time between sessions) rather than discontinuing them abruptly. Scheduling "booster sessions," much like dental checkups, can also help ensure that you continue to apply the techniques you have learned and identify any new problems before they become too disruptive. These periodic re-evaluations allow for updates of your therapy goals and revisions of your home-based practice program.

CAN COGNITIVE REHABILITATION HELP ME, EVEN IF MY MEMORY AND CONCENTRATION ARE SLOWLY GETTING WORSE?

Yes, cognitive rehabilitation is designed to maximize your cognitive functioning and develop long-term strategies to compensate for functions that are not likely to respond to restorative treatments. In the course of cognitive rehabilitation, you will learn skills that you can use now and in the future, even if your problems get worse. In fact, there is probably some advantage to learning these skills early on, when it may be easier to assimilate them. For example, you may learn strategies for better regulating your attention and limiting environmental distractions—techniques that you can continue to apply if your concentration problems get worse. Or you may learn how to use an organizer notebook or smartphone to record appointments, phone numbers, and things you need to remember to do. If your memory problems get worse, you can still use these aids and perhaps add new ones, such as a diary to record the major events of the day so that you can review them at a later time. If your cognitive problems get worse or new problems arise, you may want to return to your cognitive rehabilitation specialist to review how you can get the most out of the methods you learned in the past and identify new strategies that may be useful to you.

A FRIEND TOLD ME THAT BY CHANGING THE MAGNETIC FIELDS IN MY BRAIN, MY THINKING AND MEMORY COULD BE IMPROVED. IS THAT TRUE, AND WHERE WOULD I GO TO GET SUCH TREATMENT?

There has been increasing interest in recent years in "energy fields" and their effects on human health. Some people have hypothesized that physical and psychological symptoms can be caused by an imbalance in a person's energy fields. While it is true that in many neurologic disorders abnormalities occur in the electrical signals emanating from the brain (as measured on an electroencephalogram [EEG]), it is unclear how this relates to the concept of energy fields. At present, the concept of energy fields and trying to put them into balance using magnetic stimulation is being studied in disorders other than MS. However, there is no evidence to date that any technique related to the manipulation of magnetic fields or energy fields has any beneficial effects on cognition in MS.

MY CHILDREN KEEP ACCUSING ME OF FORGETTING THINGS THAT THEY HAVE TOLD ME. SOMETIMES I REMEMBER THESE THINGS ONCE THEY REMIND ME, BUT OTHER TIMES I DON'T RECALL THEM SAYING THESE THINGS AT ALL. I'M STARTING TO WONDER IF THEY ARE TELLING THE TRUTH. HOW CAN WE DEAL WITH THIS PROBLEM?

The first step in coming up with effective solutions is to obtain a thorough assessment of the problem. In a situation like this, it is important not only for you to have an objective cognitive assessment, but also for your family to meet with a social worker, psychologist, or other health care professional familiar with MS-related cognitive problems and their potential impact on family relationships.

If it turns out that you do have some identifiable cognitive problems, a cognitive rehabilitation specialist can work with you and your family to identify the circumstances under which these problems are most likely to occur and to modify them. For example, if your children are trying to talk with you while the television is on or while another conversation is going on in the room, the cognitive rehabilitation specialist may suggest that the television be turned off during these discussions or that you and your child seek a quieter, less distracting place to talk. If you are having trouble remembering where your children have said they were going, the cognitive rehabilitation specialist may suggest a family "memo board" in a central location for everyone to record where they have gone and when they will be back. Often, very simple changes can make a world of difference.

In some situations, however, cognitive changes are only a minor factor and the real difficulty is an underlying family issue that has been present for some time. In such cases, working with a social worker or psychologist to address the underlying family problem is critical.

RECENTLY I'VE NOTICED THAT I HAVE A LOT OF TROUBLE CONCENTRATING OR FOLLOWING CONVERSATIONS, PARTICULARLY WHEN SOMETHING ELSE IS GOING ON IN THE ROOM. IS THERE ANYTHING THAT I CAN DO ABOUT THIS PROBLEM?

It is not uncommon with MS to have difficulty ignoring background noise or distractions and, as a result, to have difficulty following social conversations. The ability to pay attention selectively to important information (i.e., what the person is saying to you) while ignoring unimportant information (such as other conversations in the room) is one aspect of information processing, commonly referred to as *selective attention*. A cognitive rehabilitation specialist can work with you to improve this skill, teach you how to compensate for this problem, or both. For example, restorative strategies might include improving your selective attention through a series of increasingly challenging exercises in which you have to ignore competing background messages and attend only to what is important. Compensatory strategies might include learning ways to alter the environment so that it is easier for you to concentrate.

Communication is a cycle of "give and take" between speaker and listener. Some people are embarrassed when they cannot keep up with a conversation, so they nod and pretend they are following it. Others simply find excuses to avoid social situations in which they will be confronted with this problem. However, it is your responsibility and right as a listener to let others know what you need to participate successfully in a conversation. There are two ways to regulate input in this type of situation—quieting the background noise or moving away from it. For most people, it will take some practice to feel comfortable making requests such as "I'd appreciate it if you could lower the volume of the TV so that we can continue our conversation" (to quiet the background noise) or "Let's go to a quieter room so that we can talk without being interrupted" (to move away from the noise).

Other types of communication breakdown can also occur. If you find that too much information is coming too quickly, or is "over your head," you might say one of the following: "Please repeat that—a little slower this time," "Tell me a little at a time," "Let's take a break and come back to this later," "Please explain that in different words or give me an example." Often, when friends or family members understand the difficulties you may be experiencing, they automatically begin to modify their speech. In the long run, it is far better to learn strategies for regulating input than to allow a breakdown in communication.

MY FRIENDS HAVE SUGGESTED THAT I TRY SOME OF THE "BRAIN GAMES" ON THE WEB TO IMPROVE MY MEMORY. DO THESE GAMES WORK FOR PEOPLE WITH MS?

The Internet has dozens of Web sites where you can find games and exercises to "boost brain power." These vary in the extent to which they are based on solid science and how easy they are to use. In addition, video game consoles and computers can host cognitive exercises and games. There is no harm in trying some of these to see what suits you and whether you experience any benefits. However, it is a good idea to have a professional evaluation first and then to work with a rehabilitation specialist to help you pick out the games and exercises that are most suitable for your situation. Keep in mind that the jury is still out concerning whether any of these games are actually beneficial to people with MS.

I USED TO ENJOY READING, BUT NOW I FIND THAT I HAVE A LOT OF TROUBLE REMEMBERING WHO THE CHARACTERS ARE AND WHAT THE STORY LINE IS. ARE THERE STRATEGIES FOR DEALING WITH THIS PROBLEM?
Problems with reading can have several different causes. First, reading requires you to see and use your eyes well. Visual problems that are common in MS—such as blurriness, double vision (***diplopia***), "jiggly eyes" (***nystagmus***), and difficulty with left-to-right scanning eye movements—can interfere with the reading process. Second, reading requires you to concentrate on the written material, understand what you are reading, and remember it later. People with MS report little or no difficulty understanding what they read. However, problems with concentration and memory result in frequent complaints such as "I cannot read for as long as I used to," "I have to reread it many times," "When I pick up a book to continue where I left off, I can't remember what I've already read."

A treatment plan can be developed following a thorough evaluation to determine the cause of your reading difficulties. If you have problems with eye movements and coordination, an occupational therapist or behavioral optometrist (an optometrist with additional expertise in eye training) can suggest eye movement exercises that may be helpful. The eye specialist will also make sure that you are fitted with the proper lenses.

If concentration and memory problems interfere with reading, a cognitive rehabilitation specialist may recommend exercises directed at the underlying attention/concentration problem, as well as specialized reading techniques such as the "four R's"—Read, Re-read, Reorganize, and Review. The first phase of the "four R's" involves scanning the headings, pictures, and first and last paragraphs (of a newspaper article, for example) to get the gist or main idea. This builds a framework to organize new information as you then read each paragraph aloud. As you proceed to reread the entire article, it is helpful to highlight the key ideas, make notes, and continually relate the information in the new paragraph to the previous one. The next step is to reorganize the information by putting various elements into your own words, developing opinions, and personalizing the information. Many people find it helpful to reorganize information into the main idea and "Who, What, When, Where, and How" details. Finally, as you review your highlights and notes, it may be beneficial to discuss the information with another person. The goal is to involve as many language modalities as possible (seeing, saying, hearing, and writing it) in order to improve your reading ability. It may take extra time to process information in this fashion, but the likelihood of recalling it later is much greater.

RECENTLY I'M FINDING THAT IT TAKES ME A VERY LONG TIME TO DO ROUTINE TASKS LIKE PAYING THE BILLS AND BALANCING MY CHECKBOOK. I EVEN MAKE ERRORS ON SIMPLE CALCULATIONS. I DON'T WANT TO HAVE TO ASK MY HUSBAND TO DO THIS FOR ME. IS THERE A SOLUTION TO THIS PROBLEM?

The skills required for effective money and checkbook management are more complex than most people realize. Not only are adequate vision and hand function important, but a whole host of cognitive skills are involved (e.g., attention to detail, calculation ability, calculator use, organization, sequencing, decision-making, problem-solving, and the ability to follow through and complete an activity). If independence in money and checkbook management is a realistic goal, the cognitive rehabilitation specialist can use treatment strategies such as devising a monthly budget, developing a flow chart for bill-paying, and teaching you how to avoid checkbook errors by "talking your way through" checkbook entries and double-checking your work with a calculator. If you are comfortable with the use of a computer, you may be instructed in the use of a money management software program.

If independent money and checkbook management is not a realistic goal, the cognitive rehabilitation specialist can work with you and a family member to develop ways for you to be involved in financial decision-making without the burden of maintaining a checkbook and paying bills. In some communities, banks and special agencies can provide automatic bill-paying services and assistance in reconciling your checkbook with the bank statement on a fee-for-service basis. As always, it is important to have a thorough evaluation of the problem in order to set realistic goals and develop appropriate solutions to problems such as these.

I'VE BEEN HAVING PROBLEMS WITH MY MEMORY, MANAGING THE HOUSEHOLD, AND KEEPING TRACK OF THINGS I HAVE TO DO. WOULD A SMARTPHONE OR COMPUTER BE HELPFUL TO ME?

A variety of compensatory aids can help with memory and organizational problems. These include the day planner notebooks that have been used for many years, smartphones such as the various Blackberries, the new crop of highly portable tablet computers such as the iPad, and computers. Dictaphones, digital voice recorders, and speech-to-text computer software can also be used if problems with hand coordination or weakness are making it too difficult to write. Taking time each day to make a "to do" list, and to check off each task as it's completed, can help keep you organized and on track. Keeping a detailed log of important events, soon after they happen, can help you recall them later. Keeping a monthly calendar for appointments, and transferring those appointments to your daily "to do" list, can help you avoid missing important engagements. Whatever system you choose to develop, keep in mind that it should be small enough to be with you always (so that you can consistently refer to it and add entries as needed). It should also have all of your important information in it, in order to avoid slips of paper here, there, and everywhere.

The disadvantage of computers and electronic gadgets is that learning how to use them can be somewhat complex. However, if you can master their operation, they are among the most powerful tools at your disposal. Smartphones can keep track of names and addresses, appointments, and to-do lists. Their built-in cameras can be used to record all sorts of visual information on the fly. Computers do all these things and more, but are less portable.

Many types of computer software also can assist your memory and organizational efforts. Personal information managers perform most of the functions that loose-leaf organizers can do, but generally also have a powerful database capability. You can type in notes on a given subject, such as "Birthday List," and later do what is called a "random search," in which all your notes on the subject are retrieved, sorted, and presented to you. Money management software can allow you to keep tabs on your checking account and reconcile your bank statement in a matter of minutes, with no need to do any arithmetical computations yourself. If you find that memory problems are requiring you to write yourself a lot of notes or lists, the computer can be invaluable. Large amounts of data can be managed and retrieved using database and/or word processing software. Sometimes relying exclusively on paper can become cumbersome as you begin to accumulate piles of notes, reminders, and other materials.

Smartphones and computers are not magic. Like all compensatory strategies, they require learning and practice to make best use of their potential. A cognitive rehabilitation specialist can help you to select the device(s) that is most appropriate to your individual needs and abilities, and to develop skill and consistency in using these modern marvels. Ideally, your response to MS cognitive changes should involve a comprehensive program that includes individual, social, paper-and-pencil, and electronic aids. A well-balanced combination of all these approaches should enable you to deal effectively with many of the cognitive changes brought about by MS.

I HAVE ALWAYS BEEN AN ORGANIZED PERSON. NOW I SEEM TO BE HAVING A LOT OF TROUBLE SCHEDULING MY TIME AND ESTIMATING HOW LONG IT WILL TAKE ME TO GET A JOB DONE. EVEN WHEN I HAVE FIGURED OUT WHAT I AM GOING TO DO, I SEEM TO HAVE A LOT OF TROUBLE GETTING STARTED. IS THERE ANYTHING THAT I CAN DO ABOUT THIS PROBLEM?

Organizational skills are extremely important for a person's independent functioning; these include goal setting, planning, scheduling, monitoring the progress of a task, and completing tasks in a timely fashion. MS can affect your ability to carry out activities efficiently, causing you to take "detours" along the way or making it necessary to backtrack and take care of a step or two that you inadvertently left out. MS can also cause you to get "stuck" while trying to solve problems that come up in daily life. Problems with these types of executive functions are thought to be due to MS lesions in the white matter connecting the front portion of the brain (*frontal lobes*) with other important brain structures.

Cognitive rehabilitation for problems with executive functions typically has the dual focus of teaching compensatory strategies and identifying environmental modifications. Helpful compensatory strategies might include using structured approaches to analyze tasks and activities, developing a checklist of steps to follow, setting realistic timetables, using an alarm on your wristwatch to signify when to begin a planned task, and using problem-solving flow sheets. Environmental approaches might include maintaining a consistent daily schedule and involving family members to guide you in planning and problem solving, or to cue you to begin an activity. Generally, the greater your problems with executive functions, the greater the likelihood that the cognitive rehabilitation specialist will emphasize addressing environmental approaches.

MY FRIENDS AND FAMILY HAVE STARTED TO COMPLAIN THAT I INTERRUPT A LOT AND SEEM TO HAVE TROUBLE WAITING UNTIL THEY'RE FINISHED BEFORE I START TO SPEAK. I'VE ALWAYS DISLIKED PEOPLE WHO INTERRUPT A LOT, AND I DON'T KNOW WHY I'M DOING THIS. CAN I LEARN TO CONTROL IT?

Conversational problems such as poor listening and interrupting others are referred to as *pragmatic communication deficits*. These deficits are thought to be executive dysfunctions caused by MS lesions that affect connections to the frontal lobes. A person who has pragmatic communication problems may be unaware of them or of subtle negative feedback from the listener. Social isolation can be a significant consequence of these communication deficits, because people tend to avoid interacting with those who dominate conversations, interrupt them when they are talking, do not listen well, or do not take turns.

A speech/language pathologist is skilled at evaluating and treating deficits in the pragmatics of communication, using both individual and group therapy techniques. The first step in learning to control these problems is for you to become aware of behaviors that you or others exhibit that can disrupt communication. Watching a videotape of yourself in conversation and getting feedback from the speech/language pathologist and others are good starting points. The speech/language pathologist can then teach you ways of improving your listening skills through the use of eye contact, verbal and nonverbal acknowledgments (e.g., saying "that's interesting" or nodding), and minimizing interruptions. To improve your speaking skills, you may learn how to take turns in conversation, be concise, limit comments, ask questions, and solicit responses from others. The goal is to change from speaking in a monologue to participating in a dialogue that includes the other person more actively in the communication process. You may be videotaped practicing these skills so that you can monitor the reactions of others to these behaviors and chart your progress. Improving your pragmatic communication skills can make a major difference in the quality of your social interactions and the enjoyment you derive from social relationships.

I SEEM TO HAVE TROUBLE COMING TO THE POINT WHEN I'M TALKING. EVEN THOUGH I KNOW WHAT I WANT TO SAY, I CAN'T FIND THE RIGHT WORDS, AND I SEEM TO GO OFF ON TANGENTS AND TALK TOO LONG. IS THERE A SOLUTION TO THIS PROBLEM?

People tend to become "wordy" and go off on tangents when they are having trouble retrieving specific words or find it difficult to organize the complex thoughts they wish to express. "My vocabulary seems to be shrinking," "It's on the tip of my tongue," or "My thoughts and speech are out of sync" are commonly heard complaints from people with MS. While these word-finding difficulties can be quite frustrating, they are typically less noticeable to the listener than to the speaker. Evaluation and treatment by a speech/language pathologist or other cognitive rehabilitation specialist are recommended for these mild cognitive/language difficulties.

Therapy may include word association techniques and self-cueing strategies to improve specific word retrieval. Learning to "impose a delay" and quietly organize your thoughts before speaking often helps verbal expression. Concise, specific expression of ideas is possible when adequate time is allotted for preplanning. Using a "Beginning, Middle, End" format can help you stay on the topic and teach you how to delete unnecessary, irrelevant comments. During therapy, it is also important to refine your self-evaluation skills to help guard against wordiness and tangential speech.

RECOMMENDED RESOURCES

READINGS

Arden JB. *Improving Your Memory for Dummies.* New York: Wiley Publishing, Inc., 2008.

Chiaravalloti ND, DeLuca J. Cognitive impairment in multiple sclerosis. *Lancet Neurology.* 2008;7:1139–1151.

Fraser RT, Kraft GH, Ehde DM, Johnson KL. *The MS Workbook: Living Fully with Multiple Sclerosis.* Oakland, CA: New Harbinger, 2006.

Gingold J. *Facing the Cognitive Challenges of Multiple Sclerosis.* New York: Demos Medical Publishing, 2006.

Gingold J. *Mental Sharpening Stones: Managing the Cognitive Challenges of Multiple Sclerosis.* New York: Demos Medical Publishing, 2008.

LaRocca NG, Kalb RC. *Multiple sclerosis: Understanding the Cognitive Challenges.* New York: Demos Medical Publishing, 2006.

National MS Society Resources—available by calling 800-344-4867 or online at www.nationalmssociety.org:

- *www.nationalMSsociety.org/Cognition*—general information about cognitive function in MS
- *www.nationalmssociety.org/AssistiveTechnology*—information and resources about tools to make computer technology more manageable and accessible
- *www.nationalMSsociety.org/Brochures*—publications related to cognition
  Solving Cognitive Problems
  MS and the Mind
    - *Hold that Thought*—a 50-page book about cognition available for downloading (www.nationalmssociety.org/HoldThatThought)

OTHER ONLINE RESOURCES

MyBrainGames: a daily "dose" of cognitive exercises available at http://www.multiplesclerosis.com/us/index.php

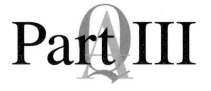

Part III

How Do Individuals and Families Cope with the Challenges of MS?

The diagnosis of multiple sclerosis (MS) is unwelcome news for everyone—the person who has the disease and family members who share its impact. In this part, we answer questions about how you and your family can adjust to life with this chronic, unpredictable disease and deal more comfortably with the stresses associated with it. The goal of these chapters is to highlight strategies and resources that can ease everyone's efforts to cope with the day-to-day challenges of MS. Because MS is diagnosed most commonly in the young adult years, when couples are making decisions about starting or adding to their families, we devote the last chapter to the questions and concerns about fertility, pregnancy, and childbirth.

Coping and Adaptation:
Making a Place for MS in Your Life

Rosalind C. Kalb, PhD, and Deborah M. Miller, PhD, LISW

No one asks to be diagnosed with multiple sclerosis (MS), and no one knows quite how to deal with it when it happens. "Why me? What did I do to deserve this? What's going to happen to me?" are common questions that run through people's minds. They wonder whether life will ever feel the same again. When and if the disease becomes more disabling, people struggle to figure out how to keep doing those things that are important to them—from walking to working, from parenting to paying for retirement, and they wonder how they will ever be able to adjust to the unpredictable changes that MS brings to their lives. In this chapter, we answer many of the most common questions people ask as they learn to cope with life with MS.

I WAS DIAGNOSED WITH MS ABOUT A MONTH OR SO AGO, AND NOTHING HAS FELT THE SAME SINCE. MY EMOTIONS ARE ALL OVER THE PLACE, AND I DON'T KNOW WHAT TO DO WITH MYSELF. PHYSICALLY, I'M FEELING FINE, BUT EMOTIONALLY I'M A WRECK—WHAT'S GOING ON WITH ME?

Being diagnosed with MS generally comes as a pretty big shock, and it can take some time to come to terms with the news. Initial reactions often include a wide range of feelings: shock and disbelief ("This can't possibly be happening to me?"); anxiety ("Am I going to end up in a wheelchair?"); anger ("This isn't fair!"); and sadness ("I just don't feel like me anymore"). It is not at all surprising that you are feeling very emotional right now, and it may be a while before all those feelings simmer down to a more manageable level. One of the best ways to regain a feeling of control is to begin learning about the disease, in whatever way feels best for you. Some people prefer to get information on their own—by reading or going online; others prefer educational programs, support groups, or chat rooms; and still others like to talk one-on-one with a health professional. Take a look at the Recommended Readings at the end of this chapter and call the National MS Society (800-344-4867) for information about helpful resources in your area.

I'VE HAD MS FOR A COUPLE OF YEARS NOW, BUT I STILL FEEL INCREDIBLY ANGRY ABOUT THE WHOLE THING. MY FAMILY AND FRIENDS ARE BEGINNING TO WONDER WHY I CAN'T JUST "ACCEPT THE MS" AND MOVE ON, BUT IT'S NOT THAT EASY FOR ME.

Maybe "acceptance" is not a reasonable goal for you—particularly if you feel that acceptance implies giving in to the disease. After all, how many people would be able to accept a perpetual earthquake that keeps shifting the ground beneath their feet? A more reasonable goal to set for yourself may be to look for ways to adapt your life to the changes that MS brings. In other words, you may never be able to accept this disruption in your life, but you can find ways to work with it and around it. Your challenge—which is one we hope this book will help you with—is how to make space in your life for MS without giving it any more time and attention than it actually needs.

HOW DO I BEGIN TO FIGURE OUT WHO I AM NOW THAT I HAVE DIFFICULTY DOING SO MANY OF THE THINGS I USED TO DO?

Your self-image—like a large jigsaw puzzle—has been built up slowly over your lifetime. Your personality, talents, accumulated skills, and life experiences have all contributed to the picture you have of yourself. MS is an additional, oddly shaped piece that somehow needs to find its way into the puzzle (see Figure 15-1). An important step in coming to terms with this unexpected change in your life is allowing yourself to grieve over the loss of the "old you" so that you begin to get more comfortable with the "new you" who has MS, and every time the disease interferes with your ability to do something important to you, or forces you to do something in a different way than you ever did before, you will need to mourn that loss as well. Because MS can affect a person in so many different ways, you may find that you are grieving over one

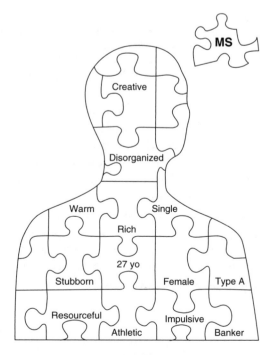

FIGURE 15-1. The puzzle of "You."

loss or another much of the time—which means that your self-image will be shifting around to incorporate these changes.

At the same time, however, you are in the process of learning new things about yourself. As you confront the challenges of everyday life with MS and learn alternative ways to do things, you will begin to identify strengths and talents you never knew you had, and these will add new dimensions to your puzzle.

If you are forced to give up one or another activity that has been important in your life, try to experiment with others that may turn out to be equally satisfying. Most importantly, look for that aspect of yourself that MS is unable to touch. For one person, it may be her sense of humor, for another his religious beliefs, for yet another her love of music. By identifying this "MS-free zone" within yourself, you can retain a sense of who you are, even in the face of stressful changes. The MS-free zone can also be an important source of emotional energy—a place within yourself that you can go to refuel when the challenges of everyday life leave you feeling drained or overwhelmed.

I STILL CAN'T BRING MYSELF TO TELL ANYONE ABOUT MY DIAGNOSIS. I DON'T KNOW HOW PEOPLE WILL REACT, AND I'M NOT SURE I'M READY TO FIND OUT. WHAT IS THE BEST WAY TO TALK ABOUT MY MS WITH OTHER PEOPLE?

Although it is never possible to predict exactly how another person will react to your MS, it is safe to assume that most people will take their cues from you. Be prepared to explain what MS is and to let the person know if you feel comfortable talking about it and answering questions. Some people will want to tell you about others they have known with MS; others will want to give you a lot of suggestions or advice. Most, however, will express shock and concern, and then wait for you to tell them what you want or need from them. Since you will want or need different things from different people, think this through before you talk to someone. Try not to jump to conclusions about that person's reactions to you. Some people may seem to withdraw a bit; this is probably a reflection more of their own anxiety about how to talk to you about the MS than any lack of caring or concern on their part. For more information about talking to your employer or colleagues about your MS, refer to Chapter 20.

FAMILY, FRIENDS, AND WORK ARE EACH IMPORTANT PARTS OF MY LIFE. NOW THAT I HAVE MS, I DON'T HAVE ENOUGH ENERGY TO DEAL WITH ANY OF THEM AS WELL AS I WOULD LIKE. HOW CAN I LEARN TO ACCEPT MY LIMITATIONS AND FEEL LESS GUILTY?

Accepting personal limitations is always difficult, but everyone—with or without MS—experiences the frustration of overload at one time or another. Try to remember that the MS is not your fault, and that doing the best you can is all that anyone can ask of you. Then, take time to think through your priorities at home and at work and look at your weekly schedule to see if the way you actually spend time matches these priorities. Most people find that they spend too much time on activities that are not really necessary or important to them. Be sure to allow yourself enough time for brief rests if you need them. The time you invest in these rest periods will help you be more productive in all your activities. Talk with the significant people in your life about the ways in which MS affects you, and share with them your concerns about limitations on your time and energy. They will be reassured to know that you care enough to discuss this with them, and you will be relieved of some of the worry about letting people down.

WHAT IS A SUPPORT GROUP, AND WHAT KINDS OF GROUPS ARE THERE FOR PEOPLE WITH MS?

A support group—or self-help group—is a form of emotional support in which people with a common problem come together to share information, feelings, and ideas—or just to listen. Some of the larger groups (anywhere from 20 to 200 people) are more educational in nature, with invited speakers coming to talk about various topics of interest. Other groups, usually with a smaller, more consistent membership (8–10 people) from one meeting to the next, place greater emphasis on mutual support and shared problem solving. While most groups take place in person, some also happen by conference call or online. Groups can be led by trained professionals, peer-led (by someone with MS who has taken on the leadership role), or have no leader at all. Some support groups are time limited while others continue on a regular basis until the membership decides that it is time to stop.

At present, the National Multiple Sclerosis Society sponsors approximately 1,500 self-help groups around the country. The Multiple Sclerosis Foundation also offers support groups. Among the most common are groups for the newly diagnosed; for those with more severe disability; and for couples, spouses, or children. There are also employment groups in which people discuss problems related to job stress, disclosure, reasonable accommodations, and retirement. There are singles groups for men and women who want to meet others with MS and share some of the problems and frustrations of life with the disease. The important thing to remember about groups is that they can vary in size, structure, focus, and quality. Call the National MS Society (800-344-4867) or visit the MS Foundation at msfocus.org/support-groups.aspx for information about the groups available in your area. A staff member will be able to help you select the group that is most suitable for you. If you try one, and it does not seem to meet your needs, try another. If you try several and cannot find what you are looking for, think about starting one of your own. These MS organizations are interested in your suggestions and ideas and will be very helpful in your efforts to find a support group or start one in your area.

I'M EMBARRASSED TO BE SEEN USING A CANE. IF I EVER GET TO THE POINT OF NEEDING A WALKER, I'M AFRAID I'LL JUST LOCK MYSELF IN THE HOUSE. WHAT CAN I DO ABOUT THIS FEELING?

Some folks are reluctant to be seen using a cane or walker because they are worried that other people will think less of them. Others are afraid that people will feel pity. The first step in dealing with these concerns is to look at your own feelings about the cane or walker. If you believe that you are less of a person or that you have less to offer others because of these aids, try discussing this with your spouse, a close friend, or a colleague. Let them remind you of the qualities and talents they value in you, whether or not you need a mobility aid. You might also think about joining a support group with others who use mobility aids. As you get to like and respect others in the group, you will gradually learn to see beyond their canes, walkers, or wheelchairs; you will find that you notice the people and not their hardware. As you begin to see beyond their mobility aids, you will also begin to see beyond your own.

The second step in adjusting to a cane, walker, or any other mobility aid is to begin to see it as an important energy-saving tool in your life (see Chapter 9). Rather than interfering with your ability to do your chosen activities, the mobility aid makes it possible for you to do them more safely, quickly, and effectively. As you start to view the aid as a tool for getting things done, others around you will begin to view it in the same way.

I GET ANGRY AT COLLEAGUES AND FRIENDS WHO TELL ME, "BUT YOU LOOK SO GOOD…" HOW CAN I EXPLAIN TO THEM THAT I ALMOST NEVER FEEL AS GOOD AS I LOOK?

Some people say that you look good because they are trying to be supportive and encouraging. Others are asking in a roundabout way why you are not being more active or more productive. Almost everybody who says it is trying to figure out what MS is and how it affects you. Try to remember that most people's experience with illness is that it makes you feel and look sick for a few days or weeks, and then you get better. It will take them quite a while to understand that MS does not go away like the flu or the measles, and that it affects how you feel and act even when they cannot see any signs of it. Be patient; answer people's questions about MS; and, whenever possible, try to explain how you are feeling in ways that others can relate to ("Because of my *optic neuritis* everything looks as though I'm seeing it through a dark mesh screen." "When I walk around it feels as though I'm slogging my way through thick mud." "I constantly feel as though I just stepped off the roller coaster and haven't got my balance back"). In addition, there are several short, easy-to-read pamphlets about MS (http://www.nationalmssociety.org/Brochures) that you can give people if they are interested.

I HAVE A LOT OF VERY SUPPORTIVE FAMILY AND FRIENDS TRYING TO HELP AND ENCOURAGE ME. BUT NO ONE REALLY UNDERSTANDS WHAT I'M GOING THROUGH WITH MY SYMPTOMS. I FEEL VERY ALONE, AND I DON'T KNOW WHAT TO DO ABOUT IT.

Perhaps the loneliest aspect of life with MS, or any other illness, is that even the most loving and supportive friend cannot "get in your shoes" and feel what you are feeling. Because so many of the *symptoms* of MS are invisible—such as fatigue, visual problems, and sensory changes—family and friends will often have a hard time understanding what is going on with you. Let them know when you are not feeling well, explain your symptoms, and offer reading materials about the illness to those who would like them. Do not expect people to be able to read your mind. Try to remember that a person does not have to be able to understand exactly what you are experiencing in order to offer you love and support.

Sometimes the best way to feel less alone is to spend some time with others who know firsthand what it feels like to live with this disease. There are a variety of ways to share experiences with others who have MS, including reading what others have written—in books or MS publications—posting messages on computerized bulletin boards, or joining a discussion group.

ALTHOUGH THERE ARE MANY THINGS I'M STILL ABLE TO DO, ALL I CAN THINK ABOUT IS ENDING UP IN A NURSING HOME. HOW CAN I LEARN TO STOP ANTICIPATING THE WORST AND GET BACK TO ENJOYING THE LIFE I HAVE?

For most people, "ending up in a nursing home" means totally losing control over one's life. While a small percentage of people with MS do require residential care or other long-term care services (see Chapter 22 for helpful information about long-term care), the reality is that the vast majority do not. Therefore, the best way to deal with the fear of loss of control is to break it down into more manageable bits. Try to identify those areas of your life in which you feel most vulnerable and least in control, and tackle them one by one. Many resources are available to help you with this problem-solving effort. Your physician can help you to manage MS symptoms as effectively as possible; an ***occupational therapist*** and/or a ***physical therapist*** can recommend tools and strategies for dealing with many aspects of daily life, a lawyer and/or accountant can help you plan effectively for the future, a support group can help you learn how to live more comfortably with the uncertainties that MS brings to your life. As you begin to tackle some of the stressful problem areas, you will find that you feel less vulnerable and therefore more able to enjoy your daily life.

MULTIPLE SCLEROSIS HAS TAKEN AWAY A LOT OF MY INDEPENDENCE. IT HAS BEEN MANY YEARS SINCE I NEEDED ANYONE TO HELP ME WITH TOILETING, EATING, AND DRESSING. HOW CAN I HOLD ON TO MY SELF-RESPECT WHEN I NEED SO MUCH HELP WITH EVERYTHING?

We all spend many years learning to be self-sufficient, independent adults, and it is painful to lose any aspect of this hard-earned independence. Because the symptoms of MS make it impossible for you to perform routine ***activities of daily living*** in the usual way, you need to rely on special equipment and/or the help of other people to get the job done. Part of the process of learning to cope with this change in your life is recognizing that you are still getting the job done. In the same way that you developed self-respect as a child by learning to master the environment, you can and should take satisfaction in meeting the challenges of life with MS. Your self-respect will come from finding solutions, identifying useful tools, and availing yourself of whatever resources might enable you to lead your life in the fullest way possible.

Loss of self-esteem is a central focus of many MS support group discussions. As people deal with the changes and compromises that MS sometimes forces them to make in their lives, they find that sharing these experiences and problem solving with other adults bolsters their sense of self-worth.

I USED TO HAVE A PRETTY ACTIVE SOCIAL LIFE. NOW I DON'T EVEN TRY TO MEET PEOPLE. WHY WOULD ANYONE BE INTERESTED IN A RELATIONSHIP WITH A PERSON WHO HAS MS?

Before you can understand why others would be interested in having a relationship with you, it is important for you to reconnect with those parts of yourself that you value. In spite of the fact that you have MS, you are still a person—complete with interests, opinions, and feelings. You may have gotten so overwhelmed by MS-related stresses and changes that you have temporarily lost sight of the rest of you. Take some time to get to know yourself again. Whether you do this in an MS support group, in counseling, or with a close friend, try to identify those aspects of yourself and your life that are independent of the MS. Then leave the rest up to others. You cannot decide for another person whether he or she will want a relationship with you. All you can do is be yourself. While some people will be put off by the MS, many others will not.

I WAS DIAGNOSED WITH MS ABOUT A YEAR AGO, AND MOST OF MY SYMPTOMS ARE NOT APPARENT TO OTHER PEOPLE. OCCASIONALLY, I NEED TO USE A CANE WHEN MY WALKING IS A BIT UNSTEADY. WHEN SHOULD I TELL SOMEONE I BEGIN TO DATE ABOUT MY MS?

As with other interpersonal issues, there is no single correct answer to this question. You must do whatever makes you feel most comfortable, given your sense of the situation and the person with whom you are dealing. The following guidelines may be helpful:

- First dates are a time for deciding whether you have any interest in pursuing the relationship further. There is no need to share any personal information with someone you do not like enough to see a second time.
- Once you have decided that the person is someone with whom you would like to develop a longer-term friendship/romance, keep in mind that half-truths and secrets make a very shaky foundation for a healthy, comfortable relationship.
- Revealing information about a chronic illness does not usually get easier as a relationship progresses; the more involved you are and the more you care about a person, the greater the potential loss.
- In deciding when to reveal significant information about yourself, think about when you would want to know similar kinds of information about the other person.
- Although some people will probably be frightened or put off by the MS, many others will not. You may be better off knowing the relationship's potential sooner rather than later.

IF THE DOCTOR COULD JUST TELL ME WHAT WAS GOING TO HAPPEN WITH MY MS, I THINK I COULD HANDLE IT. IT'S NEVER KNOWING WHAT'S GOING TO HAPPEN THAT UPSETS ME. IS THERE ANY WAY TO COPE WITH ALL THIS UNCERTAINTY?

Unfortunately, unpredictability is one of the hallmarks of MS, and you are not alone in finding this so stressful. Most people find that they gradually adjust to taking life one day at a time, making the most of good days and putting up with the bad days. If you find yourself dwelling endlessly on "what if…?" (…I get worse,…I can't walk,…I can't see,…I can't do my job), it may be helpful and reassuring to do some advance problem solving. Think through how you would deal with these changes, make contingency plans, and look into available resources. Some people find it very comforting to know that they have strategies in mind to deal with possible problems. Allowing yourself to think through the unthinkable can enable you to feel more prepared and more in control over whatever the future brings.

SINCE MY DIAGNOSIS, MY HUSBAND HAS BEGUN TO HOVER OVER ME ALL THE TIME. I KNOW HE'S WORRIED ABOUT ME, BUT I FEEL AS THOUGH I'VE TOTALLY LOST MY INDEPENDENCE. HOW CAN I EXPLAIN TO HIM THAT I NEED TO LEARN HOW TO LIVE WITH MY MS IN MY OWN WAY?

Each of you will need to learn to live with MS in your own way. At the same time that you are learning to cope with the varied and unpredictable symptoms of MS, your husband will be adjusting to his own feelings about the illness and its impact on your daily life. Your husband's protectiveness is a sign of his anxiety about your health and safety, as well as about your future together. Describe your symptoms to him so that he can understand how you are feeling. While explaining to your husband how much you value your independence, you can assure him that you will use caution and good sense, and that you will ask him for help when you need it. Invite him to come with you to visit your physician so that he can hear what the doctor has to say and ask any questions about the illness. Your physician will be able to offer reassurance and reinforce your need to be as independent as possible.

You and your husband may find it helpful to join a couples' support group. In this setting, each of you can learn from others how they have coped with the impact of MS on family life. Your husband might also enjoy a spouse group in which he can share his feelings and concerns with other husbands and wives whose partners have MS.

MY WIFE WAS JUST DIAGNOSED WITH MS. SHE KEEPS GIVING ME ARTICLES TO READ AND INSISTS I GO TO THE DOCTOR WITH HER. ALL HER SYMPTOMS HAVE GONE AWAY. WHY CAN'T WE JUST FORGET ABOUT THIS FOR NOW AND GET ON WITH OUR LIVES?

Being diagnosed with a chronic illness can be a very frightening and lonely experience. Your wife is trying to learn as much as she can about MS so that she will feel less afraid and more prepared to cope with it as time goes on. She may be asking you to share the learning process with her so that she does not feel so alone. Although MS is an unexpected intrusion in both your lives, you may have very different styles of coping with it. While talking and reading a lot about MS helps her to feel better, the same strategies might make you feel worse! The more she tries to get you to talk or think about MS, the more you will struggle to put it out of your mind. It is important to talk to each other about your different coping styles. One style is not necessarily better than the other, but she may misinterpret your reluctance to read or talk about her MS as not caring about her or her feelings. Try to reassure her, while at the same time explaining that you need to deal with her illness in your own way. Perhaps you can reach a compromise that satisfies both her need for your support and your need to focus on other things in your life.

I USED TO DEAL WITH LIFE'S FRUSTRATIONS BY EXERCISING AND PLAYING A LOT OF SPORTS. NOW THAT I'M NOT ABLE TO BE AS ACTIVE AS I USED TO BE, I'M HAVING TROUBLE DEALING WITH THE PENT-UP FEELINGS. HOW CAN I FIND OTHER OUTLETS THAT WORK FOR ME?

Most people who play a lot of sports derive satisfaction from both the physical exertion and the competition. If your primary satisfaction from sports is the exertion itself, talk to your doctor about alternative forms of exercise that might be suitable for you, such as tai chi, yoga, swimming, weight training, or a stationary bike (see Chapter 9). If what you miss most is the competitive aspect of sports, explore other forms of competition such as competitive bridge, chess, or computer games. Then remember that another way to release pent-up feelings is to talk about them. In the past, it may never have been your style to talk about feelings, but you may find at this point in your life that talking—whether it be with a spouse, a friend, or in a support group—is a satisfying relief.

SINCE MY HUSBAND WAS DIAGNOSED WITH MS A FEW MONTHS AGO, IT'S ALL HE THINKS AND TALKS ABOUT. IT SEEMS AS THOUGH OUR WHOLE FAMILY HAS BEEN TAKEN OVER BY THIS DISEASE. IS THIS NORMAL?

While each individual reacts to the MS diagnosis somewhat differently, it is not uncommon for a person to react initially by being quite preoccupied with the illness. One person might show this preoccupation by being totally unwilling to think or talk about any aspect of MS, as if ignoring it will make it go away. Another person shows the preoccupation by talking and thinking about MS to the exclusion of everything else. Whether or not they are currently experiencing symptoms, each is aware of a new and threatening problem over which he or she has very little control. Both these individuals are trying to come to terms with a diagnosis that changes the way they think about themselves, their lives, and the future.

A newly diagnosed person's preoccupation with MS can be very difficult for family members. Your husband may be experiencing a variety of strange and uncomfortable symptoms that you are unable to see or understand. At the same time that he is trying to deal with MS, you are trying to cope with your own feelings about it as well as everything else that is going on in the household. Although his feelings and concerns may be quite normal, it is still important for him to understand how his behavior affects other family members. Try to talk to him about your feelings. Ask him about going to a support group for the newly diagnosed. If, in another month or two, your husband still seems overly preoccupied with the MS, ask him if he would go with you to a therapist to talk about the impact of MS on the entire family.

I'VE BEEN HAVING A PRETTY HARD TIME ADJUSTING TO THE MS AND ALL THE CHANGES IT HAS CAUSED IN MY LIFE. MY DOCTOR SUGGESTED THAT I MIGHT WANT TO GET COUNSELING TO DEAL WITH SOME OF MY FEELINGS, BUT I'VE NEVER NEEDED THERAPY BEFORE, AND I DON'T SEE HOW IT COULD HELP ME NOW.

Your physician knows that being diagnosed with a chronic disease is a stressful and bewildering intrusion in any person's life. In short-term, problem-focused psychotherapy, a therapist who is knowledgeable about MS can help you understand and cope with your reactions to this intrusion (call the National MS Society at 800-FIGHT-MS [800-344-3867] for a referral). First, the therapist can help you work through the normal grief reaction that comes from having to alter your self-image to include a chronic illness. Second, he or she can provide you with a relaxed setting in which to ask questions and explore your options; most people find it very difficult to think of all their questions and concerns in the short time spent with the physician. The therapist can help you integrate the information you are receiving from your physician and sort through the advice and reactions of well-meaning friends and relatives. Coping with MS is an ongoing process that ebbs and flows with the changes that the disease causes in your life. As the MS follows its unpredictable course, you may find it useful to maintain intermittent contact with a therapist who can serve as a familiar resource whenever new symptoms add further stress and challenge at home or at work.

MY DOCTOR PRESCRIBED ONE OF THE INJECTABLE TREATMENTS FOR ME, TO SLOW DISEASE PROGRESSION, BUT I'M FINDING IT DIFFICULT TO CONTINUE TAKING IT. MY SYMPTOMS HAVE MOSTLY DISAPPEARED AND I'M TRYING TO FOCUS ON OTHER THINGS IN MY LIFE. GIVING MYSELF AN INJECTION IS A CONSTANT REMINDER OF THE MS, AND I FIND IT DEPRESSING.

This is a situation that is very much influenced by how you think about it. Your current view is that the injections are a reminder about your MS, something that you would rather not think about. Developing a different approach to the injections might help you see them in a different light. If you can look on the injections as something important you do to manage the disease, they may become much more acceptable. Recent studies have confirmed that irreversible damage to the *axons* can occur even in the earliest stages of MS, and it is this damage that is thought to cause irreversible disability. We also know that this underlying damage can occur in people who are not experiencing any symptoms. In other words, the disease may be active even though you are feeling fine. At present, the disease-modifying medications are the best available strategy for slowing the progression of the disease and preventing irreversible damage.

Keep in mind that you do have options in regard to medications. The injectable options vary in dosage as well as frequency and route of injection, and an oral option has also become available (see Chapter 6 for more information about treatment options). Work with your doctor to select the one that is most appropriate for your MS and your lifestyle. As you make these treatment decisions, try to imagine how you might feel down the road if you had not done everything you could to slow the progression of the MS. Will you feel better knowing that you did everything you could?

Adopting this new attitude may be something that you can do on your own, or you may benefit from working with a counselor or therapist to help you reformulate your thinking and get yourself into the habit of making the injection part of your usual routine. Many others with MS have faced the same issues that you are dealing with and have been successful in adjusting to their treatment regimen. Participation in a support group could provide you with a ready-made information network of others who have adjusted to this kind of treatment.

MY DOCTOR HAS PRESCRIBED ONE OF THE INJECTABLE DRUGS FOR ME, BUT I AM FINDING IT IMPOSSIBLE TO GIVE MYSELF THE SHOTS. I HAVE BEEN AFRAID OF NEEDLES MY WHOLE LIFE, AND THIS FEELS LIKE MY WORST NIGHTMARE. IS THERE ANYTHING I CAN DO ABOUT THIS FEAR OF MINE?

Please be assured that many people who have conditions that require injectable medication have been able to overcome the same kind of distress you are feeling. Medical personnel have worked with generations of people with diabetes—who may be required to take as many as three shots a day—overcome this needle phobia. The first thing you must do is tell your doctor or nurse about your fear and let them know that it is interfering with your ability to take the medicine. Based on that discussion, there are several different recommendations your health care provider may make to help you manage this.

- If the problem is your fear of needles in general, regardless of who is giving you the shot, it may be recommended that you work with a nurse or therapist who has specialized training to help people overcome their needle phobias. Two psychologists—David Mohr, PhD, and Darcy Cox, PhD—developed a six-session *self-injection anxiety training* for people to use with a health professional to overcome injection anxiety. You can find more information about this program on the National Multiple Sclerosis Society's Web site at http://www.nationalmssociety.org/SIAC.
- If your biggest difficulty is in giving yourself the injection, you could explore other options. Many people with MS, because of hand tremor, vision problems, or other symptoms, are not able to self-inject. In those situations, a family member or friend may give the shot. In other situations, the injections are administered in the doctor's office.
- If you are a candidate for the recently approved oral medication, your physician may offer that as an alternative.

The important thing to remember is that there are many possible solutions to this. Do not feel embarrassed or ashamed to discuss your fears with your health care providers. They can help develop a solution that matches your situation.

I'M FEELING OVERWHELMED AND CONFUSED BY THE CHOICES I NEED TO MAKE IN MY LIFE. EVERYONE'S GIVING ME DIFFERENT ADVICE—WHICH DRUG TO TAKE, WHAT TO DO ABOUT WORK, WHETHER TO HAVE A CHILD OR NOT—AND I CAN'T FIGURE OUT WHAT TO DO. ALL I KNOW IS, I DON'T WANT TO MAKE WRONG CHOICES.

The good news is that people with MS now have many options available to them that they never had before. It was not very many years ago that a person diagnosed with the disease was told that he or she would just have to go home and learn to live with it. There were no disease-modifying agents, women were told they should never have children, and both men and women were advised to quit their jobs and stay home and rest. In other words, people with MS had to live with the stress of having their choices and options taken away from them. Today's stresses are different. Now, people are being told by their physicians to make the choices that feel right for them, and they are worried about making a mistake. Fortunately, there are no right or wrong answers here. The "right" choice for one person may be the "wrong" choice for someone else. Let your choices be guided by your personal priorities and goals, keeping in mind that no one else can tell you what those should or should not be. Your best strategy for any important life decision is to:

- Think about what is important to you
- Gather as much information as you can from your physician, MS organizations, and other reliable resources such as those recommended in this book
- Seek counseling from people you trust and who have expertise in the field of MS
- Talk to others who have faced similar decisions—perhaps in an MS support group or via the Internet

Then choose the option that best meets your needs and fits with your lifestyle. Whatever choices you make, keep in mind that many resources are available to help you pursue your goals. There is no need to "go it alone."

I'M TRYING TO LEARN AS MUCH AS I CAN ABOUT MS, BUT I'M FEELING OVERWHELMED BY THE QUANTITY OF INFORMATION THAT'S OUT THERE. WITH ALL THE WRITTEN MATERIAL, WEB SITES, BLOGS, AND THE SOCIAL MEDIA, HOW DO I KNOW WHERE TO LOOK?

"Information overload" is becoming more of an issue for all of us, and sorting through the available information about MS can be particularly challenging. It will help you to begin by thinking about some of the different types of information that are available to you. Examples include information from your doctor and other members of your health care team; information written by MS specialists or MS organizations who rely on peer-reviewed data and expert opinion for their content; personal or "anecdotal" information from individuals living with MS; marketing information that is designed to sell you a product or service. Each of these types of information can be very useful to you; the key is to recognize and remember which type it is as you evaluate its relevance for you. For example, a friend's experience with a particular MS treatment may be very interesting but it is only one person's experience, and may differ significantly from your own and other people's experiences. Information about that treatment from your physician or one of the MS organizations is based on data from large numbers of people in controlled clinical trials (see Chapter 5 for information about clinical trials). Information from the company that manufactured the treatment is also based on published data, but contains marketing messaging that is designed to make you want to pick that treatment over others. As long as you are mindful of the source of the information, you can use your judgment about its relevance for you, and if you have questions about anything you read or hear, it is always a good idea to check it out with your neurologist or call the National MS Society (800-344-4867) for more information.

I'VE DONE EVERYTHING MY DOCTOR HAS TOLD ME TO DO, AND MY MS STILL SEEMS TO BE GETTING WORSE. WHAT AM I DOING WRONG—AM I JUST NOT TRYING HARD ENOUGH?

Unfortunately, we still do not know of any way to stop MS in its tracks. Sometimes, in spite of everyone's best efforts—including yours and your doctor's—the disease continues to progress. When this happens, people have a tendency to look for someone to blame. They may blame themselves for not trying hard enough, for not taking the "right" medicine, for choosing the "wrong" doctor, or for having too much stress in their lives. Or they may blame their doctor, their boss, their family members, or God. The fact is, however, that MS seems to have a mind of its own. The best strategy when MS progresses despite whatever treatment you are using is to consult with an MS specialist *neurologist*—preferably at a comprehensive MS center—to find out about any other treatment strategies that might be reasonable for you to try. The National Multiple Sclerosis Society can give you the names of specialists in your area.

RECOMMENDED READINGS

....

Blackstone M. *The First Year—Multiple Sclerosis: An Essential Guide for the Newly Diagnosed.* New York: Marlowe and Co., 2003.

Cohen R. *Blindsided—Living a Life Above Illness: A Reluctant Memoir.* New York: Harper Collins, 2004.

Farrell P. *It's Not All in Your Head: Anxiety, Depression, and Mood Swings in MS.* New York: Demos Medical Publishing, 2010.

Garr T (with H. Mantel). *Speedbumps: Flooring It through Hollywood.* New York: Hudson Street Press, 2005.

Holland N, Murray TJ, Reingold SC. *Multiple Sclerosis: A Guide for the Newly Diagnosed.* 3rd ed. New York: Demos Medical Publishing, 2007.

Kalb R. (ed.). *Multiple Sclerosis: A Guide for Families.* 3rd ed. New York: Demos Medical Publishing, 2006.

Kalb R, Holland N, Giesser B. *Multiple Sclerosis for Dummies.* Hoboken, NJ: Wiley, 2007.

Lander DL. *Fall Down Laughing: How Squiggy Caught Multiple Sclerosis and Didn't Tell Nobody.* New York: Tarcher/Putnam, 2000.

Pitzele S. *We Are Not Alone: Learning to Live with Chronic Illness.* New York: Workman Publishing, 1986.

Selected publications available from the National Multiple Sclerosis Society (800-FIGHT-MS; 800-344-4867) or online at http://www.nationalmssociety.org/Brochures:
- *Disclosure: The Basic Facts*
- *Living with MS*

Selected pages on the National Multiple Sclerosis Society Web site:
- *For people who are newly diagnosed—http://www.nationalmssociety.org/Newly Diagnosed*

RECOMMENDED RESOURCES

....

Knowledge is power: A six-week, learn-at-home program for people with a recent diagnosis of MS. Available in hard copy or by e-mail from the National Multiple Sclerosis Society (http://www.nationalmssociety.org/KIP).

Self-injection anxiety counseling: The SIAC Patient Workbook and Counselor Manual for the six-session program is available in PDF format at http://www.nationalmssociety.org/siac.asp. The materials can also be requested by your health professional from the National Multiple Sclerosis Society's Professional Resource Center at healthprof_info@nmss.org.

Social networking opportunities: The National MS Society invites you to Facebook, Twitter, MS Friends, and other options at www.nationalmssociety.org/onlinecommunity.

Emotional Changes and the Role of Stress

Nicholas G. LaRocca, PhD

Stress is no stranger to people with multiple sclerosis (MS). In fact, many of those living with the disease believe that stress may be one of the precipitating factors in the onset of MS and its progression. Although research has provided mixed evidence concerning this belief, there is no doubt that MS creates significant stress in people's lives.

Life's stresses are primarily of two types. The first is caused by major events or changes that require significant adjustment. Such stressful life events might include the loss of one's job, the birth of a new child, or the diagnosis of a disabling illness. The other type of stress, aptly termed "hassles" by some, consists of the pressures of everyday life. While these daily hassles do not call upon us to make major changes in our lives, they are still emotionally taxing. Examples of this type of stress might include fighting rush hour traffic, paying bills, or dealing with children's homework. While everyone is subject to both types of stress, having MS seems to make both types of stress feel more burdensome.

Since stress is so much a part of life with MS, it is not surprising that people report significant emotional distress. It is safe to say that adjusting to something as unpredictable and potentially disabling as MS may entail quite a bit of emotional turmoil. To experience such distress and turmoil from time to time is therefore a natural and normal reaction.

People often look for a road map to guide them in their adjustment to MS and are disappointed to find that none exists. Unlike terminal illness, in which a person's adjustment may follow a fairly consistent set of emotional "stages," adapting to life with MS follows no fixed pattern. It is impossible to map out predictable "stages" of adjustment because the disease can vary so much in the types of *symptoms* it presents and its speed of progression. However, significant emotional issues are likely to arise intermittently over the course of the illness:

- *Uncertainty* may be the first emotional challenge faced by people with MS. It begins with the initial mysterious symptom of MS, be it fleeting ***optic neuritis***, intermittent numbness, or a fall. When symptoms first appear, the person believes that something is wrong but is uncertain what it might be. Months or years may go by before a diagnosis is established, during which time uncertainty breeds a lingering feeling of anxiety. Uncertainty remains even after the diagnosis has been made. Will the symptoms get worse? Will new symptoms appear? How long will walking be possible? Will working become impossible? Creating a sense of security in one's life in the face of such uncertainty is a significant and lifelong challenge.

- *Accepting the reality* of having a ***chronic***, disabling illness is not a simple matter. Most people with MS will say that they have never really "accepted" it, any more than they would "accept" living in the middle of a battlefield. People sometimes feel a sense of relief when the diagnosis is first pronounced, simply because some of the uncertainty is resolved and many of their questions have finally been answered. However, a sense of shock and disbelief often follows—a state that may be prolonged by a person's inability or unwillingness to acknowledge what has happened. For most, this reaction is short-lived, and the reality of the diagnosis is eventually recognized even though it may never be "accepted." This recognition is an important first step toward finding ways to adapt to the presence of MS in one's life.

- *Grief* often ensues as the reality of the diagnosis sinks in. The person grieves for his or her lost sense of self (see Chapter 15). Most people think of themselves as invulnerable to disease and take for granted their physical and intellectual abilities. A chronic, disabling illness robs people of this old sense of self and may also compromise many of those physical and intellectual abilities. As people mourn these losses, they are forced to reformulate their expectations for themselves and the future.

- *Self-image* is likely to go through a transition. The person slowly and painfully lets go of the old sense of self and works gradually to build a new one that incorporates the limitations and constraints brought about by the MS (see Chapter 15).

- *Adaptation* occurs as people with MS and their families make specific changes in their life patterns in response to the disease. Such adaptation may involve using mobility aids or other forms of assistive technology, changing jobs, swapping roles within the household, making alterations in the house, and giving up certain physical activities.

- *Re-emergence* eventually occurs as people make the necessary changes in their lives. The disease may occupy a great deal of attention and effort at the time of diagnosis and during subsequent ***exacerbations***. During periods of stability, people may find that they can pay less attention to the disease and more to the business of living.

Adjustment to MS takes time. Moreover, since the disease can wax and wane, many people find that they have to adjust over and over again. They may go through a grieving process each time new disabilities appear. Because of the changeable nature of MS, people may experience dramatic fluctuations in their emotional state. They may plunge into a severe depression when a bad exacerbation begins and experience joy and relief with the onset of ***remission***. Living through this emotional roller coaster is one of the most significant challenges of MS.

Adjustment to MS is as complex as it is slow. Many factors may influence how a person copes with the illness, including disease course, personality and coping style, the availability of social supports and financial resources, and other concurrent life stresses. A very important factor influencing adjustment is one's self-appraisal. People who view themselves as ineffectual and powerless are likely to adjust differently—and less comfortably—than those who view themselves as effective and able to manage what life brings them.

EMOTIONAL ASPECTS OF MS

HOW COMMON IS DEPRESSION IN MS?

One answer to this question depends in part on what you mean by "depression." People tend to use the term casually to describe many different feelings. Everyone feels distressed, demoralized, and "down in the dumps" from time to time. When we feel that way, we say we are "depressed." However, technically, we are simply experiencing the generalized psychological distress that is a standard part of living. If this generalized state of sadness and distress is fairly constant and continues for years, it is known as *chronic dysphoria* (or *dysthymic disorder*) and probably warrants professional treatment. People may also refer to themselves as "depressed" when they are actually grieving about the loss of someone or something that is important to them. MS can bring about significant losses in people's lives, including the loss of certain abilities, expectations for the future, and employment. As a result, most people with MS go through a grieving process that may be repeated many times over the course of the illness as new losses occur.

A true depression, referred to as "clinical depression" or a "major depressive episode," is characterized by sadness that is severe and unremitting, along with a variety of other symptoms such as low self-esteem, sleep disturbance, changes in appetite, hopelessness, and sometimes suicidal thoughts. There is ample evidence that, compared to the general population, people with MS are at greater risk for depression. It has been estimated that, at any given time, one out of every seven people with MS is experiencing a major depression. Approximately 50 percent of people with MS will experience a major depressive episode during the course of their illness, compared to 5 to 15 percent in the general population.

The diagnosis of depression is complex and requires a very specific set of symptoms, along with an equally specific time frame in order for the diagnostic criteria to be met. One challenge to diagnosing depression in people with MS is that many of the symptoms of depression can easily be confused with MS symptoms and effects. For example, the symptoms of depression include fatigue, sleep disturbance, and difficulty concentrating. These symptoms are often part of the MS picture as well. It can thus be very tricky to diagnose a major depressive episode in a person with MS.

Keeping the above in mind, it is important to remember that MS is a psychologically challenging condition. People with MS are at greater risk than the general population for a variety of emotional complications. Those who deal with MS, either their own or someone else's, must be alert to the potential need for help, especially professional help. For the sake of clarity in the remainder of the chapter, the term *depression* will be used to distinguish the more severe major depressive episode or chronic dysphoria from the relatively common, episodic feelings of distress and discouragement that most people experience from time to time.

WHY DO SOME PEOPLE WITH MS GET SEVERELY DEPRESSED WHILE OTHERS DO NOT?

The intensity of a person's reactions seems to depend on a variety of factors in addition to the severity of the disease itself, including personality style and coping skills, availability of social supports, financial security, and genetic predisposition to depression. In addition, evidence suggests that depression in MS is related to *demyelination* in certain parts of the brain that play a role in the experience or expression of emotions, and to changes in the immune system. Therefore, disease severity is by no means the only or most reliable predictor of a person's emotional response. A person with less disabling disease may develop a severe depression, whereas one with greater disability may not.

IF DEPRESSION IN MS IS CAUSED BY DEMYELINATION IN THE BRAIN, WHAT WOULD BE THE POINT OF PSYCHOTHERAPY OR ANTIDEPRESSANT MEDICATION TO TREAT IT?

Demyelination as a cause of depression in MS is still the subject of intense study. One study, for example, found that, compared to people with MS who were not depressed, those who were depressed showed greater *lesion* volume in certain areas of the brain and more brain tissue loss on magnetic resonance imaging (MRI). Other studies have found a relationship between depression and either lesion volume or tissue loss, but these relationships have generally been very weak. Other types of studies have been tantalizing but inconclusive. For example, tentative evidence suggests that some persons with MS show a dysfunction in *glucocorticoids*, brain substances that play a role in regulating certain of the hormones involved in moods. One study found that both affective disturbances and neuroendocrine abnormalities were related to white cell counts in the *cerebrospinal fluid* and to *gadolinium-enhancing lesions* on MRI. Another study found that improvement in self-reported depression was related to a drop in levels of *interferon*-gamma (a naturally appearing substance that is thought by some to be associated with exacerbations of MS). One small study found that blood flow in the limbic *cortex* (an area of the brain thought to be involved in emotions) differed between depressed and nondepressed persons with MS.

MS has wide-ranging effects on the brain. It would therefore not be surprising if future research confirmed that MS-related changes in the brain play a major role in depression. Even if MS does involve such a "direct" or "biologic" influence on mood, however, it is unlikely to be the only factor involved. Depression is a complex phenomenon and, in any given person, many factors are probably at work in determining the type and severity of depressive symptoms. Some of these factors might include one's appraisal of altered life circumstances, the availability of social support, inherited predisposition to affective disturbances, and life stress. Since it is a complex problem, depression demands a sophisticated response. Even if the causes of depression involve biologic changes in the brain, psychotherapy and medication can still help to alter mood and assist people in dealing with these and other MS-related changes. Research to date has shown that both psychotherapy and medication can be effective in treating MS-related depression. As we refine our understanding of this problem, we will be able to develop increasingly effective, multifaceted treatments.

HOW CAN I TELL IF I'M HAVING A NORMAL REACTION TO BEING DIAGNOSED WITH A CHRONIC ILLNESS, OR IF I HAVE A SERIOUS DEPRESSION?
Almost everyone reacts negatively to being diagnosed with a disabling illness. Reactions may include shock, disbelief, anger, anxiety, sadness, grief, pessimism about the future, and loss of self-esteem. These reactions can at times become fairly intense and may be difficult to distinguish from depression.

However, depression does have some distinguishing characteristics. Serious clinical depression consists of more than just feeling down in the dumps. The feelings of sadness and/or irritability tend to be constant, with little or no relief for days or weeks at a time. People who are depressed may lose interest in most of the things that used to be enjoyable, such as hobbies, visiting friends, reading, work-related projects, and sexual activity. They may experience loss of appetite or gradually begin eating much more than usual. Sleep may be disturbed by early morning awakening, or they may begin wanting to sleep longer or more frequently. Depression can include feelings of worthlessness and self-blame for everything that seems to be going wrong. Individuals who are depressed may also feel guilty without knowing why, as if they had done something horrible that must be punished. A depressed person's thoughts and actions may be slowed, and behavior may appear listless. However, unlike those who are simply suffering from MS fatigue, people who are depressed do not really care about feeling listless because they are not interested in doing anything. The person who is depressed may also be plagued by thoughts of death and even suicide.

In contrast to this devastating picture of clinical depression, the reaction to having a chronic illness tends to be less severe and not as broad in its effects. For example, individuals who are reacting to MS may also feel downhearted, blue, and pessimistic, but can still be interested in life activities and forget their troubles long enough to take care of their responsibilities and engage in things they enjoy. The person who is learning to live with MS may struggle with an altered self-image that includes newly acquired limitations, without necessarily feeling useless or worthless. Thoughts of suicide are less likely to arise.

It is important to keep in mind that there can be considerable overlap at times between the "ordinary reaction" to chronic illness and a serious depression. Most people are likely to experience something in-between—a reaction to MS that occasionally has some of the characteristics of depression. Consultation with a mental health professional with experience in MS or chronic illness can help you to clarify the issues involved and identify the most useful form of treatment.

I WAS DIAGNOSED WITH MS ABOUT A YEAR AGO, AND SO FAR I SEEM TO HAVE DONE PRETTY WELL COMPARED TO SOME. I CAN'T RUN ANYMORE AND MY ENDURANCE IS LOW, BUT OTHERWISE I HAVE FEW PROBLEMS. I THINK THAT I SHOULD BE GRATEFUL THAT MY MS IS SO MILD, BUT INSTEAD I FEEL DEPRESSED. WHY SHOULD I FEEL DEPRESSED IF I'M DOING SO WELL?
There is no simple relationship between a person's physical symptoms or limitations and how well he or she feels emotionally. MS is generally progressive and can lead to increasing disability. Even though you say you are doing "pretty well," you still have

lost some physical abilities. For many people, this initial loss, no matter how mild it may seem, can be the most emotionally challenging. Everyone reacts differently to the physical changes brought on by MS. However, it has been consistently observed that the first few years after the diagnosis are often the toughest. During those early years, people are still processing the sudden shift that has taken place in their expectations for the years ahead. Most of us anticipate good health and intact physical abilities for the foreseeable future. A diagnosis of MS undermines these expectations, even if the changes have not as yet taken place. An added burden for many is a sense of guilt because they are doing well but still feel upset about having MS. For most people, these feelings slowly subside as they get used to having MS in their lives. Moreover, many find that having gone through this initial distress helps to prepare them should the MS lead to other changes in the future.

I CAN'T TELL IF I'M TIRED ALL THE TIME BECAUSE I'M DEPRESSED, OR DEPRESSED BECAUSE I'M ALWAYS TIRED. WHO CAN HELP ME FIND THE ANSWER TO THIS QUESTION?
Depression is often accompanied by a feeling of listlessness and/or a lack of interest in everyday activities. On the other hand, people who experience MS fatigue often feel "down" because they are not able to do the things they would like to do. It is not always easy to separate depression from an intense feeling of fatigue; however, people who have experienced both usually report that they feel quite different. You are probably not depressed if you are frustrated because your fatigue prevents you from getting your chores done and enjoying your hobbies and social life. However, you could well be clinically depressed if you wake up in the morning feeling tired, and find you don't really care if you get anything done or not.

Distinguishing between depression and MS-related fatigue can be difficult, especially because the two can coexist. It is important to have an accurate assessment because the treatments for clinical depression and fatigue are quite different. Consultation with your *neurologist* in conjunction with a psychiatrist or psychologist can help to identify the exact nature of the problem. Depression is treated most effectively with psychotherapy and/or medication. Exercise has also been shown to improve mood in people with MS. Fatigue is usually treated with medications such as Symmetrel (amantadine), Provigil (modafinil), or Nuvigil (armodafinil) see Appendix B—and by energy conservation measures such as schedule changes, naps, and the use of adaptive equipment. Keep in mind, however, that depression and fatigue can occur in the same person and may both need to be addressed.

WHAT IS THE BEST TREATMENT FOR DEPRESSION IN A PERSON WHO HAS MS?
Appropriate treatment requires identification of the exact nature and severity of the depression. The two major approaches to the treatment of depression are psychotherapy and medication. Psychotherapy is generally conducted individually (although it can be done in groups) by a qualified psychiatrist, psychologist, social worker, or counselor. Support groups and peer counseling may be a useful addition to treatment but are not a substitute for psychotherapy (see Chapter 15 for more information about support groups). Research has shown that certain types of psychotherapy can improve depression in MS, sometimes in just a few weeks. However, psychotherapy

generally requires several months to achieve substantial results. While there are many different approaches to psychotherapy, the important factor seems to be the ability of the therapist and the therapist–patient relationship.

Many people find that a combination of psychotherapy and medication works well; the medication helps to elevate mood while the therapy provides a supportive setting in which to explore feelings and learn more effective coping strategies.

Anecdotal reports indicate that a variety of medications have been used successfully to treat depression in MS, although research on this issue is very limited. For many years, tricyclic antidepressants such as Tofranil (imipramine), Elavil (amitriptyline), and Pamelor (nortriptyline) were the treatment of choice. In recent years, however, the serotonergic antidepressants, such as Prozac (fluoxetine), Zoloft (sertraline), Paxil (paroxetine), and Effexor (venlafaxine), have become more widely used (see Appendix B). A number of other antidepressants have been used less frequently in MS that are neither tricyclics nor serotonergic. These include Wellbutrin (bupropion HCl), Serzone (nefazodone), and Desyrel (trazodone). Each of these medications has a slightly different side effect profile. Because no two people are exactly alike in the side effects they experience, one or another of these drugs may be preferable for a given person.

These medications should be administered under the supervision of a psychiatrist who can monitor your progress and adjust the dosage as needed. It generally takes at least 4 to 6 weeks to determine if a particular medication is effective. A medication may need to be gradually increased, or combined with other medication(s) to achieve maximal treatment effects. In a study at the University of California at San Francisco, it was determined that people with MS may need as much as three times the minimal recommended dose to obtain complete relief from their depressive symptoms.

In some instances, electroshock therapy (ECT) can be very effective although there is some evidence that ECT can increase a person's risk of having an exacerbation. In rare instances in which episodes of depression alternate with periods of elevated mood and hyperactivity, a mood stabilizing drug such as Depakote (divalproex sodium), Eskalith (lithium carbonate), or Tegretol (carbamazepine) may be used in addition to or instead of an antidepressant. Whatever you are experiencing, you need not suffer alone. Getting help is a constructive and active coping strategy. It does not imply weakness or giving up. Quite the contrary, it means that you are determined to confront the emotional challenges of life with MS.

I HAVE HAD MS FOR 7 YEARS. I THINK THAT I HAVE BEEN DEPRESSED ON AND OFF MUCH OF THAT TIME. MY DOCTOR NEVER ASKED ME ABOUT MY MOOD, AND I NEVER THOUGHT I NEEDED ANY TREATMENT. RECENTLY, AT MY WIFE'S URGING, I SAW A SOCIAL WORKER WHO REFERRED ME TO A PSYCHIATRIST. I HAVE BEEN TAKING AN ANTIDEPRESSANT FOR ABOUT TWO MONTHS NOW AND SEEING THE SOCIAL WORKER ONCE A WEEK. I FEEL LIKE A NEW PERSON. IS MY EXPERIENCE COMMON?

Unfortunately, your experience is all too common. One study found that, in a sample of persons moderately disabled by MS, 80 percent had experienced a psychiatric disorder during the past year but only 60 percent had received any form of psychiatric treatment. Another study found that 26 percent of people with MS being treated by neurologists in a managed care setting met criteria for a major depressive episode, but that 66 percent of these were receiving no antidepressant medication and an additional 5 percent were receiving inadequate doses. There seem to be several reasons for this. People with MS are generally followed by neurologists, whose primary focus may be on the physical aspects of the disease. In addition, many neurologists tend to assume that a person's more general medical needs (e.g., mood disorders, gynecological problems, high blood pressure) are being addressed by a primary care physician. People with MS may also assume that feeling a little depressed is simply their lot in life, to be endured with the rest of their symptoms or problems. As you have seen, however, one does not necessarily have to go through life feeling chronically depressed. Help is available. If the doctor doesn't ask about mood, the person with MS should bring up the subject.

SOME OF MY FRIENDS WITHOUT MS HAVE BEEN TAKING ST. JOHN'S WORT FOR DEPRESSION, AND THEY TELL ME THAT IT WORKS WELL AND HAS NO SIDE EFFECTS. I HAVE MILD BOUTS OF DEPRESSION THAT OFTEN LAST FOR A FEW WEEKS. SHOULD I CONSIDER ST. JOHN'S WORT?

St. John's wort is not considered a safe or effective treatment for depression. It is an extract of a flower that grows wild in many countries, and it has been used medicinally for centuries. The active ingredient is *hypericum*. St. John's wort is currently available in drug and health food stores in the form of capsules and tea. These products vary widely in purity, consistency, and the amount of hypericum they contain.

In numerous European trials over the years, hypericum was found to be about equal in effectiveness to the tricyclic antidepressants in treating mild to moderate depression, with few side effects. No comparisons were made in the European studies to the serotonergic antidepressants (e.g., Prozac and Zoloft). Because of the growing interest in St. John's wort in the United States, and numerous scientific flaws identified in the European studies, a large-scale U.S. study was funded jointly by the National Center for Complementary and Alternative Medicine, the National Institutes of Health, and the Office of Dietary Supplements. This controlled study found hypericum to be no more effective than placebo for the treatment of major depression of moderate severity.

In two additional studies, hypericum was found to interact negatively with several drugs used in AIDS and organ transplant patients. Hypericum apparently increases the activity of the liver enzymes that metabolize and inactivate the drugs, lowering effective blood levels. In the case of the AIDS drug Crixivan (indinavir), hypericum standardized extracts at a dose of 300 mg three times a day lowered blood levels by 57 to 82 percent, rendering the indinavir therapeutically ineffective. In two patients with heart transplants, hypericum extracts in the same dosage reduced circulating levels of the anti-rejection drug cyclosporin to the point that both patients began to reject the transplanted heart. Hypericum had reduced circulating cyclosporin levels to approximately 50 to 70 percent of their pre-hypericum levels within 2 weeks.

The most serious risk associated with St. John's wort, however, is that a person's clinical depression will be inadequately treated. A person who fails to find relief from depressive symptoms may come to believe that no help is available. The best strategy for dealing with depressive feelings is to have them evaluated and treated by a psychiatrist or psychologist.

MY FRIENDS AND RELATIVES HAVE BEGUN TO NOTICE HOW NERVOUS I AM LATELY. I DON'T REMEMBER EVER FEELING THIS ANXIOUS BEFORE IN MY LIFE. WHAT IS THE BEST TREATMENT FOR ANXIETY IN MS?

A number of anti-anxiety medications such as Valium (diazepam) and Xanax (alprazolam) are classified as benzodiazepines. Because these medications (particularly Xanax) can be associated with physical and psychological dependence, they should generally be used on a short-term basis and only if other strategies such as psychotherapy have not completely resolved the problem. Recently, the U.S. Food and Drug Administration (FDA) has extended the approval of several antidepressant medications—Zoloft (sertraline), Paxil (paroxetine), Effexor (venlafaxine)—to include the treatment of some types of anxiety. No controlled *clinical trials* of these drugs have been performed in MS, so their use in this disease is based on clinical experience and studies done in other populations.

Anxiety almost always can be traced back to life circumstances. Everyday stresses, worry about the future, and financial strain can all precipitate or worsen anxiety. It may be helpful to try to identify the sources of your anxiety and evaluate your current way of handling these difficult circumstances. This can best be done through psychotherapy, counseling, or stress management training with a professional. It is often possible to reduce anxiety through a better understanding of its sources and by altering one's approach to dealing with it. Medication can at times facilitate this process by reducing anxiety to a more manageable level. However, the long-term goal is to be able to deal with the sources of anxiety without having to rely on medication.

CAN ANY OF THE MEDICATIONS I'M TAKING FOR MY MS AFFECT MY MOOD?

Yes, many of the medications used in MS can affect your mood (see Appendix B). Space does not permit a discussion of all of them, but here are some of the more important ones:

- Antidepressants are sometimes used to treat bladder problems and unpleasant sensory symptoms, generally in doses lower than those used to treat depression. However, some people find that the antidepressants may improve their mood even in these low doses.

- Valium (diazepam) is a benzodiazepine (a class of tranquilizers) that is sometimes used to treat *spasticity* (see Chapter 4). Valium may make you feel more relaxed both physically and psychologically.

- Lioresal (baclofen) is the drug most commonly used to treat spasticity in MS. When treatment is started, many people feel drowsy until their bodies get used to the drug. However, a more dramatic side effect may occur if you abruptly stop taking it, especially if you are on a very high dose. Stopping a high dose of Lioresal abruptly may cause you to experience extreme symptoms such as hallucinations (seeing or hearing things while awake that are not there), agitation or restlessness, convulsions, or mood changes. It is therefore important not to cease taking this medication abruptly, but to taper the dosage.

- *Corticosteroids* (also referred to as *steroids*) that are used to treat MS exacerbations can produce a variety of mood alterations. Some people become depressed on steroids while others become happy, euphoric, irritable, or hyperactive. This steroid "high" is often followed by a "low" when treatment ends. Individuals react differently to steroids. Moreover, the same person may have different reactions at different times. In other words, just because steroids gave you a "high" the last time you had them does not necessarily mean that you will have the same experience the next time. People who have a history of extreme reactions to steroids are sometimes treated in advance with mood-stabilizing drugs such as Eskalith (lithium carbonate), Depakote (divalproex sodium), or Tegretol (carbamazepine) to prevent these wide and upsetting swings. It is important to work closely with your physician when you are treated with steroids and to report promptly any unusual reactions (see Appendix B).

WILL I EVER STOP FEELING ANGRY AND SAD ALL THE TIME?

Many people with MS go through periods when they feel acutely and persistently distressed. This often happens when the disease is first diagnosed and when symptom flare-ups cause greater disability. At times like these, the disease (and your feelings about it) seems to fill your life, crowding out other thoughts and feelings. Most people find this to be a temporary experience. You will probably find your distress becoming less acute as you begin to get used to having MS and learn how to make a place for it in your life. This will gradually allow more space for other emotions to return. MS will no longer occupy your total attention, and you will once again become interested in your work, family, social life, and hobbies.

If you remain persistently sad and angry, despite the passage of time and despite improvement or stability in your symptoms, you probably need to seek professional help. A knowledgeable mental health professional can help you determine whether you need some psychotherapy or medication to help you get through these feelings. If and when the MS flares up, you may find that the disease once again becomes an all-encompassing emotional preoccupation. These periods of intense distress followed by relative calm are not uncommon in MS. Because of this, many people with MS find that they benefit from brief psychotherapy at several points in the course of their lives. When things get tough, they may return to therapy for a "tune-up." Adjustment to MS is an ongoing and evolving experience, not a one-time happening.

I HAVE READ THAT SUICIDE IS VERY COMMON IN MS. IS THIS TRUE?

Although precise estimates vary, suicide is at least twice as common in MS as it is in the general population, and may be as much as seven times as common. Indeed, it is one of the major causes of death among people with MS. The reasons for this are complex. Suicide is most often associated with depression, and we know from research in this area that depression is more common in MS than in the general population or in other disabling illnesses. So, prompt diagnosis and adequate treatment of depression are very important for people living with MS.

However, suicide is generally more common among people with chronic, "incurable," debilitating illnesses. Many of the so-called "assisted suicides" that have been in the news have been individuals with MS. The disease can create the sorts of conditions (e.g., financial strain, family stress, isolation, overall deterioration in quality of life, and a bleak outlook for the future) in which suicide occurs. Suicide tends to result from feelings of hopelessness rather than just depression per se.

At present a great ethical debate is raging in the United States concerning suicide, particularly assisted suicide. Many believe that one has the right to choose to end one's life. Others believe that the desire to take one's own life is by definition a psychiatric condition against which the person must be protected by society. Tragically, many individuals take their own lives while in a state of depression and hopelessness that could have been successfully treated with psychotherapy and/or medication. Depression can make a person perceive their life situation as more hopeless than it really is. However, there are people who seem to choose suicide not as a result of the distortions attending depression, but as rational adults in full command of their faculties who see clearly what they want for themselves. The debate over suicide will continue and expand during the next few years. For a variety of reasons, MS will occupy an important place in that debate.

SINCE MY HUSBAND QUIT WORKING BECAUSE OF MS, HE SEEMS TO HAVE LOST INTEREST IN MOST OF THE THINGS THAT HE USED TO ENJOY. NOW HE JUST SITS IN FRONT OF THE TV ALL DAY DOING NOTHING. WHY IS THIS, AND WHAT CAN I DO TO HELP HIM?

Lack of motivation and failure to initiate activities can be symptoms of depression, but they can also occur when extensive demyelination occurs in important brain regions responsible for planning and initiating activities. Oftentimes, the family member is more distressed by this behavior than the person with MS. If your husband left work because of MS-related physical problems but his mind is still "sharp," he could well be depressed. Depression is fairly common following a major life change, such as leaving the workforce. If, on the other hand, he was having trouble performing his job due to changes in his cognitive function, or if you know that he has had an MRI that showed a lot of MS *plaques* (lesions) in the front part of his brain, his difficulty initiating activities may be due to structural changes in his brain rather than just a result of feeling discouraged.

In either case, you should discuss your concerns with both your husband and his neurologist. The neurologist can refer you to a *neuropsychologist* or neuropsychiatrist who, through a diagnostic interview and appropriate testing, can identify the likely cause of your husband's problem. If the cause is depression, treatment may involve psychotherapy, medications, or a combination of these. If the cause is neurologic damage caused by demyelination, recommendations may include setting up a daily schedule with activities appropriate to his level of function and making sure that he has the help he needs to get started and continue working on activities. Depending on your situation, this could be carried out at home, or you might want to look into having your husband get involved in a structured activity program at a clinic or community center. You will have a clearer idea of which solutions are likely to work best for both of you once you have a better sense of the cause of the problem.

MY HUSBAND SEEMS VERY MOODY AND IRRITABLE LATELY, WHICH MAKES HIM PRETTY DIFFICULT TO LIVE WITH. IS THIS CHANGE IN HIS MOOD CAUSED BY MS, AND IS THERE ANYTHING TO DO ABOUT IT?

The issue of moodiness is one of the most common mentioned by MS families. The disease causes structural changes in the brain that may increase the risk of abrupt changes in mood and emotional expression that can occur within minutes. Some mood changes may be caused by medications, especially high-dose steroids. Many people also feel moody or irritable in response to all the changes and losses that MS has created in their lives. And research has shown that depression in MS causes irritability. Regardless of the cause, abrupt changes in mood can make family life stressful and unpleasant for all concerned. It is important to seek professional consultation and treatment for this problem.

Depending on the cause, moodiness and irritability can be handled in different ways. Mood changes caused by high-dose corticosteroids should get better once the treatment has ended. For someone who has reacted strongly to steroids in the past, the physician may prescribe some preventive treatment such as Eskalith (lithium), Depakote (divalproex sodium), or Tegretol (carbamazepine) to diminish the reaction (see Chapter 6 for more information about treatment with corticosteroids). Mood changes related to frustration may be helped by psychotherapy and/or medication. Family therapy is often extremely useful, both to help family members understand the problem and to ensure that they are not inadvertently contributing to the deteriorating emotional climate within the family. Finally, if the moodiness or irritability last significantly longer (2 weeks or more) and are accompanied by symptoms of depression, treatment typically involves a combination of antidepressant medication and psychotherapy.

SOMETIMES MY WIFE STARTS LAUGHING OR CRYING FOR NO REASON. SOMETIMES SHE EVEN SEEMS TO BE DOING BOTH AT THE SAME TIME, EVEN WHEN THERE IS NOTHING FUNNY OR SAD GOING ON. SHE THINKS HER "WIRES ARE CROSSED." WHY IS THIS HAPPENING TO HER?

Your wife is probably experiencing what is known as ***pseudobulbar affect*** (PBA or uncontrollable laughing or crying), a condition in which episodes of laughing and crying occur with no obvious precipitating event. This condition was formerly thought to be caused by damage to some of the nerves passing through the medulla oblongata (a structure in the brainstem). The current thinking is that it is associated with lesions in the *limbic system*, a group of brain structures involved in emotional feeling and expression and structures connected with it. Recent attention has also focused on the possible role of lesions in the ***frontal lobes***. To date, research on this question has been inconclusive.

For a person with PBA, the laughing or crying is totally out of proportion—or even unrelated—to what the person is actually feeling. An episode of crying may thus begin even when the person is feeling rather happy or content; laughing might occur in a situation in which nothing is funny—such as a funeral, for example. Once these laughing or crying episodes begin, the person is often unable to stop them. This symptom requires patience and understanding on the part of family and friends. The bouts of laughing and crying can be misunderstood by others, who may be offended by what they consider to be inappropriate or embarrassing behavior.

In 2010, a medication called Neudexta (dextromethorphan/quinidine) was approved by the FDA for the treatment of PBA in MS and other neurological disorders. This medication is made from a combination of dextromethorphan and quinidine. Prior to the approval of Neudexta, PBA was generally treated with the tricyclic antidepressant amitriptyline or by a selective serotonin reuptake inhibitor antidepressant such as Prozac (fluoxetine).

Many people find that the experience becomes somewhat less frightening once they get used to the fact that these uncontrolled bouts are going to happen from time to time. Again, the understanding of others is a key part of dealing with this problem.

MY HUSBAND HAS GOTTEN DEPRESSED ABOUT ALL THE CHANGES IN OUR LIVES SINCE THE MS GOT WORSE. I'VE ASKED HIM TO SEE A PSYCHIATRIST, BUT HE SAYS HE'S NOT CRAZY AND ADAMANTLY REFUSES TO GO. WHAT SHOULD I DO? I'M REALLY WORRIED ABOUT HIM AND ABOUT OUR RELATIONSHIP.

Going to a psychiatrist or other mental health professional still carries an unjustified stigma for many. You might try pointing out to your husband that depression is one aspect of life with MS that can be effectively managed, and that is likely a result of the disease process itself as well as a reaction to it. If it is okay to seek help for problems with walking or vision, why not for the emotions? Using psychotherapy and/or medication, it is possible to come to grips with depression, feel more optimistic about things, and thus put more enjoyment back into life.

Going for psychotherapy does not mean that someone is crazy. Quite the contrary, it indicates that he or she is sharp enough to know when some assistance is needed to get through a difficult life situation. You might suggest that your husband see a therapist on a trial basis. Many people resist this sort of help until they meet a therapist who makes talking seem comfortable and enjoyable.

Since you are having a hard time with your husband's depression, you might also want to tell him about your own feelings. Ask him to see a therapist for the sake of your relationship and offer to go with him. Treatment cannot be sustained over a long period of time if it is being done only for the sake of another person, but this may be a way to get him started. If all else fails, you should consider going to see a therapist yourself for assistance in dealing with the situation. Individual therapy for the non-MS partner can be quite helpful and, in many instances, the MS partner eventually agrees to join the therapeutic effort. Some adamant spouses grudgingly show up for the first session, determined never to return, and wind up staying for the duration of treatment. For you, the important thing is to get help for all who are willing to use it, even if that means only you.

I'VE READ SOME OLDER BOOKS ABOUT MS THAT TALK ABOUT THE "MS PERSONALITY." WHAT TYPE OF PERSONALITY DOES THIS REFER TO?

At one time it was thought that certain medical conditions were caused, at least in part, by specific personality types. MS was supposed to be more likely to develop in people with emotionally immature and dependent personalities. Such archaic notions of disease were abandoned long ago. Some people still believe that MS can "produce" a specific type of personality after the disease develops, but this is not the case. People with MS may find that they share similar problems, experiences, and concerns, and so have a lot in common. However, they do not have the same personality. The personality characteristics one had before getting MS are likely (for better or worse!) to be the same ones the person has after getting MS.

WHAT IS EUPHORIA, AND IS THIS A COMMON PHENOMENON IN MS?

MS-related *euphoria* is an exaggerated and unrealistic state of happiness or well-being that, to the observer, seems out of keeping with an individual's life situation. People with MS are said to be euphoric when they appear blasé and lighthearted in the face of serious or life-threatening problems. Someone who is euphoric may tend to giggle inappropriately, even when nothing funny has happened. This inappropriate giggling almost always occurs in people with severe intellectual loss. The combination of *cognitive dysfunction* and unrealistic optimism can lead to the neglect of important self-management issues, such as medical care, nutrition, and personal safety. Euphoria is thought to be the result of damage to parts of the brain involved in judgment and the control of emotions. It is sometimes confused with the uncontrollable laughing and crying that can affect people with MS, but these are more often precipitated by something that is emotionally charged, and can occur even in the absence of significant intellectual loss.

MY SISTER HAS HAD MS FOR 10 YEARS. SHE WALKS WITH A CANE AND HAS SOME VISUAL LOSS AND BLADDER PROBLEMS. THREE TIMES DURING THE PAST TWO YEARS, WE HAVE HAD TO CALL THE POLICE BECAUSE SHE HAD VIOLENT RAGES DURING WHICH SHE THREW THINGS, YELLED, AND TRIED TO ATTACK MEMBERS OF THE FAMILY. THE LAST TIME THIS HAPPENED, SHE PUNCHED A NEIGHBOR AND IS NOW UP ON CHARGES. CAN MS CAUSE THIS TYPE OF EXTREME BEHAVIOR AND, IF SO, WHAT CAN BE DONE ABOUT IT?

Just because a person has MS does not mean that every physical and psychological problem is due to the disease. There are people without MS who have rages and become violent. However, the behavior you describe can be one of the more unusual manifestations of MS. Although some of your sister's anger may arise from frustration related to her illness, it is more likely due to changes in those areas of the brain concerned with the expression and control of emotions. We all get angry from time to time, but in most cases we manage to control the expression of those emotions so that we do not physically assault other people. Your sister may have lost some of the ability to control these strong emotions. She should be evaluated by a neuropsychiatrist, a psychiatrist who specializes in conditions having both neurologic and psychiatric aspects. The type of problems your sister is experiencing can sometimes be helped with a regimen of medication and psychotherapy. Very often, the neuropsychiatrist will also teach the family to recognize the warning signs of an impending blow-up so that it can be avoided. You may never know for certain whether these symptoms are due in whole or in part to MS. Whatever the cause, the treatment is much the same.

STRESS AND MS

CAN STRESS CAUSE MS OR MAKE IT WORSE?

There is perhaps no more controversial question in MS than this one. Many investigators have attempted to show that stress can precipitate the onset of MS, trigger exacerbations, or hasten progression. Although some studies have found evidence to support one or more of these ideas, the relationship between stress and MS remains uncertain. A recent review of the research concluded that stress does not increase a person's risk of developing MS. Studies looking at stress and exacerbations of MS are somewhat contradictory. A study done in Israel during the first Gulf war found that the stress of being under almost constant attack by SCUD missiles did not increase the risk of MS exacerbations. On the other hand, a study completed in Denmark found that the loss of a child did increase the risk of developing MS. A recent systematic review of studies examining the relationship between stressful life events and subsequent exacerbations of MS concluded that most of the studies reviewed supported such an association. However, some of the studies included in the review were methodologically weak, thus rendering their findings suspect.

Recent studies have begun to focus on different questions. Some studies have attempted to determine how stress might affect the ***immune system***, and through the immune system, affect MS. Research in a variety of medical conditions and in healthy controls has shown that the immune system is sensitive to stress in a variety of ways. By understanding the links between immune function and stress, we may shed light on the possible links between stress and MS. Other studies have looked at the relationship between stress and changes on MRI. In one such study, it was found that persons with MS reporting higher amounts of stress and depression tended to show more gadolinium-enhancing lesions on MRI eight weeks later. Studies outside the field of MS have shown that stress can promote ***inflammation***. Recently investigators have been considering the possibility that stress may play a role in MS by triggering or promoting the inflammatory process associated with exacerbations. While the findings from all these studies are suggestive, they must be confirmed in larger samples.

In the meantime, we should be very cautious about attributing changes in the disease to stress. Family members sometimes feel guilty in the belief that they caused stress that worsened a loved one's MS. Such beliefs are unfounded. People with MS occasionally quit their jobs in the mistaken belief that they can slow the progression of their MS by reducing "occupational stress." Nothing is gained by such actions, and the individual loses the stimulation and satisfaction that working can provide.

Everyone is searching for explanations for this mysterious disease, and stress is one explanation that is readily available because we encounter it every day. MS adds a lot of stress to most people's lives. Thus, the real issue is not whether stress is altering the course of the MS, but how one can most effectively deal with the stresses that life and MS produce.

WHAT SHOULD I DO ABOUT THE STRESSES IN MY LIFE?
I DON'T THINK I CAN MAKE THEM ALL GO AWAY.

Sometimes people with MS are told by well-meaning people to try to "reduce the stress in your life." Nice trick if you can do it! There may be situations or relationships in your life that do not contribute much to life satisfaction but which are both stressful and avoidable. It would be worth it to try to steer clear of such situations and/or people. Unfortunately, most sources of stress in our lives are not under our control. Moreover, many times when people set out to "reduce stress," they do so by bailing out of important life activities such as work or family responsibilities. These activities provide much of the stimulation and inspiration that make life worth living. Do not withdraw from life on the basis of the mistaken notion that this will reduce stress.

The key is to learn how to cope with stress rather than to avoid it. You can learn to deal with this problem in a variety of ways, including stress management programs, psychotherapy, counseling, support groups, peer counseling, self-help books, exercise, and effective organizational strategies. The first step is to identify the sources of stress in your life and evaluate your present coping style. Try to determine how you appraise these situations and how you react to them. Next, you need to experiment with more effective coping strategies. Sometimes changing one's appraisal of a situation helps to reduce the stress growing from that situation. For example, if dealing with a certain person in your life always makes you feel stupid, you might examine why you are interpreting the interaction in that way and learn to interpret it differently. So instead of interpreting the interaction as showing you up, you might interpret it as simply a difference of opinion between two people.

Learning to deal more effectively with stress is probably best done with a professional who is trained in the requisite skills. Once you have mastered these skills, you should be able to cope on your own, perhaps returning from time to time to sharpen your skills or learn how to deal with new situations that have arisen.

RECOMMENDED READINGS

Brown RF, Tennant CC, Sharrock M, Hodgkinson S, et al. Relationship between stress and relapse in multiple sclerosis: Part II. Direct and indirect relationships. *Multiple Sclerosis.* 2006;12:465–475.

Elkin, A. *Stress Management for Dummies.* New York: Wiley Publishing, Inc., 1999.

Farrell P. *It's Not All in Your Head: Anxiety, Depression, and Mood Swings in MS.* New York: Demos Medical Publishing, 2010.

Feinstein A. Mood disorders in multiple sclerosis and the effects on cognition. *Journal of the Neurological Sciences.* 2006;245(1-2):63–66.

Feinstein A, Feinstein K. Depression associated with multiple sclerosis. Looking beyond diagnosis to symptom expression. *Journal of Affective Disorders.* 2001;66:193–198.

Feinstein A, O'Connor P, Feinstein K. Multiple sclerosis, interferon beta-1b and depression A prospective investigation. *Journal of Neurology.* 2002;249:815–820.

Fraser RT, Kraft GH, Ehde DM, Johnson KL. *The MS Workbook: Living Fully with Multiple Sclerosis.* Oakland, CA: New Harbinger, 2006.

Goldman Consensus Group. The Goldman consensus statement on depression in multiple sclerosis. *Multiple Sclerosis.* 2005;11:328–337.

James J. *One Particular Harbor.* Chicago: Noble Press, 1993.

Minden SL, Orav J, Reich P. Depression in multiple sclerosis. *General Hospital Psychiatry.* 1987;9:426–434.

Mohr DC, Boudewyn AC, Goodkin DE, Bostrom A, et al. Comparative outcomes for individual cognitive-behavior therapy, supportive-expressive group psychotherapy, and sertraline for the treatment of depression in multiple sclerosis. *Journal of Consulting and Clinical Psychology.* 2001;69:942–949.

Mohr DC, Cox D. Multiple sclerosis: empirical literature for the clinical health psychologist. *Journal of Clinical Psychology.* 2001;57:479–499.

Mohr DC, Goodkin DE, Islar J, et al. Treatment of depression is associated with suppression of nonspecific and antigen-specific TH1 responses in multiple sclerosis. *Archives of Neurology.* 2001;58:1081–1086.

Mohr DC, Hart SL, Julian L, Cox D, et al. Association between stressful life events and exacerbation in multiple sclerosis: a meta-analysis. *British Medical Journal.* 2004;328:731–735.

Pitzele S. *We Are Not Alone: Learning to Live with Chronic Illness.* New York: Workman Publishing, 1986.

Sobel RM, Lotkowski S, Mandel S. Update on depression in neurologic illness: stroke, epilepsy, and multiple sclerosis. *Current Psychiatry Reports* 2005;7:396–403.

RECOMMENDED RESOURCES

Selected publications available by calling 800-344-4867 or online at www.nationalmssociety. org/Brochures:

- *Depression and MS*
- *MS and Your Emotions*
- *Taming Stress in MS*
- *MS and the Mind*
- *"But You Look So Good"*
- *So You Have Progressive MS?*

MS Learn Online programming available at www.nationalmssociety.org/mslearnonline.

How Multiple Sclerosis
Affects the Family

Deborah M. Miller, PhD, LISW, and Rosalind C. Kalb, PhD

Multiple sclerosis (MS) has often been compared to the unexpected visitor who arrives at your house, complete with bag and baggage, and never leaves. This visitor has the tendency to spread his belongings through every room of the house, affecting the lifestyle and activities of every member of the household. MS, with its varied symptoms and unpredictable course, is an intrusion that the whole family must learn to accommodate. While a relatively small number of people with MS experience severe disability, the uncertainty and variability of the disease create their own day-to-day stresses even for those with minimal ***impairment***.

By necessity, the adjustment process is an ongoing one; as the ***symptoms*** of MS come and go, or come and stay, coping and adjustment ebb and flow as well. Since each family member will approach this challenge with his or her own particular coping style, effective communication will enhance the family's ability to work together to handle the day-to-day challenges of life with a ***chronic*** illness.

The questions in this chapter deal with the impact of MS on family life and on relationships among family members. The answers also serve to highlight the role of ongoing education, effective communication and coping strategies, and supportive counseling in a family's efforts to live comfortably and productively with this challenge in their lives.

IMPACT ON FAMILY LIFE

MY BOYFRIEND AND I ARE TALKING ABOUT GETTING MARRIED NEXT YEAR. HE KNOWS THAT I HAVE MS, AND HE SAYS IT DOESN'T MATTER TO HIM—HE LOVES ME ANYWAY. HE HAS NEVER BEEN TO THE DOCTOR WITH ME AND SEEMS RELUCTANT TO GO. I THINK IT'S IMPORTANT FOR HIM TO HEAR WHAT THE DOCTOR HAS TO SAY SO THAT HE KNOWS WHAT HE'S GETTING HIMSELF INTO. HOW CAN I EXPLAIN THIS TO HIM?

You might want to have a conversation with your boyfriend about how challenging marriage can be even under the best of circumstance. Going into it blindfolded can only make things harder. Since your MS is a challenge you will both be living with, it is a good idea to begin life together by facing it head on. Although love is an important part of a successful marriage, the ability to talk, problem-solve, and make decisions as a couple is also essential—particularly when life involves an unpredictable chronic illness. Explain to him that you would be more comfortable planning to share your life with him if you were confident that he had some understanding of what that might entail. If you are concerned that your boyfriend might be frightened by what your physician has to say, tell him so and assure him that you would rather start dealing with his fears and doubts now than be overwhelmed by them later.

WE HAVE WORKED HARD TO SAVE MONEY FOR OUR DAUGHTER'S EDUCATION. SOON MY HUSBAND, WHO IS IN A WHEELCHAIR, MAY NEED A VAN TO DRIVE HIMSELF TO WORK. HOW CAN WE POSSIBLY CHOOSE BETWEEN A COLLEGE EDUCATION AND A VAN MY HUSBAND NEEDS TO GET TO HIS JOB?
The heavy expenses related to chronic illness can drain family resources and necessitate compromise on the part of every family member. Before you start trying to choose between a van and a college education, however, be sure to look into possible funding sources for each.

- Education loans and scholarships based on financial need are often available, and chronic illness in the family is a valid and recognized financial hardship. You can start by calling the National Multiple Sclerosis Society (800-344-4867) to ask about their scholarship program, or read about it online at http://www.nationalmssociety.org/Scholarship.
- Some automobile companies also have programs to help people meet the cost of adaptive equipment.
- You might also want to consult a financial planner (see Chapter 23) who has expertise in the area of chronic illness, or call the National Multiple Sclerosis Society to learn about the free financial consultations offered through Financial Education Partners, a collaborative program with the Society of Financial Services Professionals.
- In addition, most states have an agency, perhaps called the Bureau of Vocational Services or Rehabilitation Services Commission, which is funded to provide goods and services to persons with disabilities to help them maintain or gain employment. Check to see if your state agency can help with the purchase of the van and provide other assistance.

Once you have gathered all the financial information, sit down together to review your options and decide which choices make most sense for your family.

OUR SON RECENTLY TOLD ME THAT HE DIDN'T LIKE TO BRING FRIENDS OVER ANYMORE BECAUSE THE WHOLE HOUSE IS STARTING TO FEEL LIKE A SURGICAL SUPPLY STORE. THERE'S NO SPACE TO "HANG OUT" WITHOUT TRIPPING OVER ONE PIECE OF EQUIPMENT OR ANOTHER. HOW SHOULD WE DEAL WITH THIS?
All members of the family need to feel "at home" in the house. When the needs of one person begin to crowd out everyone else, the balance is out of kilter and needs to be restored. Ideally, there should be space for all of you to relax, converse, and entertain without tripping over medical equipment or mobility devices. Have a family meeting to talk over the problem and see if together you can come up with any

space-saving, organizational ideas for managing the assistive equipment and creating equipment-free areas. The essential point to share with the whole family is that it is important for each of you to feel comfortable in the home.

You may also want to discuss with your son his feelings about MS. Depending on his age, he may be feeling embarrassed or self-conscious about having a parent with a disability who needs to use **assistive devices**. He may be concerned about what his friends will think, and he may be uncomfortable with their questions. If he seems to have difficulty talking this over with you, you can offer him age-appropriate reading materials from the National Multiple Sclerosis Society (available on the Society's Web site at http://www.nationalmssociety.org/childrensliterature) and alert him to the possibility of talking or writing to youngsters his own age who also have a parent with MS. Your local National Multiple Sclerosis Society chapter can help him to make these kinds of connections.

OUR FAMILY USED TO DO A LOT OF HIKING AND CAMPING. SINCE MY WIFE GOT MS, SHE CAN'T REALLY HIKE FOR ANY DISTANCE, AND SHE'S UNCOMFORTABLE "ROUGHING IT." I DON'T KNOW WHETHER I SHOULD TAKE THE CHILDREN CAMPING WITHOUT HER OR GIVE UP CAMPING AND TRY TO FIND ANOTHER KIND OF INEXPENSIVE FAMILY VACATION.

As with many of the other questions in this chapter, there is no one correct answer. The solution lies in talking the options over with your wife (and children if they are old enough to understand and participate) and deciding what works best for all of you. Your goal should always be to try to balance the needs and wishes of all family members. One solution may be to compromise; go on occasional father-and-children camping excursions and, at the same time, begin investigating other, less physically strenuous possibilities for the whole family. If you give up camping altogether, the less-than-desirable outcome may be that you and the children feel a bit resentful, and your wife feels guilty. Consult a travel agent who is knowledgeable about vacation opportunities for the disabled (see Appendix E). There are even camping programs for mixed groups of disabled and able-bodied people.

I'VE HAD TO MOVE BACK IN WITH MY MOTHER SINCE I CAN NO LONGER MANAGE ALONE IN MY APARTMENT. WE GOT ALONG FINE WHEN I WAS ON MY OWN, BUT NOW WE'RE BACK TO THE OLD TENSIONS FROM MY TEENAGE DAYS. HOW DO FAMILIES HANDLE THIS KIND OF PROBLEM?

Parents and children spend many years preparing to separate. By the time the children have grown up enough to leave home, they feel ready to take personal responsibility and make decisions for their own lives. Parents let them go, usually with some trepidation and a big sigh of relief. As time passes, parents and their adult children learn to relate to each other in a slightly different way, with gradually growing separateness and mutual respect. When an adult child returns home, the parent-child relationship may need to be negotiated all over again.

Your mother once again has one of her children living with her, but her parenting role is different from what it was when you were younger. You have returned to your mother's house after having spent time on your own, running your own home, making your own decisions. Presumably, you want your mother to treat you like an independent adult, free to make your own decisions and come and go on your own schedule. She, on the other hand, wants to continue to feel that her home is her own, subject to her tastes and preferences. In addition, she has always related to you as your mother, and may not know how to interact with you in any other way. Particularly when illness and/or disability are part of the picture, parents often feel an increased need to help and protect. Your mother may need time to learn how to balance your needs for help and support with your needs for freedom and independence. You may need the same time to reconcile yourself to being back in your mother's home and sphere of influence.

This is not an easy situation for any parent and adult child. You and your mother need to talk about the conflicts you are having and try to renegotiate your relationship. If you and your mother find that this renegotiation process is too difficult or stressful, a family therapist can help you communicate your individual needs and mutual expectations more effectively.

MY HUSBAND HAS HAD MS FOR SEVERAL YEARS. I KNOW THAT THINGS ARE VERY DIFFICULT FOR HIM, BUT THE MS HAS MADE THINGS TOUGH FOR ME AND THE CHILDREN AS WELL. HOW CAN I EXPLAIN TO MY HUSBAND THAT WE'RE ALL HAVING TROUBLE DEALING WITH THE CHANGES AND LOSSES IN OUR LIVES?
Some people have so much difficulty coming to terms with the impact of MS on their own lives that they have a hard time realizing how it affects other members of the family. Others feel so anxious and guilty about the impact of their disability on family members that they try not to think about it. Thus, there may be a variety of reasons why your husband seems insensitive to the feelings of other family members.

Presumably, you have tried to talk with him about the ways in which MS affects you and the children. If he feels that you are being selfish and unfeeling when you talk about your own needs, try communicating about them in a different way. For example, you might consult your local chapter of the National Multiple Sclerosis Society about family programs that you could attend together. Share with your husband some of the literature published by the National Multiple Sclerosis Society on families living with the disease. Perhaps he can hear your message more clearly if it comes from someone else. Knowing that all families living with MS find it stressful, and that family members cope best by helping one another, may enable him to feel less alone and more able to respond to you and the children. You may also consider working with a mental health professional to facilitate your conversation.

ALTHOUGH I NEED TO USE A WHEELCHAIR MOST OF THE TIME, I HAVE LEARNED TO BE QUITE SELF-SUFFICIENT IN MY OWN APARTMENT. MY PARENTS WANT ME TO LIVE WITH THEM, BUT I REALLY WANT TO STAY WHERE I AM, IN A FAMILIAR NEIGHBORHOOD, CLOSE TO MY FRIENDS. HOW CAN I CONVINCE MY PARENTS THAT I'M FINE RIGHT WHERE I AM?
Your parents are probably worrying about your physical safety and your ability to get help if and when you need it. One way to reassure them is to create a home "safety net" for yourself. This is a good idea for any disabled person living alone, whether or not Mom and Dad are worried!

A portable telephone can be carried in a pouch attached to your wheelchair. This will enable you to make and receive calls even if you cannot get to the regular phone. You might also wish to install a medical alert system that gives you immediate access to emergency help (see Appendix E). This kind of system comes in several varieties, but the general principle is that the push of a single button (worn around your neck or attached to the wheelchair) alerts a central office that you are in some kind of trouble. After determining the type of problem you are having, the central office calls one of the individuals on your emergency list: neighbor, family member, physician, police, fire department, and so on. If you were to take a bad fall, for example, and find yourself unable to get back up or reach a telephone, you could get immediate help simply by pressing the alert button.

The Medic-Alert identification bracelet is another useful safety precaution (see Appendix E). If you were unable for any reason to communicate clearly about your condition (following a serious fall, for example), the bracelet would indicate that you have MS and identify the medications you are taking. Any other important information about your health status would be available in your Medic-Alert file.

Knowing that this kind of safety net is in place may help your parents feel more comfortable with your independence. Knowing that you are looking out for your own welfare and safety may make them less inclined to feel they have to do it for you.

PARENTING

NOW THAT I'VE BEEN DIAGNOSED WITH MS, I DON'T KNOW IF I SHOULD HAVE CHILDREN. I'M AFRAID THAT I WON'T BE ABLE TO DO THINGS FOR A CHILD THAT A FATHER IS SUPPOSED TO DO. WHAT IF I CAN'T EVEN PLAY CATCH OR TEACH MY CHILD TO RIDE A BICYCLE?

Most parents, with or without MS, will tell you that their experiences with raising children were very different from what they had expected. They will also tell you that there is no single or correct way to be a "good" parent. Your decision to have children should be based on your desire to have this experience in your life as well some assessment of your ability to provide the kind of love and security that all children need.

The diagnosis of MS should not necessarily interrupt your wishes or plans for parenthood in any way. Keep in mind that it is impossible to predict with any certainty how your MS will affect you; you might not have any of the difficulties you are anticipating. You might even have a child who has no interest in playing catch! It is certainly reasonable to expect that MS will have some impact on your future family. The best way to prepare for that is for you and your wife to educate yourselves about MS, talk to the doctor about your particular symptoms and the course they are likely to take, and talk to each other about how you plan to share the parenting and bread-winning responsibilities. Ultimately, the goal is for you and your wife to feel comfortable as an effective parenting team, with consistent ideas about raising children, mutual support, and flexible ideas about what are "father jobs" and "mother jobs."

Please be sure to read Chapter 18, on pregnancy and MS, for information related to disease-modifying therapy, pregnancy, and breast-feeding.

**MY CHILDREN DON'T BRING THEIR FRIENDS AROUND THE HOUSE ANY MORE.
NOW THAT I'M IN A WHEELCHAIR, THEY SEEM EMBARRASSED ABOUT ME.
WHAT IS THE BEST WAY TO DISCUSS THIS WITH THEM?**

It is important that families living with MS do not automatically relate all the changes they experience to the disease. Otherwise, changes that occur because of normal maturation or because of some stress other than MS could be misinterpreted. For example, it is quite typical and normal for young teenagers to begin spending less time at home and more time with their friends. Or, children may bring fewer friends around if they sense that Mom or Dad is very tired or cranky a lot of the time.

Begin the conversation with your children by letting them know that you have noticed a change. It is important to do this in a very neutral way so that your children feel free to respond to the observation you have made rather than to the tone of your voice. Ask them if they have noticed that their friends are not over at the house as much as they used to be, and, if they have, ask them what they think has changed. If they do not offer any explanation, or if they offer one that you do not quite believe, let them know that you are concerned this might be related in some way to your MS. Assure them that you want to know about any feelings or concerns that they might have because it is important to you that they and their friends are comfortable in the house. If they do voice concerns about the MS or anything else, work with them to develop strategies to make the situation more comfortable.

**NOW THAT MY WIFE HAS BECOME A BIT MORE DISABLED, THE CHILDREN HAVE
A LOT MORE CHORES TO DO AROUND THE HOUSE. WILL THIS RESPONSIBILITY
BE TOO MUCH FOR THEM?**

Research has indicated that children who have a parent with MS are very much like children whose parents do not have any major health problems. They continue to develop and thrive in spite of the added stresses and responsibilities. Let your children know that you are aware that they have more responsibilities than their peers and that you appreciate their efforts. Offer your children choices about which chores they take on and give them some leeway in deciding when they will complete them. Reassure them with both words and actions that, in spite of their increased responsibility, you are there to parent, protect, and take charge. Try to make sure that your children have time in their lives to be children; they need some regular opportunities, however limited, to participate in a school activity or be with friends. If, in spite of these efforts, you notice a significant change in your children's school performance, usual moods, or social relationships, it would be best to have a consultation with a child or family therapist.

**I WENT INTO THE HOSPITAL RECENTLY DURING A PARTICULARLY BAD RELAPSE.
WE TOLD OUR 7- AND 9-YEAR-OLD CHILDREN ABOUT THE ADMISSION AHEAD OF
TIME, AND THEY SEEMED OKAY WITH IT. BUT WHILE I WAS AWAY, THE OLDER ONE
GOT REALLY UPSET AT SCHOOL AND MY HUSBAND HAD TO GO PICK HIM UP.
HOW SHOULD WE HANDLE THIS IN THE FUTURE IF I HAVE TO BE ADMITTED AGAIN?**

Children have a difficult time with the unknown, and you and your husband were right to try to prepare them in advance for your admission. In spite of parents' best efforts, however, children are often frightened by the idea of a hospital stay (since many people who go into hospitals are very sick or dying) and worried that the parent will not come home again. Having you return safely from this initial hospitalization is the first step in preparing your children for any future hospitalizations that you may need. Take the time now to describe what happened to you during this hospital stay and let them talk to you about what it was like for them while you were gone. If and when you need to be hospitalized again, ask the hospital staff if the children can accompany you during the admission process. Find out if the hospital has child-life workers on staff who can talk with them about the hospital and its procedures. Make plans with your children to talk with them by phone at a scheduled time each day—or to have a visit if that is allowed. The idea is to give your children an under-standing of what happens during the admission and how it will help your MS, and assure them that you are okay and available by telephone while you are gone.

WE HAVE TOLD OUR PARENTS AND A FEW OF OUR CLOSEST FRIENDS ABOUT MY MS. I'VE ASKED THEM NOT TO TALK ABOUT IT BECAUSE I DON'T WANT MY CHILDREN TO KNOW YET. MY HUSBAND THINKS I'M WRONG TO TRY TO KEEP THIS FROM THEM. I THINK THAT 8- AND 10-YEAR-OLD CHILDREN ARE TOO YOUNG TO HAVE TO WORRY ABOUT THIS. WHAT SHOULD WE BE TELLING THEM?

Eight- and 10-year-olds are very observant people who generally have a sixth sense when something is not right in the family. Your children are probably aware that you are having some sort of health problems, whether or not these problems are influenc-ing your usual activities with them. The ideas that children conjure up for themselves are almost always more frightening than the reality, particularly if they get the idea that the "something" is so terrible that Mom and Dad cannot even talk about it. In short, not discussing your MS with the children can, in the long run, cause them more worry than talking about it would. In addition, the longer you delay talking to them, the more you increase the risk that they will hear the news from someone other than yourselves. By openly discussing an important issue like this one in your life, you also lay the groundwork for good parent-child communication about issues that will come up in their lives.

I KNOW THAT ALL CHILDREN NEED TO TEST AND "SEE WHO'S THE BOSS" SOMETIMES. BUT SINCE I STARTED TO USE A CANE, IT FEELS AS THOUGH THE CHILDREN ARE TESTING ALL THE TIME. HOW CAN I DISCIPLINE MY CHILDREN WHEN I CAN'T EVEN KEEP UP WITH THEM?

There are many different styles of discipline. The better your negotiation and com-munications skills, and the more consistent you are in using them, the less you will have to depend on being mobile to provide discipline. Different approaches to parenting and discipline are described in the parenting literature (see Recommended Readings). In addition, many community centers and schools offer parent effective-ness programs designed to help you build confidence and consistency in using these techniques. Keep in mind that being a good parent does not mean doing it all on your own. Enlist your spouse or other adults to help you learn and use these different approaches. In the meantime, remember also that children sometimes "test" in order to reassure themselves that the adults in their lives are still in charge and can still take care of them. Your children may be expressing their fears about MS and whatever effects it is having on you. Be alert to their questions and worries, and read or talk with them about the MS whenever it seems appropriate.

I ALWAYS USED TO ENJOY DOING THINGS WITH MY CHILDREN AFTER SCHOOL OR IN THE EVENING BEFORE THEIR BEDTIME. NOW I'M SO EXHAUSTED BY THE TIME THEY GET HOME THAT I AM EITHER ASLEEP OR SO CRANKY THAT THEY WISH I WERE ASLEEP! IS THERE ANY WAY TO DEAL WITH THIS PROBLEM?

Fatigue is a common MS symptom that is usually best managed by prioritizing your activities and budgeting your energy. In some cases fatigue may also be helped with medication (see Chapter 4). At your first opportunity, discuss the fatigue with your physician, who can help sort out its cause(s). The physician may also refer you to a *physical therapist* or *occupational therapist* who can design a personalized exercise program to increase your energy, as well as work simplification and energy conservation strategies to help you make effective use of the energy you have (see Chapters 9 and 10). Your best day-to-day strategy is to find a time to recoup some energy before the children come home so that you can resume some of the activities that you and they are missing. Since MS-related fatigue is most noticeable in the late afternoon, try to work in a brief rest just before the children arrive home. You may want to rearrange your daily routine so that you do more of your physically demanding chores earlier in the day and then have a chance to rest. If you are returning from work late in the day, schedule a regular rest time for yourself and make a "date" with the children for some special time together before they go to bed. Brainstorm with the children about some new "quiet time" activities that you could enjoy doing together.

SINCE MY WIFE BEGAN HAVING DIFFICULTY GETTING AROUND THE HOUSE AND DOING THINGS FOR HERSELF, SHE'S ALWAYS AFTER THE REST OF US TO DO, OR GET, OR GO. THE CHILDREN AND I WANT TO BE HELPFUL, BUT WE DON'T LIKE BEING CONSTANTLY ON CALL. HOW CAN I MAKE HER UNDERSTAND HOW WE FEEL?

There are two very difficult aspects to the situation you are describing in your family: how frustrated and out of control your wife must be feeling; and how unappreciated and burdened you and your children are feeling. One key to making home life more satisfying and comfortable for all of you is to develop some ways of talking about what is happening so that you can start building solutions together. The best way to start talking with others about your own feelings and needs is to show some understanding of theirs. This helps to build mutual respect, to facilitate open communication and cut down on everyone's tendency to become defensive. Then you can begin to tackle specific areas of stress and conflict one at a time. Let your wife know that the family wants to meet her various needs, but that you each have needs and commitments of your own to deal with as well. Family members should speak openly about how they would like requests to be made, and how they feel when their own needs and activities are ignored. If you find that these conversations become too difficult because of all the issues that seem to emerge, keep in mind that lots of emotions may need to be sorted out. You may want to enlist the help of a family therapist who is knowledgeable about chronic illness to get you started on this process.

MY 12-YEAR-OLD HAS HAD TO HELP ME UP FROM THE FLOOR A COUPLE OF TIMES WHEN I HAVE FALLEN. NOW HE'S AFRAID TO BE AT HOME ALONE WITH ME. HOW CAN I HELP HIM WITH THESE FEELINGS?

Your son's feelings may be difficult for him to describe, but are probably related to a fear that he cannot do enough to help you, or that he is having to deal with a problem that is bigger and stronger than he is. For both your sakes, do everything you can to protect yourself from falls. Arrange for the two of you to have a session with an occupational therapist or physical therapist in your home. This professional can point out ways to maximize your stability and safety, perhaps by removing area rugs, installing bathroom safety equipment, or recommending a mobility aid. The therapist can also show you different ways of performing transfers and teach your son techniques for helping if you do fall. You might also consider having a medical alert system installed in your home that enables you to notify family, neighbors, or community safety officials that you need help. These steps will reduce your son's fears by demonstrating to him that you are doing everything you can to protect yourself and that you do not expect him to be solely responsible for your safety.

OUR YOUNGEST DAUGHTER WILL GRADUATE FROM HIGH SCHOOL NEXT YEAR. RECENTLY, SHE STARTED TALKING ABOUT GETTING A JOB RATHER THAN APPLYING TO COLLEGE. MY HUSBAND AND I ARE AFRAID THAT SHE FEELS WORRIED ABOUT LEAVING ME NOW THAT I'VE BECOME SO MUCH MORE DISABLED. SHOULD WE PUSH HER TO GO TO SCHOOL?

Your daughter's second thoughts about college could be caused by any number of factors. As her parents, you should certainly discuss her plans with her and share your feelings about her going away to college. However, it would do little good to force her into a decision about leaving home; her reasons for deciding against college at this point could be very well thought out and unrelated to your illness. If her change in plans does seem to stem from anxiety or guilt about your MS, let her know what steps you and your husband have taken to manage your increasing disability. Remind her that, just because she is the youngest child, it does not mean that her role in life is to take care of you. If finances are her major concern, share with her your plans for balancing medical costs and any help you plan to give her with her educational expenses. Be prepared to help her explore options for attending college away from home or locally. The goal of the conversation should be to let her know that her needs and priorities are important to you and that you can, as a family, come up with a plan that addresses the needs of all the members of the family.

SOMETIMES MY SON OR DAUGHTER HAS TO HELP ME WITH GETTING DRESSED OR GOING TO THE BATHROOM. I DON'T LIKE THIS ANY MORE THAN THEY DO, AND I'M WORRIED ABOUT HOW THIS WILL AFFECT THEM.

Your concern about having the children help with your personal care activities is very understandable and appropriate. Providing that kind of intimate assistance can be very confusing for youngsters who are developing their self-concepts and working to attain more independence from their parents. In addition, your children's involvement in personal care sends a strong message that you would be "lost" without them—a message that could have a significant impact on their plans for the future.

Some of the tasks that you need help with happen at the same time each day. Try to develop a schedule with adults in your family to help with your morning routine. Talk to your chapter of the National Multiple Sclerosis Society about the possibility of getting help from a home health agency. If, despite your best efforts, you can find no other helpers, consider involving your children in individual or family counseling.

An opportunity to sort out their feelings about their caregiving role could relieve some of the stress on all of you.

MY HUSBAND HAS BEEN VERY UPSET AND ANGRY ABOUT THE WAY HIS MS IS GETTING WORSE, AND HE SEEMS TO TAKE A LOT OF IT OUT ON THE CHILDREN. THEY TRY SO HARD TO PLEASE HIM, BUT HE YELLS A LOT AND CRITICIZES EVERYTHING THEY DO. WHAT IS THE BEST WAY TO TALK TO HIM ABOUT THIS?

While your perception is that your husband's relationship with the children is very strongly affected by his MS, he may not recognize the ways in which his reactions to the disease are spilling over onto the family. The sooner you begin to talk this over with him, the better it will be for all of you. He must begin to understand the impact of his behavior on the children. It is best to start this process by talking about a particular situation rather than about his general attitude or the way he is coping with MS. Discussing how to improve on the outcome of a specific, recent event will be less threatening. Undoubtedly, one conversation will not reverse the pattern that has developed; it will, however, lay the groundwork for future conversations.

It is not unusual for people to take out their uncomfortable feelings on those closest to them. As MS interferes with a person's sense of independence and personal control, the natural tendency is often to try to take control in other ways—perhaps by bossing people around or "trying to organize the raindrops." Children often feel that they get the brunt of this type of behavior. The most effective way to deal with this problem is often to help the person talk about the loss of control and brainstorm about more effective ways to restore a sense of order and independence in daily life. It is also appropriate to let the children know you understand how difficult and unfair this can sometimes feel.

Keep in mind, as well, that mood swings, irritability, and depressive feelings are common in MS (see Chapter 16). While the exact relationship between these emotional changes and the illness is not well known, they appear to be part of the illness itself as well as a reaction to it. Regardless of the specific cause(s), however, the resulting behaviors can have a significant impact on family life. If you feel that your husband is behaving very differently from his "usual self," you could ask him to mention it to his *neurologist* and think about going with you to a mental health professional who is familiar with MS to talk over these changes.

MOST OF MY MS PROBLEMS DON'T SHOW ON THE OUTSIDE; FATIGUE AND VERTIGO ARE MY WORST PROBLEMS. HOW CAN I HELP MY CHILDREN UNDERSTAND HOW I AM FEELING? THEY ARE ANGRY ABOUT THINGS I CAN'T DO ANY MORE, AND DON'T SEEM TO APPRECIATE THE THINGS I STILL MANAGE TO DO FOR THEM.

It is difficult to describe to children symptoms that they cannot see and have probably never experienced. Try to describe your symptoms in terms that they can readily understand. For example, you might have your children experiment with ankle and wrist weights to learn how your body feels when you are fatigued. Or, you might tell them to spin themselves around a bit and then try to walk from one room to another. Reading together about MS will let them see that other parents experience very similar symptoms. The National Multiple Sclerosis Society has several excellent booklets written for children in different age groups. Many chapters of the Society also offer special programs to help children learn about the disease and its symptoms and provide ways for them to get in touch with other children who have a parent with MS. Contact your local chapter (800-344-4867) to learn more about these services. Your physician can also be a valuable resource. For example, the children might sit in during one of your office visits to learn about the neurologic exam and the ways in which your physician tests those "invisible" symptoms. He can also refer you to a child or family therapist who can help your family develop more effective ways to talk about MS and the ways it is affecting each of you.

As you try various strategies for teaching your children about MS, keep in mind that no two children learn in exactly the same way. What seems to work with one of your children may be of no interest to the other(s). One child might be interested in reading or talking with you about MS, while another might want to attend a meeting and talk with other children who have a parent with MS. Some children want simply to be reassured that you will continue to be able to take care of them.

SHOULD I LET MY CHILDREN'S TEACHERS KNOW ABOUT MY MS?
Under most circumstances, it is very helpful to let your children's teachers know about your diagnosis. School can be a very important source of stability and self-confidence, and the teacher is a primary player in any child's day-to-day experiences. If they are aware of the MS, teachers can be very helpful to you in gauging how your children are responding to your illness and the changes it is causing in your family. In addition, awareness of your situation will enable the teachers to be attentive to any changes in your children's school performance and social relationships, and be prepared to provide help and support as needed.

THE CAREGIVING EXPERIENCE

EVERYONE IS ALWAYS ASKING HOW MY HUSBAND IS. HOW DO I LET THEM KNOW THAT MY LIFE HAS CHANGED ALMOST AS MUCH AS HIS AND THAT I NEED THEM TO ASK ABOUT ME TOO?
Your feelings are shared by many well spouses. There is no reason to feel embarrassed, selfish, or in any way inadequate because you have needs of your own. Over the course of the illness, you will need support just as much as your husband does, but you may have to look for it from different sources. Having one special friend or relative with whom you are comfortable sharing your feelings can be much more meaningful than expressions of concern from people with whom you have a more casual relationship. Many chapters of the National Multiple Sclerosis Society sponsor spouse groups that provide the opportunity to meet with others who are sharing your experiences. The National Well Spouse Foundation (see Appendix D) is another organization that provides support to caregiving spouses through newsletters, local support groups, and annual national meetings. An increasing amount of reading matter is available to inform, support, and empower you in your role as the spouse of someone with a chronic illness (see Appendix C).

MY WIFE CAN'T PLAY TENNIS ANYMORE. SHE GETS UPSET WHEN I GO AND PLAY, AND I FEEL GUILTY ABOUT WANTING TO PLAY. SHOULD I GIVE UP THE ACTIVE THINGS THAT I LIKE TO DO BECAUSE SHE CAN NO LONGER DO THEM WITH ME?

There are likely to be a variety of changes that you and your wife will have to face together in dealing with MS, and responding to changes in her level of disability is a very significant one. Before making any decisions about continuing to play tennis, try to talk the situation over with her. Your wife's distress may stem from feelings of loss and envy; she may simply find it very painful to know that you are doing something that she loves but can no longer do. Or she may be concerned that the two of you will have less time together if you continue to play without her. She may also worry that she will miss out on the social contacts the two of you had with other players. Identifying the sources of her distress will help the two of you decide the best way to deal with the situation. Make sure that your wife understands how important it is for you to keep playing tennis, while reassuring her that you are interested in finding other activities that you can do together. Support her own efforts to find satisfying and enjoyable hobbies to replace those that she can no longer do. It is important that family members not rush to give up any and all activities that the person with MS is unable to do. The eventual cost in resentment and guilt is too great.

I'VE STARTED TO FEEL MORE LIKE A CAREGIVER THAN A HUSBAND. I AM COMMITTED TO MY WIFE, AND HAVE NO WISH TO LEAVE HER, BUT I REALLY MISS THE COMPANION WHO SHARED SO MUCH WITH ME. HOW DO OTHER PEOPLE COPE WITH THE LONELINESS AND LOSS OF COMPANIONSHIP?

The feelings of loss you are describing are particularly common for couples who have always shared many interests and activities but now increasingly spend time simply managing the consequences of MS. In the same way you have partnered each other in other aspects of your life, try to become partners in the management of MS. An important goal of this partnership is to be able to communicate effectively about ways to integrate MS-related care activities into your lives in such a way that there is still time and energy left for other enjoyable activities. This will help both of you to feel that you are managing the MS rather than the other way around. It will also help you regain your feelings of togetherness so that each feels less alone with the burdens imposed by the disease. Discussing your concerns at a couples' support group could benefit you and your wife in several ways: You will be reassured to learn that other couples are living with, and finding solutions to, the kinds of stresses and strains you are describing. The group can brainstorm together on ways to solve commonly shared problems and find substitute activities for those that you can no longer do because of the MS. You may also find that the group becomes a social outlet as well.

I FEEL AS THOUGH MY WHOLE LIFE IS CONTROLLED BY MS, AND I DON'T EVEN HAVE THE DISEASE. HOW CAN I REGAIN MY LIFE AND STILL MAKE SURE MY HUSBAND HAS THE CARE HE NEEDS?

When life with MS becomes so overwhelming that you feel you are losing yourself in the disease, it is time to take a step back from the situation and find ways by which it can be made more manageable. The first step in this process is to begin to think of yourself as your husband's *care partner* rather than caregiver; the responsibility for managing the MS and the needs that it generates rest on both of you.

In as objective a way as possible, the two of you should make a list of his needs and yours. Try to identify the specific ways in which the MS-related needs have infringed on yours, paying particular attention to those times when you feel especially burdened or overwhelmed. Finally, write down those activities that you personally are missing and want to regain in your life. The goal of this process is to help you think in more specific terms than "MS" and "my whole life." The more specific you are able to be, the more likely it is that you and he will be able to identify strategies for regaining a sense of independence and control in your lives.

While it will not be possible for you to free your lives totally of MS, you will be able to adopt strategies and identify resources to help both of you meet your needs. This kind of problem solving requires good communication and a lot of creativity. Working with a family therapist can help with the process if you find that, individually or together, you are feeling too overwhelmed or emotionally overloaded to be able to discuss the issues. Also keep in mind that MS support groups can be a helpful resource, particularly those designed for couples.

MY WIFE IS DESPERATE TO FIND A CURE FOR HER MS. EVERY TIME A NEW TREATMENT IS MENTIONED IN THE NEWSPAPER, SHE IS READY TO FLY AROUND THE WORLD TO GET IT. I GET ANGRY WHEN SHE IS READY TO SPEND OUR RETIREMENT MONEY ON EVERY QUACK GIMMICK THAT COMES ALONG. HOW CAN I GET HER TO UNDERSTAND THAT THE MONEY WE SAVED IS FOR BOTH OF US AND THAT WE NEED TO AGREE ON HOW TO SPEND IT?

This commitment to trying every publicized MS "cure" can be especially frustrating to family members. In addition to making them feel as if their own needs have become unimportant, it tends to keep the entire family on an uncomfortable emotional roller coaster as hope is repeatedly replaced with disappointment. Your wife may be responding more with emotion than with reason to these reported "cures." To give her some background on the great number of these that have turned out to have no real value, you may want to read together a book entitled *Alternative Medicine and Multiple Sclerosis* (2nd ed.) by Dr. Allen Bowling (see Appendix C). This book describes most of the proclaimed treatments and cures, the ways that each was thought to work, the quality of the scientific research done to evaluate their effectiveness, and benefits and risks associated with each.

Another way to help your wife feel satisfied that she is doing everything possible to treat her MS is to encourage her participation in a ***clinical trial*** of one of the very promising drugs that are now being scientifically tested (see Chapter 5). If your wife continues to want to use your retirement savings to pursue untested "cures," the two of you might consider a consultation with an accountant or tax attorney (see Chapter 23) to determine how her spending will affect your retirement and how to establish a financial plan that will protect your retirement funds.

MY HUSBAND HAS BECOME QUITE DISABLED BY HIS MS, AND HE DOESN'T GET OUT OF THE HOUSE MUCH ANY MORE. FRIENDS HAVE STOPPED INVITING US TO DO THINGS BECAUSE HE IS NO LONGER ABLE. HOW CAN I LET THEM KNOW THAT I STILL NEED TO SEE PEOPLE AND HAVE A SOCIAL LIFE EVEN THOUGH HE CAN'T COME WITH ME?

You are wise to take the initiative with your friends rather than waiting for them to take the initiative with you. They may simply need to hear from you that you want to maintain your social relationships and continue to be active. You may start by inviting one friend or couple over for dinner and saying that your husband will join you for part of the evening but excuse himself if and when he becomes too tired. Or, invite them to join you at a restaurant for dinner and let them know that, although your husband will not be coming, he is pleased that you are arranging an evening out. During the evening, after you have had a chance to catch up with one another, ask your friends to tell other members of your circle that you are still looking to socialize with them. You may want to let them know, if it is indeed the case, that you and your husband have talked this over and are both comfortable with the idea that you will continue to make plans even if he is not always able to be with you. It is by your own example that your friends will become comfortable seeking you out for social engagements, even if your husband cannot always participate.

I'VE BEEN ABLE TO DEAL RELATIVELY WELL WITH MY WIFE'S SIGNIFICANT PHYSICAL PROBLEMS BUT THE COGNITIVE CHANGES AND MOOD SWINGS HAVE BEEN MUCH MORE DIFFICULT FOR ME. AT TIMES SHE SEEMS LIKE A DIFFERENT PERSON, AND I BEGIN TO FEEL AS THOUGH I HAVE LOST MY LIFE PARTNER. HOW CAN I LEARN TO ACCEPT THIS LOSS?

As painful as it is to recognize the cognitive changes that your wife is experiencing, it is fortunate that you understand their possible relationship to her disease. Many spouses and family members, who don't know that MS can directly cause these memory and behavioral changes, tend to misinterpret the problems and believe that the person with MS is being deliberately difficult or forgetful. With a more complete understanding of the situation, you can begin to deal with it more realistically. Chapters 14 and 16 provide an orientation to the ***cognitive impairment*** and emotional changes that can occur in MS, and describe how these problems are assessed and managed.

The changes your wife is experiencing are undoubtedly having a major impact on you and your relationship. First, you are probably assuming more of those household responsibilities your wife used to manage, as well as providing more care and supervision for her. Finding the time and energy for this can be a challenge given the many responsibilities you already have at work and at home. Even more importantly, the changes your wife is experiencing are literally taking her away from you. You may be missing her sense of humor, her intellect, her interest in your work and the comings and goings of your children, or her ability to participate with you at social gatherings with family and friends. In a very fundamental way, she is not the person you married.

This idea of having "lost" your spouse while she remains in your home and under your care can be very difficult to accept, and requires a unique kind of grieving process. It is important that you begin to think of your relationship as being very different from most marriages. This grieving process will help you acknowledge the help your wife needs, while allowing you to let go of the woman you married and accept the wife who is now so dependent on your care. The grieving process will also help you shift your expectations for the relationship and prepare for your new responsibilities.

Although family, friends, and support group members can be helpful and sympathetic, few will have any experience with the loss you are experiencing in your marriage. For that reason, it is very useful to work with a mental health professional experienced in dealing with the grief of your ever-changing relationship with your wife. The therapist can help you deal with the losses you are experiencing, the paradox of having to care for that person who is in many ways no longer your spouse, and in sorting out how you and the rest of your family can continue with your lives.

There is no one correct way to manage this situation that suspends you between being partner and nurse. A mental health professional can be an important ally as you find your way in managing this very difficult situation. This can include exploring ways to maintain relationships and activities that you used to share with your wife, or developing new ones. Just as importantly, working with a therapist can help you identify and hold on to those parts of your relationship with your wife that remain intact.

MY HUSBAND INSISTS ON DRIVING A CAR EVEN THOUGH SOME OF HIS MS SYMPTOMS ARE MAKING HIM AN UNSAFE DRIVER. WE ADDED HAND CONTROLS TO THE CAR 2 YEARS AGO, WHEN LEG WEAKNESS WAS HIS MAJOR PROBLEM. BUT NOW HIS VISION IS VERY BAD, AND I'M AFRAID THAT HIS CONCENTRATION IS JUST TOO POOR FOR HIM TO BE SAFE. HE HAS ALREADY HAD ONE ACCIDENT, AND I'M AFRAID THAT SOMEONE WILL BE HURT THE NEXT TIME.

People find it very difficult to give up driving because it represents a tremendous loss of independence. However, as you have indicated, the consequences of severely impaired driving skills can be life threatening. Trying to convince your husband by yourself that he should stop driving might be difficult. If you are uncertain about his driving competence, or if you believe that your husband will resent your suggestions, you might accompany him to his next medical appointment and raise the issue with his physician. Explain your concerns to the doctor and ask about the availability of a driving evaluation. This kind of evaluation, which should test both physical and cognitive skills, is often available at *rehabilitation* facilities. With your husband present, ask about the doctor's responsibility for reporting unsafe drivers to the state bureau of motor vehicles (this responsibility varies from state to state). If your husband insists on continuing to drive, and you are certain in your own mind that he is an unsafe driver, let him know that you and your other family members will not ride in the car when he is driving. Help him to make arrangements for rides to those places he is accustomed to going on his own. Many communities have door-to-door transportation services that can help him remain independent. You might also encourage him to consult a psychotherapist for help with the feelings of loss and helplessness that accompany this kind of major life adjustment.

MY HUSBAND WANTS OUR SEXUAL RELATIONSHIP TO BE THE WAY IT USED TO BE. BUT I AM EXHAUSTED AFTER A FULL DAY OF WORK AND TAKING CARE OF HIM. IT'S HARD FOR ME TO FEEL ROMANTIC AFTER HELPING HIM WITH HIS PERSONAL NEEDS. HOW CAN I DISCUSS THIS WITHOUT HURTING HIS FEELINGS?

A couple's sexual relationship is important because of both the physical pleasure it provides and the emotional intimacy that it expresses. At different times over the course of every marriage, the sexual relationship is influenced by how the couple is getting along, their family responsibilities, and their physical and emotional health. Remaining close and intimate with each other during these times is an important part of sustaining a good marriage. Before discussing your sexual relationship with your husband, you may want to spend some time sorting out your own feelings. As you have described, your sexual feelings for your husband have been affected by your own physical exhaustion as well as changes in how you feel emotionally. It is also possible that some of your husband's MS-related physical changes are interfering with your sexual activities or your sexual response to him. It will probably make your conversation easier if you have sorted through some of these feelings in advance and perhaps talked them over with a therapist.

The next time your husband talks about your sexual relationship, try sharing some of your feelings with him. As with any important conversation, be sure to put as much effort into hearing him as in expressing yourself. By being honest with him about the way you are feeling and open to his response, you are initiating an important and satisfying form of intimacy. The two of you might also consider talking with a therapist who specializes in sexual relationships. That person can help you talk about your feelings and concerns, explore ways of being sexual that accommodate your husband's disability, and otherwise enhance the intimacy in your relationship. The sexual relationship in MS is discussed in detail in Chapter 11.

I HAVE ALWAYS LOVED MY WIFE AND, UNTIL HER MS CAME ALONG, WE SELDOM EVEN ARGUED. I WOULD NEVER HAVE BELIEVED THAT I COULD INTENTIONALLY BE HURTFUL TO HER. BUT NOW THAT SHE IS AT HER MOST VULNERABLE, MY TEMPER IS BECOMING SHORTER AND SHORTER. LAST NIGHT SHE WOKE ME THREE TIMES TO HELP HER TO THE BATHROOM. THE SECOND TIME, AT 3:00 IN THE MORNING, I FOUND MYSELF SHOUTING AT HER THAT I HAD TO BE UP AT 5:30 AND SHE COULD WAIT UNTIL THEN. WHEN SHE CALLED ME AGAIN A HALF-HOUR LATER, IT WAS BECAUSE SHE HAD HAD AN ACCIDENT. EVEN THOUGH I KNEW IT WAS A BOWEL ACCIDENT, I LET HER LAY IN THE SOILED BEDCLOTHES WHILE I TRIED TO "COOL DOWN" AND GET CONTROL BEFORE GOING TO HELP HER. I WAS AFRAID I MIGHT HURT HER. THESE BAD FEELINGS AND REACTIONS ARE VERY FRIGHTENING TO BOTH OF US, AND THEY ARE COMING MORE OFTEN AND MORE POWERFULLY. I AM FRIGHTENED FOR HER AND FOR ME. WHAT CAN I DO?

Fortunately, you have begun to recognize your need for help in managing the reactions you are having to your wife and her care needs. We know from research and clinical practice that couples who have no history of domestic violence can become hurtful to each other in the course of living with a chronic disease like MS. This hurtfulness is often a reaction to the physical stress and emotional strain of living with the illness. We also know that this kind of aggressive behavior is more likely to occur when the illness involves personality and behavioral changes or bowel or bladder incontinence. This is by no means an excuse for becoming either emotionally or physically abusive. It is an alert that anyone can become abusive and that income, gender, and level of disability are no protection when the stress of the situation becomes too much.

You are right to be worried about your reactions. This is the kind of situation that will only become more stressful and dangerous if you try to manage it on your own. Counseling with a mental health professional is a useful and essential strategy for dealing with emotions that are beginning to feel out of control. The professional can help you and your wife to develop a short-term plan to relieve the immediate pressure related to her care, and a long-term strategy to prevent future occurrences. If you do not know a therapist, ask for a referral from your physician or the local chapter of the National Multiple Sclerosis Society.

It is important to let your wife's doctor know immediately that the caregiving has become too much for you, and that you need help in caring for her. You can also ask the National Multiple Sclerosis Society (800-FIGHT-MS; 800-344-4867) for information about local options for respite care, in-home nursing care, and a variety of other strategies (see Chapter 22). It is fortunate that you have had the courage to recognize the danger that you and your wife are facing. It is now essential that you find the strength to get professional help to correct the situation.

**I KNOW THAT ELDERLY COUPLES HAVE TO FACE THE POSSIBILITY OF
NURSING HOME PLACEMENT WHEN THEY CAN NO LONGER CARE FOR
EACH OTHER ANY MORE, BUT MY HUSBAND AND I ARE IN OUR 40S
AND FACING THAT POSSIBILITY NOW BECAUSE OF HIS SEVERE DISABILITY.
HOW CAN WE BEGIN TO TALK ABOUT THIS FRIGHTENING TOPIC?**

One of the most difficult aspects of facing nursing home placement at this time in your lives is that it is such an unanticipated event. Few, if any, people in your immediate circle can appreciate the practical, emotional, and financial issues you are facing. You may be feeling guilty that your husband's care needs have become overwhelming in spite of any assistance you have been able to enlist from friends, relatives, or professionals. In addition, you are probably concerned about the likelihood of finding a facility that has other young adults. You may also be concerned that your family and friends will think you are "abandoning" your husband.

To deal with these issues, it is important to step back from the jumble of overwhelming thoughts and feelings and take an objective look at your situation. The fact that you and your husband are considering residential care for him means that you feel you have exhausted all the other long-term care options. You can refer to Chapter 22 for a detailed discussion of long-term care to determine if this is indeed the case. As you and he examine the positive and negative aspects of each long-term care strategy, you can choose the one that best meets the needs of everyone in the family.

Your husband's ability to participate in this discussion, and the subsequent planning involved, will depend on his cognitive abilities—in particular, his ability to recognize and appreciate his care needs. Because this is a decision that will significantly affect both of your lives, it is important that he be included in this decision to the greatest extent possible.

The starting point for this kind of planning and decision making is the acknowledgment that you, your husband, and your children each have needs that must be met, and each person's needs are just as real and valid as everyone else's. Much of the anxiety and guilt surrounding this difficult issue results from the mistaken belief that family members ought to be able to care for a loved one at home no matter what. However, research has demonstrated that the physical and emotional health of caregivers can be severely compromised by the extraordinary demands of caregiving. The goal is to arrive at a plan that ensures the health and well-being of the entire family, and allows family members to love and care for one another in the most comfortable way possible.

If your husband is not able to participate meaningfully in this decision because of cognitive impairment, you may want to discuss your options with members of his family. Family members, friends, a clergyman, and a caregivers' support group can all be valuable sources of help and support during this difficult time. It may also be helpful to work with a mental health professional who can provide a "reality check" concerning the options you are considering, guide your efforts to select a facility and arrange placement, and be a source of support as you advise family and friends about your decision.

RECOMMENDED READINGS

Chatman L, Chatman C. *The Art of Living with Multiple Sclerosis (Six Secrets for Managing MS as a Team)*. Jacksonville, FL: Two-Hearts Publishing, 2006.

Cohen MD. *Dirty Details: The Days and Nights of a Well Spouse*. Philadelphia, PA: Temple University Press, 1996.

Cristall B. *Coping When a Parent Has Multiple Sclerosis*. New York: Rosen Publishing, 1992. (Written for teens.)

Kalb R. *Multiple Sclerosis: A Guide for Families*. 3rd ed. New York: Demos Medical Publishing, 2006.

Mintz SG. *Love, Honor, and Value: A Family Caregiver Speaks Out About the Choices & Challenges of Caregiving*, 2002. Available on the Web site of the National Family Caregivers Association (NFCAcares.org).

Sherkin-Langer F. *When Mommy Is Sick*. St. Louis, MO: Fern Publications, 1995. (P.O. Box 16893, St. Louis, MO 63105; Fax: 314-994-0052. Recommended for children ages 2–8.)

Strong M. *For the Well Spouse of the Chronically Ill*. 3rd rev. Mainstay, NY: Little, Brown, 1997.

Selected publications available from the National Multiple Sclerosis Society (800-344-3867), or online at http://www.nationalmssociety.org/Brochures:
- *What Everyone Should Know about Multiple Sclerosis*—an overview of MS, suitable for the whole family (available only in a print version)
- *Someone You Know Has MS: A Book for Families*—for children 5–12
- *Keep S'myelin*—a colorful newsletter for children ages 5–12, available in a print version or interactive, online version at http://www.nationalmssociety.org/KS
- *Keep S'myelin Activity Book*—for children 5–12 (available only in a print version)
- *When a Parent Has MS: A Teenager's Guide*—a booklet designed for teens
- *A Guide for Caregivers: Managing Major Changes*—a booklet for families dealing with caregiving challenges

Fertility, Pregnancy, Childbirth, and Gynecologic Care

Barbara Giesser, MD*, Maria Teresa Benedetto-Anzai, MD, and Michael A. Werner, MD

A person living with multiple sclerosis (MS) has an additional piece of bewildering information to add to the common concerns—such as the stability of the marriage, financial security, and the commitment to raising children—that all adults must take into account when thinking about starting a family or adding another child.

Regardless of the person's level of disability, a joint decision by prospective parents is vital. Specific questions about conception, pregnancy, and delivery are only the beginning; parenthood's bigger picture stretches many years into the future. Important long-range considerations include the possibility of increasing physical disability, the threat to financial security if income were to be lost due to that disability, the availability of adequate support from friends and extended family, and the ease or comfort with which the mother and father could share parenting and wage earning roles if needed. No single decision is "right" for everyone, and a couple may find that agreement on family planning decisions does not come quickly or easily. Proactive ways to become more comfortable with these decisions might include working together as a couple to make an honest assessment of your family situation—including the emotional, financial, and medical aspects of your daily life; asking your doctor to participate in a thorough discussion of present disease activity and possible disease progression; talking to other families in which one of the parents has MS; and seeking information from the National MS Society. Included in this chapter are answers to some of the most commonly asked questions about family planning, fertility, pregnancy, childbirth, and nursing, as well as suggestions for well-woman care. So often, those with a chronic condition do not receive basic screening tests, wellness strategies, and health care recommendations that are routinely offered to those without an illness.

---

*With grateful acknowledgment of materials from previous editions written by Kathy Birk, MD.

FAMILY PLANNING AND FERTILITY

I AM A 25-YEAR-OLD WOMAN WITH MS. WHAT TYPES OF CONTRACEPTION ARE SAFE FOR ME TO USE UNTIL MY HUSBAND AND I DECIDE THAT IT'S TIME TO START A FAMILY?

Contraceptive choices should be made after considering such factors as personal preference, manual dexterity and coordination, other medications being used, and the possible risk of infection.

- *Barrier contraceptives*, including the diaphragm, spermicides, and condoms, are safe and effective, but require manual dexterity and control or a partner who is willing and able to provide assistance. Using a diaphragm may increase your risk of bladder infections. In addition, the diaphragm requires the application of a spermicide prior to each act of intercourse and should be removed eight hours after insertion. For maximum reliability, it is recommended that a condom be used in conjunction with the diaphragm. Some women find it easier to use a spermicidal suppository that is inserted 10 minutes prior to intercourse. Used in combination with a condom, the spermicide is just as reliable as a diaphragm. The condom, alone or in combination with another birth control method, reduces the risk of sexually transmitted diseases.

- *Birth control pills* are generally considered a safe and highly effective means of birth control. However, the use of certain drugs, such as ***corticosteroids***, antibiotics, Dilantin (phenytoin) and Tegretol (carbamazepine), may reduce the pill's effectiveness (see Appendix C). Women who are taking any of these medications should discuss with their physician the need for additional protection, such as a condom or other barrier-type contraceptive. Birth control pills should be used with caution by any woman with high blood pressure. They should be avoided by women over the age of 35 who smoke, due to the increased risk of heart disease, and by women with very limited mobility because hormone-based contraceptives increase the risk of deep vein thrombosis.

- *Long-acting medications* are also safe and effective options. A progesterone shot (Depo-Provera) is effective for 12 weeks and is not known to be affected by those drugs that may alter the pill's effectiveness. Depo-Provera is also a safer method of birth control for women who are unable to stop smoking or have limited mobility. In addition, a long-acting, implantable progesterone device called Implanon was introduced in the summer of 2007. This device, which is simple to implant and remove, is more than 99 percent effective for up to 3 years. Each of these methods may be associated with side effects (including weight gain and irregular bleeding) and must be carefully reviewed and understood before a woman opts to use them.

- *The intrauterine device* (IUD) is also a safe, effective, and convenient form of birth control for women with a mutually monogamous relationship who are not planning to get pregnant but are not ready to consider an irreversible procedure such as tubal ligation. IUD insertion is a simple, reversible office procedure. Some concern exists that the use of antibiotics or immunosuppressive medications could decrease the effectiveness of the IUD, so women who are taking any of these medications should discuss with their physician the possible need for additional birth control protection. The two types of IUD currently available in the United States are the ParaGard (a copper device that is effective for up to 10 years) and the Mirena (a device that releases progesterone and can remain in place for up to 5 years).

- *Vasectomy*, a safe, effective sterilization procedure for men, is usually performed in a physician's office. Since reversal of a vasectomy requires delicate microsurgery that is only sometimes successful, it should be undertaken only after careful deliberation.
- *Tubal ligation*, a sterilization procedure for women, is typically done in the hospital under general anesthesia. This procedure must also be considered irreversible.

Although some of these contraceptive choices require visits to the health care provider, keep in mind that those visits do not replace the routine health care assessments that everyone should have. It is important to continue seeing those practitioners who do your regular exams, and to find out from them how often you need to be seen and what screening procedures are recommended for your age group.

WILL MY MS MAKE IT DIFFICULT FOR ME TO GET PREGNANT?

The disease itself does not cause infertility. The lower pregnancy rates that have been reported among women with MS result from a variety of factors: some of the medications used to treat MS may lead to problems with regular ovulation; women sometimes delay becoming pregnant because they are reluctant to stop taking medications that are important in the management of their MS, but are not safe for use during pregnancy; and some couples decide not to have children, or to have fewer children, because of the illness.

MY HUSBAND HAS RECENTLY BEEN DIAGNOSED WITH MS.
WILL THIS DISEASE MAKE HIM STERILE?

MS does not affect sperm production. Unless your husband had a pre-existing and unrelated problem with sperm production, there is no reason why he would become sterile in the future as a result of the disease.

Because some medications may compromise sperm quality, any woman who is trying to become pregnant should discuss with her physician all the medications her husband is taking. Although there are no published data on the interferon medications (Avonex, Betaseron, Extavia, and Rebif), Copaxone (glatiramer acetate), Tysabri (natalizumab) or Gilenya (fingolimod), men who are taking any of these medications might want to discuss with their physician the possibility of stopping the medication while trying to conceive. Men who are prescribed Novantrone (or any of the other chemotherapy agents that are sometimes used to treat MS—including Cytoxan (cyclophosphamide), Imuran (azathioprine), and Rheumatrex (methotrexate)— should consider freezing some of their sperm prior to starting the medication. In addition, some men with MS experience difficulties with intercourse and ejaculation that can interfere with conception, despite having normal sperm counts. Thus it may be worthwhile for some men to consider sperm banking at the first signs of erection or ejaculation issues.

SOMETIMES I HAVE DIFFICULTY GETTING OR KEEPING AN ERECTION DURING INTERCOURSE. WILL THIS PROBLEM PREVENT ME FROM BEING ABLE TO FATHER A CHILD?

It is important to distinguish between the ability to have intercourse and the ability to ejaculate sperm and ultimately father a child. Many men who have difficulty maintaining an adequate erection for neurologic or non-neurologic reasons are still able to ejaculate. If you are able to ejaculate, even though you sometimes have difficulty maintaining an erection that is firm enough for intercourse, your doctor can teach you how collect the ejaculate in a cup, and then use a syringe to place it directly in your partner's vagina. There is no truth to the commonly held belief that ejaculation outside the woman's vagina in any way affects the quality of the sperm or their ability to fertilize an egg. Refer to Chapter 11 for a discussion of MS-related erectile problems and available treatments.

I AM A 28-YEAR-OLD MAN WITH MS. FOR THE PAST SEVERAL MONTHS I HAVE HAD DIFFICULTY EJACULATING DURING INTERCOURSE. MY WIFE AND I HAVE BEEN TRYING TO HAVE A BABY FOR SEVERAL MONTHS WITHOUT ANY LUCK. HOW WILL WE BE ABLE TO HAVE A CHILD IF I CAN'T EJACULATE?

If you are able to ejaculate on some occasions but not others, you have the option of banking your sperm for insemination during your wife's fertile period. The disadvantage of this type of banking is that the quality of the sperm does deteriorate somewhat when frozen and thawed. If you are unable to ejaculate even intermittently, there are medications that can be used to try to stimulate you to ejaculate. The most commonly used drugs are pseudoephedrine and Tofranil (imipramine). These are prescribed by a fertility specialist who will closely monitor your ejaculation in order to adjust dosage levels. Some men who seem to have no ejaculation actually experience a "retrograde" or backward ejaculation. These same medications can convert a backward ejaculation to a forward ejaculation.

If you are unable to ejaculate even with the use of these medications, a reflex ejaculation can sometimes be induced through vibratory stimulation of the underside of the penis. This technique is effective for those individuals whose ejaculatory mechanism is impaired because of faulty nerve transmissions between the brain and spinal cord. Your doctor can show you how to use a vibrator effectively to achieve a sufficient level of stimulation. The ejaculate can be placed in your wife's vagina for attempted fertilization if the timing is appropriate, or stored for insemination at a later time.

Some men are unable to ejaculate with either medications or vibratory stimulation. A third technique, which completely bypasses the spinal cord and directly stimulates the nerves that release the ejaculate, is called *electroejaculation*. During a day hospital admission, under general anesthesia, the man is given a brief series of electric shocks through a probe placed into the rectum. The electric stimulation produces an ejaculation that can then be used for insemination or in vitro fertilization (IVF). This technique has been used for some time in men with spinal cord injury, but has also been used successfully in individuals with MS.

If electroejaculation is not successful, or is too unappealing, sperm can be taken directly from the testis with a biopsy needle. However, this procedure can only be used in conjunction with IVF, combined with injecting the sperm directly into the egg in the lab. It is important to note that with vibratory stimulation or electroejaculation, the poor quality of the sperm often requires IVF anyway.

MY DOCTOR HAS TOLD ME THAT VARIOUS KINDS OF TREATMENTS ARE AVAILABLE FOR IMPOTENCE CAUSED BY MS, INCLUDING MEDICATIONS AND SURGICAL IMPLANTS. WOULD I BE ABLE TO FATHER A CHILD USING ANY OF THESE TREATMENTS?
Impotence does not lead to infertility. As long as you are able to ejaculate, at least intermittently (with or without the medical interventions described in the previous answer), none of the treatments for erectile dysfunction will interfere with your ability to conceive (see Chapter 11).

I AM HAVING DIFFICULTY IN CONCEIVING, AND MY DOCTOR HAS SUGGESTED FERTILITY DRUGS. WILL THESE HAVE ANY EFFECT ON MY MS?
A few small studies have reported an increased relapse rate during the use of assisted reproductive techniques, including IVF. The decision to use this technology needs to be made on an individual basis by the woman and her gynecologist and neurologist.

PREGNANCY, LABOR, AND DELIVERY

DO I NEED TO STOP THE MEDICATIONS I AM TAKING BEFORE I START TRYING TO GET PREGNANT? I'M WORRIED THAT MY MS WILL GET WORSE IF I'M OFF THE MEDICATIONS FOR TOO LONG.
As a general rule, the use of any medications while a woman is pregnant or trying to become pregnant, including those bought over-the-counter, must be done with caution and under the advice of a physician who is familiar with their use during pregnancy. Medications used to treat MS fall into two groups—those that treat symptoms and those that are used prophylactically to reduce disease activity. Some drugs used to manage symptoms are safe to use during pregnancy; others are not. It is always advisable to check with your obstetrician prior to taking any medication while you are pregnant or trying to become pregnant.

None of the approved disease-modifying therapies—the beta-interferons (Avonex, Betaseron, Extavia, and Rebif), Copaxone (glatiramer acetate), Gilenya (fingolimod, Tysabri (natalizumab) or Novantrone (mitoxantrone)—are approved for use during pregnancy.

- All of the beta-interferon medications, Gilenya, and Tysabri have been given a Category C rating by the U.S. Food and Drug Administration (FDA), indicating that they should not be used during pregnancy because they have been shown in animal studies to produce harm to the animal fetus. However, recent data from the pregnancy registries maintained by the manufacturers of the interferon-β products have shown that the majority of patients who were accidentally exposed to beta-interferon in the first trimester and chose to continue the pregnancy delivered healthy infants.
- Copaxone has a Category B rating, meaning that no harm has been demonstrated in animal studies, but no data in humans demonstrate their safety. Given this B

rating, some neurologists and obstetricians feel comfortable allowing a woman to continue taking Copaxone until she becomes pregnant.

- Novantrone (mitoxantrone) is a category D medication because it is known to cause fetal damage. It should never be used by a woman who is pregnant; in fact, women are encouraged to take a pregnancy test before taking Novantrone. Because of the unknown effects of chemotherapy agents on eggs and sperm, men and women with MS who are prescribed Novantrone—or any of the other chemotherapy agents that are sometimes used to treat MS, including Cytoxan (cyclophospha-mide), Imuran (azathioprine), and Rheumatrex (methotrexate)—should consider harvesting and preserving their eggs or sperm prior to starting the medication.

Fortunately, treatment with a disease-modifying medication is not as necessary during pregnancy because the pregnancy itself produces a decrease in immune activity (to prevent the mother's body from rejecting the "foreign" fetus), which in turn reduces disease activity during that time.

It is generally recommended that women who are taking a beta-interferon medication or Copaxone stop their medication at least one or two menstrual cycles before trying to conceive, since a fertilized egg begins to develop before a woman realizes she is pregnant. Because Fingolimod stays in the body longer, it is recommended woman stop this medication at least 2 to 3 months before trying to conceive. Because there are no published data for Tysabri, women who are taking this medication need to work with their physician to determine how long before trying to conceive they should stop taking the medication. In general, it takes approximately 10–11 days for Tysabri to disappear from the body once a person stops taking it. However the effect on the immune system is much longer, so the best strategy is for a woman to talk with her gynecologist about how long she should wait before trying to conceive.

A disease-modifying therapy can be resumed within a week or two after delivery if the woman chooses not to breast-feed her baby.

I AM AFRAID TO TELL MY GYNECOLOGIST THAT I HAVE MS. I DON'T WANT ANYONE TO TELL ME THAT I SHOULDN'T HAVE A BABY. WHAT SHOULD I DO?
There is now ample evidence that a woman should not be discouraged from becoming pregnant simply because she has been diagnosed with MS. The major factors in the decision to become pregnant for couples affected by the disease are the same as for most other couples: How will adding a child to their lives work for them, and is this the right time?

Historically (and occasionally even now), couples have found that some members of the medical profession discourage pregnancy, and even parenting, for a woman who has MS. We now know that there is no medical reason for women with MS to avoid pregnancy. In fact, a woman's risk of having a relapse actually falls during pregnancy—particularly in the later months. Although her risk goes up significantly during the three to six months postpartum, it then drops again to her pre-pregnancy level shortly thereafter. Most important, research has shown that women who do choose to become pregnant and deliver a child do not develop more disability over their lifetime than women who never become pregnant.

In spite of these changes in medical opinion about pregnancy in women with MS, many couples find that they are discouraged from becoming pregnant by their physicians or well-meaning friends and family members. Women who are considering becoming pregnant should seek information and support from the National MS Society and consult a physician who is knowledgeable and willing to discuss their questions and concerns in a supportive manner. The decision to start a family or add additional children is a very personal one that must be made with careful attention to current and future emotional, medical, and financial factors. If you do not feel that you can discuss this subject comfortably with your present physician, perhaps you should find another with whom you are more at ease. An open and trusting relationship with your doctor is vital to your pregnancy and childbirth experience.

I RECENTLY FOUND OUT THAT I AM PREGNANT. MY HUSBAND THINKS WE SHOULD TERMINATE THE PREGNANCY BECAUSE OF MY MS. I CAN'T MAKE HIM UNDERSTAND HOW MUCH I WANT THIS BABY. HOW DO I DECIDE WHAT IS THE RIGHT THING TO DO?

As already mentioned, pregnancy itself has not been shown to contribute to long-term disability. The strength of the desire to raise and share life with a child should be the major factor in the decision for both you and your husband. As a couple, you need to weigh your feelings about parenting against a thoughtful assessment of your existing disability and possible future limitations that the disease might impose. Encourage your husband to share his concerns with you, think about his own desire for fatherhood, and perhaps contact the National MS Society to talk with others who have faced the fear of future parenting when MS is part of the picture.

The decision to have a child, as well as the lifetime of parenting that follows, should be a team effort. You and your husband both need to be comfortable with the decisions that you make. If the two of you are finding it difficult to communicate openly and effectively about this important life decision, you might consider talking together with your physician or with a knowledgeable psychotherapist.

CAN A WOMAN WHO HAS MS HAVE A NORMAL PREGNANCY?

MS does not appear to affect the course of pregnancy, labor, or delivery. Studies reviewing hundreds of pregnancies have found no evidence of an MS-related threat to the fetus. For many women, the risk of relapse or worsening of MS is lower during pregnancy, with the result that many women feel particularly well during this period. However, the fatigue that is so common in MS may be temporarily worsened by the normal fatigue associated with pregnancy. Women who are experiencing difficulties with balance must be particularly careful as the pregnancy progresses because their center of gravity will shift somewhat as their body changes shape. Problems with weakness or *flexor spasms* in the legs are manageable with assisted deliveries (forceps or vacuum device) and with an epidural type of anesthesia during the labor and delivery.

I RECENTLY HAD A MISCARRIAGE IN MY SECOND MONTH. WILL THIS MAKE MY MS WORSE?

Some increase in relapse rate may occur in the months following any pregnancy, whether the pregnancy ends in delivery or earlier because of spontaneous abortion (miscarriage) or elective termination. This possible disease worsening is likely to be temporary; studies have found no differences in long-term disability in women having no pregnancies, one pregnancy, or two or more pregnancies. Miscarriage during the first trimester of pregnancy is more common than most realize (occurring in 15 to 20 percent of all pregnancies) and is not caused by MS.

I FEEL SO MUCH BETTER WHEN I'M PREGNANT THAT I WISH I COULD JUST STAY PREGNANT ALL THE TIME. WHAT IS IT ABOUT BEING PREGNANT THAT MAKES MY MS FEEL BETTER?

The condition of pregnancy causes a woman's body to be in a mildly immunosuppressed state to ensure that the "foreign" fetus is not rejected by the mother's body. Therefore, during pregnancy, you are experiencing naturally the immunosuppression that certain medications can provide artificially for people with MS and some other *autoimmune diseases* (e.g., rheumatoid arthritis). This natural immunosuppression is probably responsible for the reduced disease activity during pregnancy. The most recent research indicates that a woman's relapse rate decreases progressively over the course of a pregnancy, hitting its lowest point in the third trimester.

The precise reason for this helpful reduction in immune activity is not clear. It has been demonstrated in *experimental allergic encephalomyelitis*, the animal model of MS, and in a small pilot study in women with MS, that estriol (a hormone that is only produced in pregnancy) can reduce inflammation and reduce disease activity. Based on these findings, estriol is now being evaluated in a large study for its ability to reduce the relapse rate in women with *relapsing-remitting MS*.

WHAT DRUGS ARE SAFE FOR ME TO TAKE WHILE I AM PREGNANT?

One should assume that all drugs could affect the fetus. Notable exceptions include certain antibiotics and sulfa drugs used to treat bladder infections. This is important because bladder infections are fairly common in individuals with MS and are also more likely to occur during pregnancy. Principen (ampicillin) is commonly used to treat these infections and is very safe during pregnancy and for nursing mothers. Increasingly, however, some of the infections are found to be resistant to this medication, as well as to some of the commonly used sulfa drugs, so other, safe alternatives may be utilized by the doctor.

Steroid medications can be used during acute *exacerbations* of MS. Fortunately, as noted above, such disease activity is decreased during pregnancy. Intensol (prednisone) is a steroid that has been used fairly commonly in pregnant women with a variety of illnesses, including MS, asthma, and arthritis. In the event of a significant exacerbation that requires treatment, your *neurologist* and obstetrician should discuss the appropriate dosage and timing of steroid treatment to avoid any negative impact on your baby.

IF NEW DRUGS FOR MS BECOME AVAILABLE WHILE I AM TRYING TO GET PREGNANT, IS IT SAFE FOR ME TO TAKE THEM?

No. Extreme caution is necessary when new drugs are approved before any research has been done on their use during pregnancy. The impact of a new drug on the newborn is often learned gradually, as women who are using the medication become pregnant and choose not to terminate the pregnancy. The long-term effects on an infant's development, function, and cancer risk are not clear at the time of birth or for many years to come.

HOW WILL MY LABOR AND DELIVERY BE AFFECTED BY MY MS? IS THERE ANYTHING SPECIFIC MY DOCTOR NEEDS TO KNOW TO HELP ME HAVE A SAFE DELIVERY?

Your labor is unlikely to be significantly different from what other women experience. Although MS does not increase the chance of having your delivery by cesarean section, you should be aware that all women face a 15 to 20 percent possibility of delivery by C section. Take advantage of available prenatal classes that will teach you and your partner about the stages of labor, delivery routes, and pain management strategies, and acquaint you with birthing alternatives available at the hospital.

It is important to meet with someone from the anesthesia department to discuss your MS and the options for pain control during labor. All forms of anesthesia, including epidural, spinal, and general, are considered safe for women with MS. An epidural can be particularly beneficial for women who have difficulty with leg control and spasms caused by *spasticity*. If fatigue or muscle weakness occurs after two hours of pushing to deliver the baby, the delivery may be assisted using forceps or a suction device on the baby's head.

POSTPARTUM AND BEYOND
....

WHAT IS THE LIKELIHOOD THAT THE MS WILL GET WORSE AFTER MY BABY IS BORN? IS THERE ANYTHING THAT I CAN DO TO DECREASE THIS LIKELIHOOD?

While virtually all studies have found that women with MS are less likely to experience relapses or worsening during the nine months of pregnancy, the disease does tend to be more active during the three to six months following delivery. About 10 percent of women experience relapses during the nine months of pregnancy, while 29 percent may have an exacerbation during the first six months after delivery.

For many women, a more significant concern than the experience they might have during pregnancy or postpartum is whether the decision to have a child will increase their long-term disability. Most research has found no difference in long-term disability between women with MS who had pregnancies and those who chose to remain childless. A recent, long-term study in Sweden even suggests that women who become pregnant after being diagnosed with MS may be less likely to develop a progressive course than women who do not become pregnant after the diagnosis. Another study has reported that women who had children before being diagnosed with MS had a later onset of the disease.

No specific treatment has been advocated to reduce the risk of postpartum relapse. Given the increased risk of disease activity in the postpartum period, you and your doctor may decide to start or restart one of the disease-modifying treatments (Avonex, Betaseron, Copaxone, Extavia, Gilenya, Rebif, or Tysabri) within a week or two after you deliver.

Studies have indicated that the best predictor of the likelihood of a post partum relapse is the pre-pregnancy relapse rate. In women who are considered "high risk" for a post partum relapse based on their pre-pregnancy level of disease activity, a few studies have shown that prophylactic post partum administration of intravenous steroids or intravenous immunoglobulin may reduce the relapse rate.

While the extreme exhaustion that characterizes new motherhood may mimic the fatigue so common in MS, that symptom alone should not warrant new medication use. Your postpartum lifestyle should allow you to focus on caring for yourself, resting, and feeding the infant. This will require that other household tasks be attended to by others, including some infant care, shopping, and social events. If you are employed, find out now how much maternity leave your employer will allow. Six to eight weeks of leave time is typical in the United States. Ideally, women with MS should have a longer leave since postpartum relapses can occur any time within the first six months following delivery.

I ALWAYS HOPED TO BREAST-FEED MY BABIES. NOW THAT I HAVE MS, WOULD NURSING BE SAFE FOR ME AND THE BABY?

Historically, neurologists usually discouraged women with MS from nursing, feeling that it posed an additional physical burden to a woman already at increased risk for an exacerbation. However, nursing is now widely encouraged if you have adequate dexterity, strength, and stamina. It eliminates the effort involved in bottle preparations and provides your baby with the best possible food. One small study has reported that women with MS who breast feed exclusively may be at lower risk for post partum relapse than women who do not nurse, or supplement nursing with formula, however this finding needs to be confirmed in additional, larger trials.

Certain medications are unsafe for a nursing infant because they are secreted into the breast milk. Because of the increased risk of relapse postpartum, some women may consider using one of the disease-modifying medications (Avonex, Betaseron, Copaxone, Extavia, Gilenya, Rebif, or Tysabri) to reduce the likelihood of an attack. Since it is not known if these medications are secreted into the breast milk, you should not take any of these medications if you plan to nurse your infant.

The high doses of ***corticosteroids*** that are prescribed for exacerbations of MS do result in significant concentrations of the steroids being present in breast milk. Since most postpartum relapses are likely to resolve spontaneously, any decision you make to use steroids must include the possible risk to the nursing baby. Because the immunomodulating drugs and the high doses of steroids prescribed for exacerbations do raise concerns about suppression of the newborn's ***immune system*** (as well as the mother's), nursing should be stopped if these drugs become necessary.

The new mother's postpartum lifestyle, as well as the care and support available to her, may help to avoid disease worsening. Caring for a newborn is an exhausting experience for all new parents. In an effort to assure yourself adequate, uninterrupted sleep, try to have someone else do at least one of the night feedings. If you are breast-feeding, do all of the feedings yourself during the first 2 weeks to build up steady and sufficient milk production. After that initial 2-week period, someone else can take over the nighttime feedings with formula or pumped and stored breast milk.

CAN I START TAKING MY REGULAR MS MEDICATIONS AS SOON AS MY BABY IS BORN?
The only limitation to medication use is whether a woman is nursing. If you are not planning to breast-feed, you may resume whatever medications you and your physician feel are best.

WHAT IS THE LIKELIHOOD THAT I WILL PASS MY MS ON TO MY CHILDREN?
The lifetime risk of MS in a child born to a person with MS has been estimated to be in the range of 2 to 5 percent (2 to 5 in 100), compared to the 0.1 percent lifetime risk (1 in 750) for the general population. In other words, while there is an increased risk to children with a family history of the disease, the actual risk is small (95 percent chance that MS will not occur). Within that range, the risk is higher for girls than for boys. We do not know if the risk is higher for children of mothers or fathers with MS. At present, there is no way to diagnose MS or assess the MS risk in a particular infant before or after birth.

I WAS ABLE TO GET PREGNANT WITH NO DIFFICULTY. NOW I'M WORRIED ABOUT HOW I'LL BE ABLE TO TAKE CARE OF MY BABY ONCE IT'S BORN. I'M EXHAUSTED ALL THE TIME AS IT IS. WHAT SHOULD I DO?
Planning ahead is essential to a successful start at parenting. If you are employed, start by trying to arrange time off from work after your delivery. Maternity leave for at least 8 weeks is in your best interest and your child's. The new father should also look into the possibility of family-leave time under the Family Medical Leave Act (see Chapter 20) or temporarily arranging his schedule to be home somewhat earlier in the day. The exhaustion of new motherhood will gradually increase throughout the day. This fatigue, coupled with the possible worsening of MS symptoms postpartum, means that you are likely to need a significant amount of help and support. Good parental teamwork will make these early days go more enjoyably and comfortably.

As you shop for baby furniture and equipment, look for things that are easy and convenient to manipulate. Choose such items as a highchair, car seat, and bath equipment with an eye to both safety for your baby and energy conservation for yourself. Create child-friendly play areas in your home where you can watch and interact with your baby as easily and comfortably as possible. Try to arrange for some hours of baby care each day so that you can get uninterrupted rest. You might consider a consultation with an ***occupational therapist*** (see Chapter 10) who can recommend energy management strategies for home and at work. Of course, couples who are planning a family can never know for sure what might happen to impact their parenting abilities. To the extent that you can brainstorm ahead of time about possible problems that might arise, you will feel more confident of your ability to manage in the days ahead.

GYNECOLOGIC CARE

DO I NEED ANY SPECIAL CARE FROM MY GYNECOLOGIST WHEN I AM NOT PREGNANT?
All women, including those with MS, must be educated about their contraceptive options and knowledgeable about sexually transmitted diseases. Women who are

managing the problems associated with a chronic illness sometimes neglect their routine medical care; regular checkups, Pap tests, and mammograms are as essential for those with MS as they are for anyone else.

Women who have used any of the disease-modifying medications to treat their MS should have a Pap test once a year. Abnormal results on tests that screen for pre-cancerous changes in the cervix are more common when the immune system is less able to discourage the formation of abnormal cells, including those on the cervix. All women should have a mammogram on the schedule recommended by the American Cancer Society: an initial screening mammogram at age 40 (or earlier if there is a family history of breast cancer), and annually after that.

I HAVE BEGUN EXPERIENCING HOT FLASHES NOW THAT I AM AT MENOPAUSE. GETTING SO WARM MAKES THE NUMBNESS AND TINGLING I HAVE FEEL SO MUCH WORSE. IS THERE ANYTHING I CAN DO ABOUT THAT?

This is an important question to discuss with your gynecologist and neurologist. While hormone replacement therapy (HRT) is effective in relieving hot flashes and may reduce the risk of bone loss (*osteoporosis*), long-term HRT may be associated with an increased risk for breast cancer and heart disease. As a result, many physicians are no longer recommending long-term use of HRT or are recommending a short course in the early menopausal years to reduce symptoms and increase your overall comfort.

Together, you and your physicians will weigh the possible benefits of HRT against the known risks, given your personal and family medical history. In the meantime, you may also find that cooling strategies—such as drinking a cold glass of water or using a cooling scarf or hat—will reduce your discomfort during hot flashes. (See Chapter 10 for more information about cooling garments.) Other strategies that may be helpful include vitamin E, up to 400 IU a day, and soy (drink, powder, or tofu). The herbs typically recommended for menopausal symptoms (evening primrose oil, black cohosh, and dong quai) have not been found to yield consistently positive results. If you do opt to try these, be sure to inform your physicians and start with low doses.

OTHER THAN USING HRT, ARE THERE ANY OTHER STRATEGIES I CAN USE TO REDUCE MY RISK OF OSTEOPOROSIS?

A very significant predictor of risk for osteoporosis and osteoporotic fracture is reduced bone mass. Women with MS have been found to have lower than average bone density of the hips and spine, probably due to their reduced mobility and increased use of steroids. The amount of reduction in bone density found in women with MS can be expected to increase their risk of fracture by two to seven times that of a person with normal bone density. A simple bone density test can alert you and your doctor if you are at risk for osteoporosis.

All women, starting when they are very young, should be certain they are getting at least 1,000 mg of calcium every day. Dairy products (milk, yogurt, and cheese) are the easiest way to get this amount through the diet (three servings every day of a dairy product). If one does not eat a lot of dairy products, calcium-fortified orange juice is a good substitute, and calcium supplements are also acceptable. Once postmenopausal, all women should increase their calcium intake to 1,200 mg per day if they are taking HRT, and 1,500 mg per day if they are not using hormones.

Recently, women with MS were found to be at higher risk for vitamin D deficiency. This, too, can contribute to the development of osteoporosis. Although this deficiency may simply be due to inadequate intake of the vitamin, it may also result from insufficient exposure to the sun. People with MS who stay out of the sun to avoid becoming overheated, may be depriving themselves of the 10 minutes or so of sun exposure per day that provides adequate amounts of vitamin D. To ensure that you are getting an adequate amount of this important vitamin, you can take it in pill form (600–800 IU is the recommended daily dose; 4,000 is considered the safe upper limit). Unfortunately, vitamin D is not found in many foods other than fortified milk. In addition to adequate amounts of calcium and vitamin D, it is important for women to engage in weight-bearing exercise to reduce their risk of bone loss.

Fosamax (alendronate), Actonel (risedronate), and Boniva (ibandronate) are non-hormonal medications for postmenopausal women that prevent thinning of the bones; decrease fractures of the spine, hip, and wrist by up to 50 percent; and treat existing osteoporosis. Evista (raloxifene), an osteoporosis prevention drug that works like estrogen, was approved for postmenopausal women in 1997. This drug increases bone mass (although not as significantly as estrogen does), reduces the risk of spinal fractures (but not hip fractures), and lowers low-density lipoprotein ("bad" cholesterol) serum levels. Unlike estrogen, Evista does not stimulate the uterine lining, so there is no need for progesterone, the second hormone that is often combined with estrogen in HRT. In addition, Evista does not increase breast cancer risk, and may even reduce it. It does, however, slightly increase a woman's risk for blood clots and may cause hot flashes to recur during the first few months of use.

RECOMMENDED READINGS

Birk K, Giesser B. Fertility, pregnancy, and childbirth. In R. Kalb (ed.). *Multiple Sclerosis: A Guide for Families* (3rd ed.). New York: Demos Medical Publishing; 2006: 81–92.

Birk K, Morrison EH. General health and well-being. In R. Kalb (ed.). *Multiple Sclerosis: A Guide for Families* (3rd ed.). New York: Demos Medical Publishing; 2006: 181–194.

Boston Women's Health Book Collective. *Our Bodies Ourselves: Menopause.* New York: Simon & Shuster, 2006.

Haseltine FP, Cole SS, Gray DB. *Reproductive Issues for Persons with Physical Disabilities.* Baltimore, MD: Paul H. Brookes Publishing, 1993.

North American Menopause Society. *Menopause Guidebook.* Tel: 440–442-7550. Automated Consumer Request Line: 800-774-5342; Website: www.menopause.org; E-mail: info@menopause.org. A comprehensive 50-page booklet published by the leading organization devoted to improving women's health through menopause and beyond.

Rogers J. *The Disabled Woman's Guide to Pregnancy and Birth.* New York: Demos Medical Publishing, 2006.

Resources for Rehabilitation. *A Woman's Guide to Coping with Disability* (4th ed.). Lexington, MA: Resources for Rehabilitation, 2003.

Selected publications available from the National Multiple Sclerosis Society (800-344-4867) or online at www.nationalmssociety.org/Brochures:

- *Genes: The Basic Facts*
- *MS and Pregnancy*
- *Hormones: The Basic Facts*
- *MS and Intimacy*
- *Fatigue: What You Should Know*

RECOMMENDED NEWSLETTERS

Environmental Nutrition
(Web: www.environmentalnutrition.com)

Harvard Women's Health Watch
(Tel: 877-649-9457;
E-mail: hhp_info@health.harvard.edu;
Web: www.health.harvard.edu/newsletters/Harvard_Womens_Health_Watch.htm)

Nutrition Action Healthletter
(Web: www.cspinet.org/nah/)

Tufts University Health and Nutrition Letter
(Email: healthletterhelp@tufts.edu;Web: http://www.tuftshealthletter.com)

Children Get MS, Too

Network of Pediatric MS Centers of Excellence*

Yes—children as well as adults get multiple sclerosis (MS). Although *symptoms* of MS were recognized in children shortly after Jean-Martin Charcot first described the disease in the latter part of the 19th century, it took more than 50 years for the medical community to acknowledge that MS can occur in childhood. Today, clinicians and researchers are working collaboratively to figure out how best to meet the needs of youngsters diagnosed with MS and their families, while looking for clues to why and how the disease occurs so early in this small segment of the MS population. It is their shared hope that learning more about pediatric MS will also help answer some of the unanswered questions about adult-onset MS.

In this chapter, members of the Network of Pediatric MS Centers of Excellence, which is under the auspices of the National Multiple Sclerosis Society's National Clinical Advisory Board and Research Programs Advisory Committee, answer the most commonly asked questions about children and adolescents with MS. The network is made up of clinicians with expertise in MS—including adult and child *neurologists*, nurses, psychologists, and social workers from sites around the United States. Like MS in adults, the disease in children is highly variable and unpredictable—which means that no one knows how any one child's MS is likely to manifest itself or progress over time. Therefore, the goal of this chapter is to explain what we currently know about pediatric MS, including how it is diagnosed and treated and the kinds of symptoms it can cause, and to describe the resources available to help children with MS and their families.

HOW MANY KIDS HAVE MS?

MS affects approximately 400,000 people in the United States and more than 1 million worldwide. Although MS is generally considered an "adult" disease, the National MS Society estimates that as many as 8,000 to 10,000 American children younger than 18 years have the disease, and another 10,000–15,000 have

---

*With grateful acknowledgement of materials from the fourth edition written by Nancy Kuntz, MD.

experienced a single episode of neurologic *symptoms* that are suggestive of MS. Some of these children will go on to develop MS—most likely as adults—while others will not.

Literature from countries including Argentina, Austria, Canada, Finland, France, Germany, Israel, Italy, Japan, Russia, Thailand, Turkey, and the United Kingdom—as well as the United States—confirms that pediatric MS occurs in many areas around the world. However, it is not known at this time if the geographic distribution in children is the same as it is in adults (see Chapter 3 for more information about the geographic distribution of MS in adults).

WHY DID MY CHILD GET MS?

As is the case with adults, we still do not know why one person gets MS and another person does not. We have not identified any specific factor that could have triggered this event in your child, and we know of nothing you could have done that would have prevented it from happening. Research indicates that the chances of a person developing MS are influenced by genetic and environmental factors. In other words, a child with a certain genetic disposition comes into contact with some kind of environmental trigger during the early years, but the MS does not become active in most people until adulthood (see Chapter 2 for more information about the *etiology* of MS). We still do not know what causes MS to become active in some young children and adolescents.

IS MS IN CHILDREN SIMILAR TO MS IN ADULTS?

In general, the disease process is similar in children and adults—episodes of neurologic changes or symptoms are caused by *inflammation* and damage to the *myelin* and *axons* in the *central nervous system (CNS)*. This process of *demyelination* is believed to be caused by an *autoimmune* process in which the body's *immune system* mistakenly attacks CNS tissue. Pediatric MS almost always begins as *relapsing-remitting MS (RRMS)*, consisting of *acute* episodes (referred to as *relapses*, exacerbations, or attacks) that are usually followed by periods of improvement and *remission* (see Chapter 2 for more information about the MS disease courses). *Primary-progressive multiple sclerosis*, which is progressive from onset without any acute relapses along the way, has rarely been described in children.

Compared with adult-onset MS, the disease in children appears to progress more slowly, at least during the first two decades following the diagnosis. Although children with MS have been observed to have more frequent exacerbations or relapses than adults with MS, the duration of these episodes is usually shorter in children, with a higher proportion of children experiencing complete recovery of function.

Additional long-term follow-up of children with MS is needed to determine whether they, like most adults, eventually transition from RRMS to *secondary-progressive MS (SPMS)*. The limited data we have so far suggest that fewer children make the transition to SPMS and, when they do transition, it is generally in adulthood, after a longer interval than is typically seen in people with adult-onset MS. See Chapter 2 for more information about disease progression in adults.

Overall, many symptoms and *signs* of MS are similar between the different age groups. Problems with vision, walking, thinking and memory, and bladder and bowel function, as well as *sensory* disturbances such as numbness and tingling or pain, can occur among children and adults with MS. The particular ways in which pediatric and adult-onset MS are the same or different is an active area of current research.

HOW IS MS DIAGNOSED IN CHILDREN?

At present, the diagnostic criteria are the same for children and adults. The doctor must be able to find evidence of *plaques* (also called *lesions* or *scars*) in the myelin of the CNS that have occurred in two separate locations at two different points in time. In addition, all other possible explanations for these plaques and the symptoms they are causing must be ruled out (see Chapter 2 for more information about the diagnosis of MS).

Just as in adults, the neurologist relies on the medical history, findings on neurologic examination, and various tests to help make the diagnosis. Tests may include *magnetic resonance imaging (MRI)*, *lumbar puncture* (also referred to as a *spinal tap*), and *visual evoked potentials*. One aspect of the diagnostic process that can differ between adults and children is the types of non-MS conditions the doctor must rule out to be sure that the culprit is MS. Because different conditions must be excluded in children, different blood tests may need to be performed. Nonetheless, the basic steps for making the diagnosis in children and adults with MS are similar.

IS MS MORE DIFFICULT TO DIAGNOSE IN CHILDREN THAN ADULTS?

MS can be more difficult to diagnose in children than in adults for a couple of reasons. In the first place, children are not as likely as adults to notice or report odd sensations or changes in their vision or balance—particularly if the changes last only one to several days—and they may not report these symptoms as quickly or clearly as adults might. This makes it more difficult for the physician to identify episodes that would meet the criteria for a diagnosis of MS.

In addition, children can experience a single episode of neurologic symptoms that is characteristic of demyelination in the CNS without it being caused by MS. *Acute disseminated encephalomyelitis* (ADEM) may follow a viral illness or some other event such as an immunization, or occur as a reaction to a medication. So, when a child comes to the doctor with neurologic symptoms, the doctor's challenge is to figure out whether this is a one-time event, or the first episode of what will eventually turn out to be MS. This distinction is important, because ADEM does not require the kind of ongoing treatment generally recommended for anyone with MS.

The doctor's challenge is further complicated by the fact that ADEM can sometimes cause recurrent symptoms that may be difficult to distinguish from MS symptoms. Efforts to distinguish ADEM from MS are continuing among clinicians and researchers in the hopes of being able to diagnose MS more quickly and easily.

Although ADEM causes some neurologic symptoms and signs that are very similar to those of MS—such as optic neuritis or other vision problems, and difficulties with balance, sensation, or strength—others are quite different. For example, children with ADEM more frequently experience fever, headache, nausea, and vomiting before the onset of neurologic symptoms. They may also develop seizures or become very irritable or sleepy.

In addition, there are a number of *leukodystrophies* (disorders involving abnormal formation of myelin in the brain and spinal cord that cause progressive loss of neurologic function) that can appear during childhood and imitate an initial acute episode of MS. Careful evaluation of each child's symptoms, physical examination, and MRI findings is necessary to determine if one of these other rare disorders might be responsible for the symptoms that are occurring.

WHAT ARE THE MOST COMMON SYMPTOMS THAT KIDS EXPERIENCE?

Demyelinating lesions caused by MS can occur at any site in the brain and spinal cord. Children frequently have a combination of symptoms during an exacerbation (which by definition lasts more than 24 hours). Common symptoms include visual loss or blurred vision, poor ***coordination*** or imbalance, numbness or tingling, and weakness. Coordination problems that affect speaking and eating can also occur. Most clinical symptoms respond to treatment and resolve over a number of weeks, although it is not uncommon for similar or different symptoms to occur later. In addition, emotional changes and problems with thinking and memory can occur in children with MS just as they do in adults. It is particularly important to be on the lookout for these emotional and cognitive changes because they can impact a child's academic performance and interactions with friends and classmates.

WHAT KINDS OF DOCTORS TREAT CHILDREN WITH MS?

The reality is that very few physicians have had much experience with young MS patients. General neurologists may or may not have many patients with MS of any age in their practice, and many pediatric neurologists have never treated a child with MS. Among neurologists around the world with MS expertise, some have seen children with the disease, while others have not. So, although children with MS are receiving treatment from their pediatricians, family doctors, general adult and pediatric neurologists, and neurologists who specialize in MS, you may or may not have anyone near you who is familiar with pediatric MS. You can call the National Multiple Sclerosis Society (800-344-3867) to find out what resources are available in your community.

To address the needs of children and teens with MS, the National Multiple Sclerosis Society established the first-of-its-kind network of Pediatric MS Centers of Excellence in 2006. The centers were established in six locations around the country, in order to be accessible to as many children and families living with MS as possible. They are staffed by teams of pediatric and adult neurologists, as well as nurses, psychologists, social workers, and other clinicians with the expertise to help children and their families manage this disease. The Center locations are

● Center for Pediatric-Onset Demyelinating Disease at the Children's Hospital of Alabama, University of Alabama at Birmingham (Project Director, Jayne Ness, MD, PhD)

- Pediatric MS Center of the Jacobs Neurological Institute, State University of New York at Buffalo (Project Director, Bianca Weinstock-Guttman, MD, Co-director, Ann Yeh, MD)
- Pediatric MS Clinic at Mayo Clinic Rochester, Minnesota (co-Project Directors, Moses Rodriguez, MD and Marc C. Patterson, MD)
- University of California, San Francisco Regional Pediatric MS Center (Project Director, Emmanuelle Waubant, MD, PhD)
- National Pediatric MS Center at Stony Brook University Hospital, Long Island, NY (Project Director, Lauren Krupp, MD)
- Partners Pediatric MS Center at the Massachusetts General Hospital for Children in Boston (Project Director, Tanuja Chitnis, MD)

More information about each of the centers is available at http://www.nationalms society.org/PediatricMS.

In addition to providing comprehensive care for children with MS, the pediatric MS centers have a shared goal of learning more about pediatric MS and sharing this information with pediatricians, neurologists, schools, and the public. To this end, the network centers are engaged in research studies, and the sites have agreed to share their research data (with all names removed) to ensure that they have the numbers necessary to conduct good prospective studies and clinical trials.

WHAT KINDS OF CARE ARE AVAILABLE AT THE PEDIATRIC MS CENTERS?

Most importantly, the pediatric MS centers are multidisciplinary referral centers where specialists have experience diagnosing, treating, and developing comprehensive treatment plans for children and teens with MS and related disorders. Because each child's MS is unique, the most appropriate treatment team will be different for each individual and will include many, but perhaps not all, of the following pediatric-trained specialists: neurologists, neuropsychologists, *urologists*, ophthalmologists, orthopedic surgeons, psychiatrists, nurses, *physical therapists, occupational therapists, speech/language pathologists*, and social workers.

In addition, all children with MS benefit from having someone—perhaps the social worker, nurse, or a child life specialist—who acts as a liaison between the health care team and the school system. This person helps ensure that the child's teachers have an adequate understanding of MS symptoms, the ways in which they may be impacting his or her performance and participation at school, and the accommodations that may be needed to promote optimal comfort, interaction, and achievement.

All of the strategies described in Chapter 2 and Part II that help with the diagnosis and treatment of adults with MS are necessary to provide care for children and teens with MS. In addition, some of the procedures (such as MRI, lumbar puncture, and evoked potentials) may require sedation of younger children for the testing to be accomplished with minimal risk and high technical quality. Pediatric referral centers, including pediatric MS centers, have protocols available to provide necessary sedation to children undergoing these tests.

HOW IS MS IN CHILDREN TREATED?

Relapse Management

As with adults, MS relapses in children are generally managed with intravenous corticosteroids (see Chapter 6). In the case of severe relapses that do not respond to corticosteroids, intravenous immunoglobulin may be used. Use of *plasmapheresis* is reserved for only the most severe relapses that have not responded to any other treatment intervention.

Disease-Modifying Therapies

The disease-modifying medications (see Chapter 6) that are delivered by injection—Avonex (interferon beta-1α), Betaseron (interferon beta-1β), Copaxone (glatiramer acetate), Extavia (interferon beta-1β) and Rebif (interferon beta-1α)—are generally considered the first-line treatment options to help slow the progression of MS in children. Although the randomized, controlled **clinical trials** of these medications only included participants older than 18 years, the consensus among MS specialists is that these treatments appear to be safe and well tolerated in children. Side effects in kids appear to be similar to those in adults, and may include abnormal liver function, injection-site reactions, fever, and flu-like reactions.

Other options for treating MS are available if a child does not gain sufficient benefit from the first-line medications. Tysabri (natalizumab) is the one most often used; Novantrone (mitoxantrone) and Rituxan (rituximab) are also used. Because the second-line options are associated with significantly greater long-term risks (see Chapter 6), they are generally used in children only at MS specialty centers. No randomized, controlled trials of these medications have been done in children with MS, but there are published reports describing the use of Tysabri in children. A decision to use a second-line medication is made on an individual basis considering each child's disease state and general health.

An oral medication, Gilenya (fingolimod) was approved to treat MS in 2010. No studies of this drug have been done in children and to date, there are no published reports of its use with this younger group. Like the second-line medications just described, Gilenya may be associated with greater long-term risks than the injectable medications, but the drug is too new to know what those might be.

Symptom Management

Symptom management strategies are also extremely important for children with MS. Treatments for problems such as fatigue, weakness, pain, mood disturbance, memory problems, sleep problems, and adjustment difficulties are all available—including both nonpharmacologic interventions (such as **rehabilitation** strategies for fatigue and weakness, counseling for coping and adjustment difficulties or behavior problems, and cognitive remediation [also called **cognitive rehabilitation**] for problems with thinking and memory) and medications (such as antidepressants for mood problems, **anticholinergic** medications for bladder problems, and antispasticity medications for muscle stiffness). The chapters in Part II of this book provide answers to questions about the various types of management strategies that are commonly used in adults with MS—virtually all of which are being adapted for use in children when and if the need arises.

THE DOCTOR JUST TOLD MY HUSBAND AND ME THAT OUR DAUGHTER HAS MS. I'M WONDERING IF IT'S A GOOD IDEA TO TELL HER WHAT SHE HAS—I THINK IT WILL BE TOO SCARY FOR HER TO HANDLE.

Although it is natural to want to protect your child from having to worry about MS as long as possible, there are several good reasons for talking openly about it with her:

- Children and teens know when they are not feeling well, and they also know when you are worried or upset about something. Without the information they need to understand what is going on, children typically use their own imaginations to come up with an explanation. And when children's imaginations get involved, they almost always come up with something more frightening than the actual problem.

- Many children, particularly younger ones, do not know how to put their worries into words or ask the questions lurking in their minds. When parents talk about the MS in a simple, honest way, they are letting their kids know that it is okay to ask their questions, while at the same time giving them the words the youngsters may need to express themselves. They are also giving the clear message that MS is not too scary to talk about.

- When you talk openly with your children about what is going on, you promote a feeling of trust within the family and set the stage for open communication and effective problem solving. This kind of openness eliminates the need for secrecy and helps to ensure that your children will feel comfortable talking to you about what is on their minds—in relation to MS, or anything else that comes along.

- Children feel more secure and less afraid when their parents can discuss diagnosis and treatment issues openly with them. This kind of openness helps them feel that you and their doctors are doing everything you can to take the best possible care of them.

- As with adult-onset MS, the general recommendation is to begin treatment as soon as possible to reduce the number of exacerbations and slow progression. Children and teens who are included in discussions about their treatment will find it much easier to understand and comply with whatever treatment strategies are recommended by the doctor.

- Youngsters with MS will be involved in ongoing relationships with doctors, nurses, and other health care professionals, and undergoing periodic examinations, medical tests, and evaluations of various kinds. Parents who encourage open, comfortable communication with these professionals—which is geared to the child's age and level of understanding—are helping to promote the kind of trusting relationship that can make these experiences less frightening.

MY SON IS NOW 14. JUST LIKE ANY OTHER TEENAGER, HE DEFINITELY HAS A MIND OF HIS OWN. NOW THAT MOST OF HIS SYMPTOMS HAVE CLEARED UP, HE DOESN'T WANT TO TAKE HIS MEDICATION OR THINK ABOUT HIS MS. I KNOW THAT HE'S SUPPOSED TO TAKE HIS SHOTS REGULARLY, BUT I DON'T KNOW HOW TO CONVINCE HIM.

No one—child, teenager, or adult—likes to take medication when he or she is feeling fine. One of the biggest challenges for any person with MS is getting used to the idea of taking an injectable medication on an ongoing basis, particularly since the disease-modifying therapies do not cure the disease or make people feel better. In reality, they are an investment in the future—a way to slow the disease as much as possible—which is a concept that children and teens may find very difficult to buy into. So, a child or teen whose symptoms have remitted may have a hard time understanding why it is important to take a medication that is injected and may cause uncomfortable side effects as well; and teenagers may not like doing what their parents want them to do under the best of circumstances!

This is one of those situations that do not have a one-size-fits-all answer. But the best strategy may be to ask your child's neurologist to sit down with your son to talk over the treatment plan. A conversation like that can accomplish a couple of things: By engaging your son in a conversation about the goals of treatment, the doctor is helping him to feel more ownership of the process—so that the treatment is something he is planning and implementing rather than having done to him. In addition, the plan becomes something between your son and his doctor, rather than something his parents are pushing. Most teenagers will respond better to recommendations that come from adults other than their parents!

HOW IS MY CHILD'S MS LIKELY TO PROGRESS?

The long-term outcome of MS is very difficult, if not impossible, to predict for an individual adult or child. This unpredictability is, in fact, one of the most stressful aspects of the disease. If your child's MS appears to be particularly active early on—including, for example, frequent exacerbations, significant loss of function, and marked changes on the MRI—the neurologist may recommend more aggressive treatment in an effort to slow the disease process.

Identifying tests that can better predict the outcome of MS is an active research area for investigators who study children and adults with the disease. In the meantime, children and adults with MS share the challenge of living with a disease that is unpredictable from day to day and year to year (see Chapter 15 for some suggestions on how to cope with this uncertainty).

WHAT ARE THE CHANCES THAT MY OTHER CHILDREN WILL GET MS?

Although the presence of MS in one family member increases the risk in other close family members, the chances are relatively small that another person in your family will get MS. While the frequency of MS in the general population is about 0.13 percent (or 1 in 750), the risk of MS in siblings or first-degree relatives of a child with MS increases to between 2 and 5 percent. The highest observed risk of recurrence is in an identical (or *monozygotic*) twin, in which the risk in the other twin has been observed to be 25 to 30 percent after the first twin has been diagnosed with MS. Studies have estimated that about 20 percent of MS is seen clustered in certain families that also have increased frequencies of other ***autoimmune diseases*** (such as rheumatoid arthritis, myasthenia gravis, or thyroiditis, for example).

The fact that the risk of MS in an identical twin of someone with the disease (25–30 percent) is less than 100 percent underscores the fact that nongenetic, as-yet-unidentified environmental factors are probably involved in the etiology of MS in both children and adults.

WHAT DO WE TELL THE SCHOOL ABOUT OUR CHILD'S MS?

Teachers and school personnel play a vital role in the life of a child with MS or related conditions. It is important to educate your child's teachers and school personnel about pediatric MS and how it affects your child when he or she is in school. Children with MS should be encouraged to participate in normal school activities as much as possible. They may, however, be affected in the following ways:

- Fatigue, which is the most common symptom, is likely to be most noticeable toward the end of the day. It can, however, occur at any time.
- Handwriting and other tasks involving manual dexterity may become affected due to numbness and tingling, weakness, or lack of coordination of the hands.
- Children may have a sense of bladder urgency with MS, and may feel the need to urinate frequently.
- Learning may be affected by problems with memory, reasoning, processing speed, and attention.

Other things that teachers need to understand include the following:

- MS is not a life-threatening disease.
- MS is not contagious.
- The symptoms in MS can vary a lot from day to day, or even from one time of day to another.
- People with MS can experience relapses (also called "attacks" or "***exacerbations***") that result in new or worsening problems with strength, balance, vision, sensation, bladder functioning, or cognition. Often, MS relapses are treated with ***corticosteroids*** to hasten recovery but it may still take weeks to improve.
- Many patients with MS, including children and teens, are treated with injectable medications that may be given once a week (Avonex), three times per week (Rebif), every other day (Betaseron or Extavia), or every day (Copaxone) to help decrease the frequency of the relapses. Some of these medications (Avonex, Betaseron, Extavia, and Rebif) can cause flu-like symptoms in the first hours following the injection, but these symptoms should improve after several weeks and should not interfere with school attendance.
- If a child is having significant learning difficulties or the symptoms are significantly interfering with a child's ability to learn, a parent may request that the child be evaluated for special services. This could result in a child needing an individualized education plan or a 504 plan. If a child has a prolonged absence from school, home tutoring can help him or her stay connected to the class and maintain a normal routine. The child, school personnel, parents, and other students can benefit from a planned school reentry program that can enable a better transition back into school, especially if a child is having difficulty with academics or peer relationships. The program can be a presentation about pediatric MS or the related condition presented by a teacher, school nurse, the child's parent, the child or adolescent, or a combination of these people.

Input from the child about the approach he or she is most comfortable with is essential.

WE FEEL VERY ISOLATED. ARE THERE SUPPORT SERVICES AND PROGRAMS FOR KIDS AND THEIR FAMILIES?

Children with MS have unique needs, and everyone in the family may need a variety of support services and programs as they deal with this chronic, unpredictable illness. We are happy to report that many resources are available to help you and your child. The National Multiple Sclerosis Society and Multiple Sclerosis Society of Canada offer services and programs both nationally and locally for young people with MS and their families. The *Young Persons with MS: A Network for Families with a Child or Teen with MS* (go to http://www.nationalmssociety.org/PedNetwork for more information)—a collaborative effort of the Multiple Sclerosis Societies in the United States and Canada—provides opportunities for children and teens with MS and their parents to interact and connect with others who are dealing with similar challenges. Since its inception in 1990, the program has provided opportunities for networking via telephone, letters, chat rooms, e-mail, or one-to-one peer support with other children and families in similar circumstances. In this forum, the families receive much-needed support.

The *Young Persons with MS Network* also offers a variety of programs (including occasional teleconferences) on issues of importance to families with a child with MS: working with the schools, MS research, managing symptoms, handling the transition from high school to college, among others. Staff members are available to answer questions related to MS and assist with referrals. They also work with families on school and social issues related to MS, and with plans and strategies for the future. To contact the Network, send an e-mail to childhoodms@nmss.org, or call the Society's Information Resource Center at 800-344-4867.

Across the country, many chapters of the National Multiple Sclerosis Society offer programs specifically designed for young people with MS and their families. These programs may take various forms, from a 1-day event to a weekend camp. The National Pediatric MS Center at Stony Brook University Hospital, Long Island, NY, offers a 4-day, weekend camp for teens with MS. The campers come from all over the United States and Canada for a few days of recreation. Although there is no formal "education" at the camp, the kids can talk to one another about their experiences, and staff members are available to answer questions. The recreational activities (such as a ropes course, swimming, or sailing) are facilitated by a group called A2A (Access to Adventure), an outdoor adventure group that has experience working with people with disabilities. For more information about the camp, call (631) 444-7802.

Similar camps are held in other areas around the country.

WHAT DO SCIENTISTS AND CLINICIANS HOPE TO LEARN BY STUDYING PEDIATRIC MS?

The study of pediatric MS has the potential to provide important information in many different areas:

● Research has shown that a person's lifetime risk of MS is somehow established during his or her childhood. Research efforts to identify environmental factor(s) that cause MS in adults have not been successful. The study of children and young adults with pediatric MS may provide an ideal opportunity to understand what triggers demyelination in the CNS. One unique aspect of studying pediatric MS is that the period from birth to the onset of MS is much shorter than in adult MS—which means that there are fewer events or factors to consider as possible culprits.

- The Pediatric MS Centers of Excellence have created a standardized way to analyze each child's medical history (immunizations, infections, newborn factors, and environmental exposures) from birth, with the goal of identifying those factors that may precipitate a demyelinating disease.

- Another unique aspect of pediatric MS is the more frequent development of ADEM early in life. The study of children with MS may provide an answer to ADEM as a risk factor for the further attacks of demyelination that are typical of MS.

- It is also unknown whether the disease-modifying agents (***interferons***, glatiramer acetate) established in the treatment of adult MS are equally effective in pediatric MS, or if these medications have potential long-term complications of which we are currently unaware. We also do not know whether these drugs affect a child's normal development in any way. The only way to evaluate these medications systematically in children is to closely follow a large number of children over a long period of time.

- Pediatric MS appears to present more frequently than adult-onset MS with behavioral or cognitive changes. It will be very important to determine if pediatric MS results in permanent cognitive deficits that may affect school performance or normal cognitive development.

- The recent development of a biologic assay (laboratory test) for the diagnosis of neuromyelitis optica, also known as *Devic's disease*, provides the opportunity to determine the frequency of this disease in children and learn how it presents in this younger age group. Devic's disease had previously been considered a form of demyelinating disease that targeted the optic nerves and spinal cord. Now referred to as *neuromyelitis optica*, this disorder has been shown to affect ***white matter*** more widely throughout the brain and spinal cord by producing ***antibodies*** that disrupt water pores in cell membranes. This mechanism of disease is different from that of MS, and it responds to somewhat different treatments. Future MS research will likely identify additional disease-producing mechanisms and allow treatments to be more specifically and effectively targeted for individual patients.

RECOMMENDED READINGS

Holland N, Murray TJ, Reingold SC. *Multiple Sclerosis: A Guide for the Newly Diagnosed.* 3rd ed. New York: Demos Medical Publishing, 2006.

Kalb R, Holland N, Giesser B. *Multiple Sclerosis for Dummies.* Hoboken, NJ: Wiley Publishing, 2007.

Kalb R, Krupp L. Parenting a child with MS. In: R Kalb, ed. *Multiple Sclerosis: A Guide for Families.* 3rd ed. New York: Demos Medical Publishing, 2006.

RECOMMENDED RESOURCES

From the National Multiple Sclerosis Society (800-344-4867):
- *Kids Get MS Too: A Guide for Parents Whose Child or Teen has MS.* An informational handbook written by specialists in pediatric MS and offered by the Young Persons with MS Network (e-mail: childhoodms@nmss.org), which contains a wide range of information pertaining to pediatric MS.
- *Mighty Special Kids.* A 20-page activity book for children with MS that contains games and age-appropriate articles to help kids understand the disease. Available by calling 866-KIDS-W-MS or online in an interactive version at http://www. nationalmssociety.org/mskids.
- *Students with MS and the Academic Setting: A Handbook for School Personnel.* An international guide for educating school staff. Available in hard copy (e-mail: childhoodms@nmss.org) or in electronic format at www.nationalmssociety.org/ pedsupport.
- *Managing School-Related Issues: A Guide for Parents with a Child or Teen Living with MS.* A resource to help parents who have a child with MS deal with the school and school-related issues. Available in hard copy (e-mail: childhoodms@nmss.org) or in electronic format at www.nationalmssociety.org/pedsupport.
- *MS Learn on Line: Pediatric MS: Partnering with Your Child's School,* found on the Society's Web site: www.nationalmssociety.org/mslearnonline.
- *Keep S'Myelin—An Interactive Children's Newsletter,* also found on the Society's Web site.

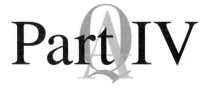

Part IV

What Are the Recommended Financial and Life Planning Strategies?

A chronic, unpredictable disease like MS makes planning for the future more important than ever, even while making it more challenging. In this part, we start by answering the most commonly asked questions about the impact of MS on employment. In the remaining chapters, we deal with questions relating to insurance issues, life planning to maximize your financial security and independence, and long-term care needs in the event that MS becomes more disabling.

Maximizing Employment Options

Phillip D. Rumrill, Jr., PhD, CRC, and
Steven W. Nissen, MS, CRC*

The working role is one of the most valued in American society. A person's work not only determines what he or she does on a day-to-day basis but also helps to define who that person is. The work that provides a person's income and economic stability also defines his or her role in the community, and a significant part of one's self-esteem is tied to occupational status.

Most adults spend at least half of their waking hours on work-related activities, making work the single most time-consuming task in their lives—and they spend much more time working than in any other life role, including that of spouse, parent, or friend. So, when a disease like multiple sclerosis (MS) affects job performance, it threatens not only the person's economic and social status, but personal identity as well.

In this chapter, we describe what is known about the impact of MS on employment, explain the disability rights legislation that has been enacted to help people remain in the workforce, and answer the most common questions surrounding employment issues. Keep in mind, however, that this information should not be used in place of personal legal advice; it is intended only to provide a background for your own personal planning and problem solving. If and when you have questions about your particular employment situation, your best strategies will be to:

- Consult the literature and other resources listed at the end of the chapter
- Consult with the National Multiple Sclerosis Society (800-344-4867)
- Seek any additional advice from an attorney who specializes in labor law and disability rights

HOW COMMON IS IT FOR PEOPLE WITH MS TO LEAVE THE WORKFORCE BEFORE RETIREMENT AGE?

People with MS are a qualified, experienced, and capable group of workers. In fact, more than 90 percent of people with MS have worked at some time in their lives,

*With grateful acknowledgment of materials from the 4th edition contributed by Mary L. Hennessey, PhD, CRC.

and approximately two-thirds were still employed at the time of diagnosis. As the illness progresses, however, a sharp drop occurs in labor-force participation. At present, approximately 40 to 45 percent of Americans with MS are employed.

It should be noted that the vast majority (as many as 80 percent in some studies) of unemployed people with MS voluntarily made the choice to leave the workforce. Upon further reflection, once they have stopped working, however, some 75 percent of unemployed people with MS feel that they would like to return to work, and more than 80 percent believe that they are able to work. So, the pattern is that these experienced and productive workers tend to voluntarily disengage from the labor force—often prematurely—and then find themselves regretting the decision to stop working.

The good news is that the current 40 to 45 percent rate of labor-force participation among people with MS is higher than rates reported during the 1980s and 1990s. This could be due to greater legal protections, improved treatment options and symptom management techniques, and advances in technology.

WHAT CAUSES PEOPLE WITH MS TO LEAVE THE WORKFORCE?

A number of research studies have been conducted over the years concerning employment and MS, but we still do not have a clear understanding of why one person with MS keeps his or her job while another, with a similar degree of disability, leaves the workforce. Factors that have been identified as predictors of employment difficulty and/or job loss for people with MS include

- Cognitive impairment
- Female gender
- Limited formal education
- Employed spouse
- Job requiring significant physical exertion
- Poor relationship with one's employer
- Negative attitudes on the part of coworkers
- Progressive course of the illness
- Job requiring out-of-doors labor
- Severe physical symptoms that affect mobility
- Workplace discrimination

WHAT RESOURCES EXIST TO HELP A PERSON WITH AN ILLNESS OR DISABILITY REMAIN IN THE WORKFORCE?

Given the negative impact that job loss can have on a family's economic circumstances and overall sense of well-being, it is important to identify ways to help people with MS continue working as long as they wish to do so. The first step is to remind people who are working while coping with MS that the decision to leave the workforce is theirs and theirs alone. There is no reason for a physician to prescribe unemployment as part of a person's treatment regimen; no evidence suggests that removing oneself from the workforce has a positive impact on health status. If and when a person is considering disability-related retirement, the choice should be made in consultation with significant others, including health care professionals.

Before making the important decision to work or not to work, people with MS will want to be fully informed about the laws, services, and resources that can assist them in maintaining their employment. Comprehensive psychosocial services, the state vocational rehabilitation (VR) program, occupational therapy, job retention programs, and consumer advocacy strategies have all been developed to support people's efforts to continue on the job while coping with MS. The Job Accommodation Network (JAN), a program funded by the U.S. Department of Labor Office of Disability Employment Policy, is also an invaluable source of information on legal rights, accommodation strategies, and disability employment issues for people with disabilities and the employer community. JAN can be reached at 800-526-7234 or online at http://askJAN.org. For information regarding the Americans with Disabilities Act (ADA), readers should contact their regional ADA Centers at 800-949-4232 or http://www.adata.org. Education for people with MS and their employers and coworkers, proactive approaches to legal rights, and legislative initiatives are also vital means of keeping people with MS in the workforce.

WHAT IS THE AMERICANS WITH DISABILITIES ACT?

The ADA of 1990 was the first comprehensive legislation passed by any country in the world to prohibit discrimination on the basis of disability. As amended in 2008, the ADA guarantees full participation in society for people with disabilities in much the same way that the Civil Rights Act of 1964 guarantees the rights of all people regardless of race, gender, national origin, and religion. The four areas of social activity covered by the ADA are employment, public services, public accommodations, and communications (telephone systems).

WHAT ARE THE PROVISIONS OF THE ADA RELATING TO EMPLOYMENT?

As it pertains to employment, the ADA requires employers with 15 or more employees to provide reasonable accommodations for qualified employees with disabilities. For people with MS, reasonable accommodations may include (but are not limited to):

- Modifications to the work schedule as a means of combating fatigue (e.g., an abbreviated work week or an extended lunch break during which to rest)
- Flexibility in the manner or location in which work is performed (e.g., home-based employment)
- Provision of equipment (e.g., a closed-circuit magnification machine for a person with a visual impairment, a motorized scooter for a person with a mobility impairment, a fan for someone who is hypersensitive to heat)
- Renovations of the work environment (e.g., modification of rest rooms to accommodate a motorized scooter)

It should be noted that reasonable accommodations are determined on a case-by-case basis, and that employers are *not* required to do any of the following:

- Eliminate a primary job responsibility from a person's job description
- Lower production standards that are applied to all employees
- Provide personal use items (e.g., a cane, wheelchair, eyeglasses) unless those items are required only for work purposes

- Excuse a violation of conduct rules
- Provide accommodations that constitute an undue hardship (i.e., changes or modifications that would prove too costly or disruptive to the operation of the business)

Before becoming eligible for a reasonable accommodation, the worker or applicant must disclose his or her disability status to the employer and make a request for the accommodation in question. This does not mean, however, that the person must initially disclose his or her underlying diagnosis or disabling condition. If your employer requires additional information, including diagnosis, to document your disability status, you may need to provide medical verification of your accommodation needs.

Although reasonable accommodations are an important part of the ADA, the employment protections available to people with disabilities go far beyond on-the-job accommodations. Under Title I of the ADA (the employment section), people with disabilities have the civil right to enjoy the same benefits and privileges of employment as their nondisabled coworkers. This means that personnel decisions (e.g., hiring, promotion, layoff, termination) must be made without regard to the person's disability status. Workers may not be harassed on the basis of their disabilities, and the compensation they receive must be commensurate with their qualifications and productivity irrespective of disability.

WHAT ARE THE KEY TERMS IN THE ADA THAT I NEED TO UNDERSTAND?

- *Individual with a Disability.* Individuals who (1) have a mental or physical impairment that substantially limits one or more life activities, or (2) have a history of such an impairment, or (3) are perceived (even erroneously) as having such an impairment.
- *Qualified Individual with a Disability.* Under Title I of the ADA, the term "qualified" applies to an individual with a disability who meets the skill, experience, education, and other job-related requirements of a position held or desired and who, with or without reasonable accommodations, can perform the essential functions of the job.
- *Essential Job Functions.* Essential job functions are narrowly defined to include fundamental job duties, as opposed to marginal ones. A job function is more likely to be "essential" if it requires special expertise, if a large amount of time is spent on that function, and/or if that function was listed in the written job description prepared before the employer advertised for or interviewed job applicants.
- *Reasonable Accommodations.* These refer to an employment-related modification that an employer must make to ensure equal opportunity for an individual with a disability to (1) apply for or test for a job; (2) perform essential job functions; and/ or (3) receive the same benefits and privileges as other employees. The employer is required to provide a reasonable accommodation for known disabilities (e.g., where the disability is obvious or the applicant/employee informs the employer of the disability). Although each case must be evaluated individually, some common examples of on-the-job accommodations include:
  - Restructuring of existing facilities
  - Restructuring of the job

- Modification of work schedules
- Reassignment to another position
- Modification of equipment
- Installation of new equipment
- Provision of qualified readers and interpreters
- Modification of application and examination procedures and/or training materials
- Flexible personal leave policies

- *Undue Hardship.* An accommodation might prove to be an undue hardship for the employer if its implementation resulted in a significant difficulty or expense. Factors to be considered in making this determination include (1) the nature and net cost of the accommodation; (2) the impact of the accommodation on the operation of the facility involved, taking into account the facility's overall resources and number of employees; and (3) the manner in which the employer's business operates, taking into account its size and financial resources. In asserting that an accommodation is an undue hardship, an employer must rely on actual, not hypothetical, costs and burdens.

I'M INTERVIEWING FOR A NEW JOB. DO I NEED TO TELL A POTENTIAL EMPLOYER ABOUT MY DIAGNOSIS? IF I DO NEED TO DISCLOSE, WHAT AM I REQUIRED TO SAY?

The issue of disclosure is one of the most important, and potentially complicated, employment concerns for people with MS. As a matter of law, you have no obligation to disclose anything about your disability status or underlying diagnosis during a job interview unless you require an accommodation for the interview itself. A prospective employer does not have the right to know your diagnosis, and people with MS and other disabilities are generally encouraged to leave medical information out of any discussion with a prospective employer.

The only time you need to disclose the fact that you are a person with a disability is when you believe that you will need a reasonable accommodation to perform one or more of the job's essential functions. If your disability is obvious, and if you are certain that you would need on-the-job accommodations, you may wish to mention your accommodation needs during an interview. If you opt for that strategy, it is important to focus on the skills and techniques you use to overcome disability-related work limitations—not on how difficult it would be for you to perform a particular function.

People are also encouraged to accompany disclosure of their disability status with a specific plan for the accommodations that would be most beneficial in performing the job. That way, you take all the uncertainty out of the accommodation process; employers are much more likely to approve a strategy that you have identified than they are to engage in the process of identifying what your needs are, especially during a job interview.

If your condition is not obvious to the employer, and you do not foresee any need for reasonable accommodations in your current health situation, there is generally no reason to mention disability at all. If your symptoms do not affect your job performance, think of it as you would any other circumstance in your life. If the fact that you are having marital problems does not affect your job performance, is it any of your employer's business? How about your credit history? What church you go to? These issues have no bearing on your ability to do your job, so you probably would not bring them up in an interview. Think of your disability in the same manner, and always err on the side of maintaining your right to privacy. You can always add more information about your disability status if the situation calls for it, but you can never recapture your privacy if you make a full disclosure during a job interview.

The National MS Society offers an online tool to assist with disclosure decisions. For help in deciding whether to disclose, how much to disclose, and whom to tell, go to http://www.nationalMSsociety.org/DisclosureTool.

WHEN CHECKING MY REFERENCES, CAN A POTENTIAL EMPLOYER ASK HOW MS HAS AFFECTED MY WORK IN THE PAST?

Absolutely not. Again, the prospective employer does not have the right to know that you are a person with MS. Even if you disclose your MS diagnosis, he or she cannot inquire about it with your references. The employer may ask for an assessment of your ability to perform the job for which you have applied, or an explanation of the kind of worker you were for the referencing employer. If you do not wish to disclose your MS or disability status to a prospective employer, it is important to ask your references who might be aware of your diagnosis not to mention any medical or disability-related information. Ask them to focus on your characteristics as a worker, not on personal issues that have no bearing on your employability. At a more basic level, having MS makes it more important to follow the generally accepted etiquette of asking permission to use former employers, colleagues, and friends as references before giving their names to prospective employers.

AFTER BEING OFFERED A JOB, I WAS TOLD THAT I NEED TO PASS A PHYSICAL EXAMINATION. WHAT SHOULD I DO?

Take the physical, and be honest with the physician. He or she may not disclose any diagnostic information to the employer. In addition, the ADA makes other important provisions:

- Physical examinations must be job specific. In other words, if you have applied for a job as a telephonic nurse case manager, for which the requirements are primarily sedentary in nature, the employer may not test you to determine whether you can lift 50 pounds over your head. In fact, medical examinations can include only the physical tasks required for the particular job in question.
- Physical examinations must be conducted on a post-offer basis; in other words, the employer must first make a determination that he or she wants to hire you before requiring the physical examination.
- Employers may not require physical examinations on a selective basis. They must require physical examinations for all applicants who have been tendered job offers if they require you to submit to a physical examination.

Although the job-specific and post-offer nature of physical examinations enhances your protection as a person with a disability, the employer may withdraw the job offer if the examining physician determines that you are physically unable to perform the job. Of course, the employer would be legally required to consider reasonable accommodations to overcome your physical limitations, but the accommodations must enable you to do the job or else you would not be deemed qualified for that particular position.

I HAVE BEEN OFFERED A JOB, AND THE QUESTION OF MEDICAL BENEFITS ARISES. CAN I BE DENIED COVERAGE UNDER MY EMPLOYER'S HEALTH INSURANCE PLAN BECAUSE OF A DIAGNOSIS OF MS?

Title I of the ADA prohibits employers from entering into contracts that discriminate against people with disabilities. This includes contracts related to health insurance. Employees with disabilities must be given the same coverage available to all other employees. In addition, an employer cannot refuse to hire you because his or her insurance company will not cover you, or because covering you increases the employer's health care premiums. However, an employer may offer health insurance coverage that contains preexisting condition exclusions or limits certain procedures, provided that those exclusions or limitations pertain to *all* employees.

The Health Insurance Portability and Accountability Act of 1996 (see Chapter 21) provides some protections for employees with disabilities who change jobs. The Act enables a person with a preexisting medical condition to join his or her new employer's health insurance plan and be exempt from preexisting condition exclusions, as long as the employee does not interrupt his or her insurance coverage.

The best advice for people with MS who leave a job is to continue their health insurance benefits as long as is allowable and then transfer their coverage to the new employer's plan. This continued coverage is made possible by the 1996 Consolidated Omnibus Budget Reconciliation Act (COBRA), which enables employees who leave their jobs to purchase ongoing coverage from their employer's insurance company for up to 18 months. Remember, COBRA requires the former employee to pay the entire premium (employee share and employer share) to the insurance carrier, so the cost of this benefit can be expensive.

Given the complexity of health care coverage in the United States, it might be tempting to conceal your MS from an insurance company during your enrollment process. This is not advisable because any insurance company can discontinue your coverage if it learns that you have falsified your medical history on application forms. Remember also that your employer has no right to read any medical information that you submit to insurance companies.

I HAVE JUST BEEN TOLD THAT I HAVE A DEFINITE DIAGNOSIS OF MS. SHOULD I QUIT MY JOB?

There is no reason to quit your job just because you have been diagnosed with MS. No evidence suggests that unemployment will have a positive effect on your health status; in fact, many experts believe that people who work are psychologically and physically healthier than those who do not. With advancements in assistive technology, medical treatment, and societal attitudes toward people with disabilities, people with MS and other potentially disabling conditions are able to maintain their jobs longer than ever before.

Keep in mind, as well, that laws are in place, including the ADA and the Family Medical Leave Act (see p. 309) to help you keep working as long as you wish to do so. If and when you decide to stop working, it is important that you weigh all relevant factors (e.g., family circumstances, financial needs, health status) with input from significant others, health care professionals, and your employer. The fact that you have been diagnosed with MS should not be the determining factor in this exceedingly important decision, and you will know better than anyone else when and if it is time to stop working.

I HAVE BEEN WITH THE SAME COMPANY FOR 3 YEARS AND HAVE RECENTLY BEEN DIAGNOSED WITH MS. HOW DO I DECIDE WHETHER OR NOT I NEED TO DISCLOSE THIS INFORMATION?

In general, the best reason for disclosing your disability status is that you foresee a need for a reasonable accommodation on your job. If you have been missing considerable time from work, if symptoms of your illness are obvious to others, if they have begun to interfere with your job performance, and/or if you have been receiving feedback from your employer that there are problems with your performance, you may want to approach your employer about possible accommodations. Although you do not have to disclose the underlying cause of your disability (i.e., your MS), it is important to frame your disability status in functional terms: "I am a person with a disability, and I have been having difficulty performing X and Y on my job. I would like to discuss some ways to accommodate these difficulties—some strategies that will enable me to continue being a productive employee."

It is also important to note that you need not reference the ADA specifically in your discussions with your employer. In fact, the National Multiple Sclerosis Society advocates a win-win approach to on-the-job accommodations, in which the employee with MS keeps his or her legal protections out of the dialog with the employer to every extent possible. The best rationale for reasonable accommodations is that they will help you to maintain or enhance your productivity on the job. The win-win approach benefits both you and the employer, and demonstrates your willingness to engage in a cooperative, nonadversarial process of identifying and implementing cost-effective accommodations. Approaching the conversation in this way is almost always more effective than invoking your civil rights or threatening to sue your employer if he or she does not meet your needs. The best advice about disclosure and the accommodation request process is to:

- Be direct but friendly
- Frame your disability-related work limitations in functional terms
- Focus on your accommodation needs rather than your medical diagnosis
- Emphasize the mutual benefits of providing you with on-the-job accommodations
- Use your legal rights and recourses under the ADA if, and only if, your employer refuses to provide an appropriate accommodation to meet your stated needs

The National MS Society has a Web-based disclosure decision tool (http://www.nationalMSsociety.org/DisclosureTool) that can be useful.

IF I DECIDE TO DISCLOSE AT WORK, WHO SHOULD BE THE FIRST TO KNOW, AND HOW MUCH INFORMATION SHOULD I BE PREPARED TO OFFER?

Your immediate supervisor is usually the person to whom you should first disclose. The supervisor may wish to involve other representatives of the employer, particularly a human resources specialist or a department manager. Your coworkers have no legal right to know anything about your disability status, but you may wish to let them know what is going on as a courtesy. Communications to coworkers about your disability should come from you, not your employer, and should include only the information needed to help them understand your circumstance. Even though supervisors are prohibited by law from sharing information about your disability status with your coworkers, it might be a good idea to ask your immediate supervisor to keep the information you share with him or her confidential, realizing, of course, that this confidentiality applies to your coworkers but not to other company officials.

In any disclosure, it is important to focus on the symptoms or effects of your disability that specifically affect your job performance. It is usually best to refrain from providing clinical, medical descriptions of any kind. Even if you choose to disclose your MS, avoid using such terms as exacerbation, attack, progressive, and disease. You may wish to write out your disclosure statement and rehearse how you will say it with a friend or advisor. The National MS Society (1-800-344-4867) can also help you in determining whether, how, and to whom you should disclose.

ALL MY MS SYMPTOMS ARE INVISIBLE. DO I HAVE TO TELL MY EMPLOYER THAT I HAVE BEEN DIAGNOSED WITH MS?

No. The only time it is necessary to disclose the fact that you have a disability is when you feel that you might need an on-the-job accommodation. If your symptoms are invisible, and if they do not pose any problems for you in doing your job, there is neither a need nor any advantage for you to mention anything about this personal aspect of your life.

MOST OF MY SYMPTOMS ARE NOT VISIBLE TO OTHERS. FATIGUE AND MEMORY PROBLEMS POSE THE GREATEST DIFFICULTIES AT WORK FOR ME. ARE THESE INVISIBLE IMPAIRMENTS COVERED BY THE ADA?

Yes. Physical or mental impairment need not be visible or obvious to substantially limit functioning in one or more major life activities, as per the ADA's definition of disability that was cited in the beginning of this chapter. The important standard regarding your symptoms is whether they pose problems for you in doing your job. Remember, a qualified person under the ADA is one who possesses the minimum credentials required for the job and who can perform essential functions of that job—with reasonable accommodations if required. Fatigue and cognitive impairments are among the most common symptoms of MS, and there are a number of proven strategies to help people overcome those symptoms while doing their jobs. Contact the Job Accommodation Network (JAN) at 1-800-526-7234 for additional information on easy-to-implement job accommodations.

IS EVERY EMPLOYEE COVERED UNDER THE ADA?

Only those employees who have disabilities, have records of disabilities, or are perceived as having disabilities, are protected by the ADA. Having a diagnosis of MS usually qualifies one as a person with a disability under the ADA. The prevailing standard involves the functional aspects of the disease—that is, whether the impairment substantially limits functioning in one or more major life activities.

More specifically, only those employees with disabilities who work for a covered employer are protected under the ADA. Title I of the ADA covers employers with 15 or more employees in both the public and private sectors. Native American tribes, the federal government, and tax-exempt private membership clubs are not required to comply with the ADA's employment provisions. The Rehabilitation Act of 1973 prohibits the federal government and employers receiving federal funds from discriminating against workers on the basis of disability, but the ADA's protections are farther reaching and more stringent.

WHO IS RESPONSIBLE FOR DECIDING WHAT ACCOMMODATIONS I NEED— MY DOCTOR, MY EMPLOYER, MY UNION, MY LAWYER, OR MYSELF?

Ideally, you and your employer make a joint and mutually acceptable decision regarding which accommodations to implement. Title I of the ADA requires that employee and employer engage in a cooperative dialog to assess the worker's needs, identify accommodation options, and implement a reasonable accommodation that is agreeable to both parties. In that process, input can be sought from medical professionals, unions, and—if the collaborative process has broken down—attorneys. In general, the accommodation process works best when most of the decision-making is done by the employee and employer, with a minimum of assistance from partisan advocates. Other resources that might be enlisted in identifying cost-effective accommodations include rehabilitation counselors, assistive technology specialists, rehabilitation engineers, ergonomists (specialists in the study of workplace design and safety), JAN, and *physical therapists* or *occupational therapists*.

WHO DECIDES IF A REQUESTED ACCOMMODATION IS REASONABLE?

When a qualified individual with a disability requests an accommodation, the employer must make a reasonable effort to provide an accommodation that is effective for that individual. An accommodation does not have to be made if it presents an undue hardship to the employer. *Undue hardship* refers to accommodations that would be too expensive or disruptive for a particular business to handle. The employer's determination of undue hardship can be challenged in court or before the Equal Employment Opportunity Commission (EEOC).

WHO PAYS FOR THE ACCOMMODATIONS THAT ARE MADE (E.G., ADAPTIVE EQUIPMENT, BUILDING RENOVATIONS, SCHEDULE CHANGES)?

In most cases, the employer will be required to pay the costs of the accommodation unless it presents an undue hardship. In determining whether an accommodation represents an undue hardship, the cost to be considered is the actual cost to the employer. Specific federal tax credits and deductions are available to employers who make accommodations required by the ADA, and research indicates that the majority of on-the-job accommodations used by people with MS cost nothing or very little to implement. A VR counselor in your area can tell you about local funding sources that might help pay for some accommodations.

MY BOSS SAYS THAT THE ACCOMMODATIONS I HAVE REQUESTED ARE TOO EXPENSIVE. WHAT SHOULD I DO NOW?

Before developing a plan for appeal, it is important to understand that the courts in ADA lawsuits have given the employer considerable discretion in determining what constitutes an undue hardship. Your best bet is to meet again with your employer. In that meeting, discuss possible alternatives to your desired accommodation that might be less expensive; the ADA entitles you to a reasonable accommodation, not necessarily your first choice.

If you simply cannot reach an agreement, your next step is to file a complaint with the EEOC, which oversees ADA Title I enforcement. Not only does the EEOC investigate complaints and make a determination about the legal merits of the complaint but it also attempts to resolve employee-employer conflicts in a non-litigious manner. Should you proceed with a formal complaint to the EEOC, it is advisable to retain an attorney who specializes in disability and/or employment law. If the EEOC complaint does not result in a satisfactory resolution to your concern, you may wish to file a lawsuit against your employer in civil court. Remedies available to people with disabilities under Title I of the ADA include hiring, reinstatement, punitive damages, compensatory damages, and court orders to stop discriminatory conduct.

I HAVE REQUESTED SEVERAL ACCOMMODATIONS THAT HAVE BEEN DENIED ON THE BASIS THAT THESE CHANGES WOULD SUBSTANTIALLY ALTER MY JOB DESCRIPTION. WHAT RECOURSE DO I HAVE?

Your employer is not required to provide accommodations that would substantially alter your job description. Restructuring of the job, one of the types of reasonable accommodations listed in ADA regulations, applies only to minor, or marginal duties of the job. Essential functions of the job, which are delineated on a written job description, are not subject to restructuring.

MY COWORKERS RESENT THE ACCOMMODATIONS THAT HAVE BEEN MADE FOR MY DISABILITY. HOW CAN I IMPROVE THE SITUATION?

Many experts would recommend that you educate your coworkers about MS and how it affects you. While that is certainly an option, remember that you have absolute rights to privacy under the ADA. You have no legal obligation to let your coworkers know what is going on, but informing them about your condition may, in some cases, help them understand that you are not receiving preferential treatment. As with any form of disclosure, the standard you should apply in deciding whether to inform your coworkers about your MS is how much information they need in order to understand your situation.

I HAVE REQUESTED A PROMOTION AT WORK, BUT I WAS TOLD THAT THEY ARE HESITANT TO PUT ME IN A MORE RESPONSIBLE POSITION BECAUSE I COULD HAVE AN EXACERBATION. IS A COMPANY ALLOWED TO TAKE THAT POSITION WITH ME?

An employer cannot limit, segregate, or classify a person with a disability in any way that negatively affects him or her in terms of job opportunity and advancement. Promotion and other personnel decisions must be based on factual evidence about the person's ability to do the job, not on any assumption, speculation, or stereotype about the worker's disability status.

Given that your employer already knows you have MS, your best strategy in this situation may be to try to reduce your supervisor's concerns about your job performance. The supervisor has a responsibility to the company to ensure that any position is filled by a person who is capable of handling the work. If your supervisor is concerned that you might miss work because of *exacerbations*, review your prior work history and attendance record with him or her. If your MS is of the relapsing-remitting type, discuss with your supervisor how you would plan to handle the work load during a period of active symptoms. If you have not experienced frequent exacerbations in the past, your supervisor may be basing his or her judgment about you on inaccurate information regarding MS. As a courtesy to the supervisor (although you have no legal obligation to do so), you might want to ask your physician to write a letter on your behalf explaining that exacerbations are not necessarily part of the MS picture.

In addition, the National Multiple Sclerosis Society has literature designed to answer employers' questions about the disease. If the company continues to deny you a promotion, and you believe that you are qualified to do the job despite your symptoms, you might want to contact the EEOC or consult an attorney.

I FEEL LIKE I AM BEING DISCRIMINATED AGAINST ON THE JOB. WHAT OPTIONS DO I HAVE?

If you believe your rights under the ADA have been violated, the U.S. EEOC is the enforcer of Title I of the ADA. You can contact the EEOC at 800-669-4000 to begin the process of filing a complaint. Even if your employer is not legally required to follow the ADA, you may have protections at the local or state level. If that is the case, you can contact your local civil rights agency/state fair employment practice agency. Before making a formal complaint to any government agency, you may wish to contact a disability employment attorney.

UNDER WHAT CIRCUMSTANCES CAN I BE FIRED FROM A JOB BECAUSE OF MY MS?

You can be terminated from your job if you can no longer perform the essential functions of the position even with the help of reasonable accommodations. You can also be terminated if the accommodations you need to perform essential job functions are too expensive or would pose an undue hardship for the employer. However, the employer is required to make an effort to find more suitable, alternative positions for you within the company. In other words, you cannot be terminated because of your inability to perform essential job functions until every reasonable effort has been made to accommodate your limitations.

WHAT IS THE FAMILY AND MEDICAL LEAVE ACT?
The Family and Medical Leave Act (FMLA) of 1993 is another federal law with important implications for employed people with MS and other disabling conditions. The FMLA has enabled thousands of American employees to retain their jobs while taking unpaid leaves of absence to attend to important family health concerns. The law requires employers in the public and private sectors to hold workers' jobs open and continue paying health insurance premiums while employees take time off to treat and/or recover from illnesses or injuries. It also provides leave for employees who must attend to the health care needs of their family members. For example, a person whose spouse has MS and needs transportation to medical appointments, or extra care following an exacerbation of the illness, could request unpaid leave to attend to the spouse's needs.

WHAT ARE THE PROVISIONS OF THE FMLA?
Any employer who has 50 or more employees residing within a 75-mile radius of the work location is covered by the FMLA. Employees are eligible for protection under this law if they have worked at the job for at least 1 year (no fewer than 1,250 hours within the 12 months preceding the requested leave date) and have (or have a family member who has) a serious health condition. Under this law, a serious health condition is defined as any illness, injury, impairment, or course of treatment that renders a person unable to perform essential job functions. The term is broader and more inclusive than the ADA's definition of disability, which means that someone with MS could be considered to have a serious health condition under the FMLA but not meet the ADA's standard for disability. Unlike the term *disability, serious health conditions* pertain to both temporary and permanent conditions (e.g., pregnancy, birth or adoption, surgery, relapse of a chronic illness).

Under the FMLA, employers are required to provide up to 12 weeks of unpaid leave per calendar year for an eligible employee who is coping with a serious health condition. The 12 weeks need not be taken consecutively, and the employer must allow the worker to return to the same or a similar, equivalent position. The right to return to work following unpaid leave can be denied only to key employees—those earning the highest 10 percent of salaries—and only when holding open the jobs of these employees would create substantial and grievous long-term economic injury to the employer's operations. The employer's burden of proof for this exception is more stringent than for the ADA's defense of undue hardship.

HOW DO I GO ABOUT REQUESTING FMLA LEAVE?
The first step is to notify your employer, preferably in writing, that you need the leave time. You must state that you have a serious health condition, but you do not need to tell your employer that you have MS. Be specific about the dates of your leave, keeping in mind that you can take as many as 12 weeks off during each calendar year. If the need for your leave is foreseeable (e.g., elective surgery, birth of a child), the law requires you to give 30 days advance notice. If the need for the leave is unforeseeable (e.g., an unexpected exacerbation of your MS), the FMLA requires that you provide "reasonable notice," but leaves that term undefined in the regulations.

Once you have issued your request for leave, the employer has two business days to respond to your request. If your employer does not respond within 2 days, you are automatically considered eligible for the leave you have requested. Your employer may ask for documentation of your serious health condition from a health care provider. In submitting this verification, the provider should adhere to the following conditions as a means of safeguarding your privacy:

- The statement should verify the need for a medical leave without disclosing the underlying medical condition.
- The information reported should be job related (e.g., need for, length of, and timing of the medical leave).
- The statement of verification should avoid any discussion of the possible future effects of the serious health condition.

To further protect your privacy, the following conditions apply within the workplace:

- Leave requests should be processed by a designated, knowledgeable person so that discussion with the employee's supervisors and coworkers is limited.
- Supervisors should be notified of facts related to the circumstances of the leave, not about specific aspects of the employee's (or a relative's) serious health condition.
- Records related to medical leave must be maintained in a file separate from the employee's personnel records.

MY EMPLOYER HAS ACCOMMODATED ALL MY REQUESTS, BUT I AM STILL HAVING DIFFICULTY DOING MY JOB. I HAVE BEEN OFFERED A POSITION IN ANOTHER DEPARTMENT, BUT IT WOULD MEAN A DEMOTION AND A CUT IN PAY. DO I HAVE TO TAKE THIS POSITION? IF I DON'T, CAN MY EMPLOYER FIRE ME FROM MY PRESENT POSITION?

According to the law, an employee with a disability can be reassigned to a different position that is equivalent in terms of pay and job status, assuming that he or she is qualified for the position and that such a position is vacant or will be vacant within a reasonable amount of time. If no such equivalent position is available, and if no accommodations would enable you to remain in the current position, your employer can reassign you to a lower-grade position. In such a situation, your employer does not have to maintain your salary at the level of your former position unless the same is done for other employees who are reassigned to lower-grade positions. Finally, your employment can be terminated if all requested accommodations have been provided, no equivalent position is available, and you cannot perform the essential functions of your current job.

I FEEL THAT I CAN NO LONGER DO MY JOB THE WAY I USED TO DO IT. HOW WILL I KNOW IF AND WHEN IT'S TIME FOR ME TO RETIRE?

It is time for you to look into other options if you have researched and requested all possible accommodations to assist you in doing your job, yet still find you cannot adequately perform the essential job functions. Be sure to investigate other positions that may be available within your company. Other options include job retraining that would enable you to continue working in some other field, volunteer work, Social Security Disability Insurance (SSDI), and long-term disability.

HOW DO I FIGURE OUT IF I AM ELIGIBLE FOR SOCIAL SECURITY DISABILITY INSURANCE OR SUPPLEMENTAL SECURITY INCOME?

Both SSDI and Supplemental Security Income (SSI) are programs run by the Social Security Administration. The medical requirements for disability payments are the same under both programs, and disability is determined by the same process. For a person with MS, the recognized areas of impairment include gait, vision, cognition, and fatigue. Eligibility for SSDI is based on prior work history, whereas SSI disability benefits are made solely on the basis of financial need. Applications for SSDI require a 5-month waiting period from the determination of disability to the start of benefits. Twenty-four months after the initial waiting period, the person becomes eligible for Medicare insurance coverage (see Chapter 21). There is no similar waiting period for SSI benefits; individuals eligible for SSI based on financial need are covered by Medicaid (see Chapter 21).

To be eligible for SSDI, a person must (1) have worked and paid Social Security taxes (FICA) for enough years to be covered under Social Security and to have paid at least some of these taxes in recent years; (2) be considered medically disabled (i.e., too disabled to work); and (3) not be working or working but earning less than the substantial gainful activity (SGA) level of $1,000 per month ($1,640 for beneficiaries who are blind). In determining a person's gross earnings, certain employment-related expenses will be deducted from the calculation if the person is paying expenses out of pocket and not otherwise being reimbursed for them. These deducted expenses include some types of attendant care services, transportation-related costs, medical and nonmedical equipment costs, medication costs, and some types of residential modifications.

The SSDI payment amount is based on a worker's lifetime average earnings covered by Social Security. The payment amount will be reduced by worker's compensation payments and/or public disability payments. Those individuals who are receiving payments from private disability insurance companies may find that these payments are reduced by whatever amount they subsequently receive from SSDI. The SSDI payment amount is not affected by other (nonwork) income or resources.

To be eligible for SSI based on a medical condition, a person must (1) have little or no income or resources, and (2) be considered medically disabled (i.e., too disabled to work). As with SSDI, certain out-of-pocket employment related expenses will be deducted from the calculation of the person's gross earnings.

Once you begin to receive SSI benefits, work activity will not bring an end to SSI eligibility as long as you remain medically disabled. Even if you cannot receive SSI income maintenance checks because the amount of money you earn exceeds the SGA, eligibility for Medicaid may continue indefinitely. The SSI payment amount is based on the amount of other income, your living arrangements, and the state in which you reside. The basic payment is known as the *federal benefit rate*; this rate is adjusted each year to compensate for inflation, and cost of living increases. Most states pay an additional amount known as a *state supplement*. The amount and qualifications for these supplements vary from state to state.

I CAN NO LONGER WORK FULL-TIME AND AM RECEIVING SSDI. WHAT WOULD HAPPEN TO MY SSDI IF I RETURNED TO WORK ON A PART-TIME BASIS?

As long as you earn under $1,000 per month (the established cutoff for SGA) or $1,640 per month if you are considered blind by Social Security Administration, you will continue to receive SSDI. However, if your earnings are greater than SGA, you will be considered gainfully employed and your SSDI payments will be stopped following your trial work period. Keep in mind that in calculating your gross income, the Social Security Administration will deduct certain types of employment-related expenses that directly affect your ability to get to and perform your job and that you have personally paid for without other reimbursement. Community work incentive coordinators are available for consultations through local Work Incentive Planning and Assistance (WIPA) programs to determine the impact work could have on your benefits. For more information about WIPA services, and a directory of providers, visit http://www.socialsecurity.gov/work/wipafactsheet.html.

WHAT IS VOCATIONAL REHABILITATION, AND HOW DO I FIND OUT IF I AM ELIGIBLE FOR THIS TYPE OF PROGRAM?

The Rehabilitation Act of 1973 provides for services designed to enable people with disabilities to become or remain employed. Although this is a program mandated by federal law, it is carried out by individually created state agencies. Each state agency has its own name and slightly different program. VR services are defined as an *eligibility program* rather than an *entitlement program*. This means that you must demonstrate eligibility by having a physical or mental impairment that results in a substantial handicap to employment. There must also be a reasonable expectation that VR services can help you to become more employable. As can be seen in the wording of these criteria, there will obviously be some variation from agency to agency in determining a person's eligibility. Many VR agencies operate under an order of selection mandate, whereby services are prioritized for those applicants who have the most severe disabilities. Your first step is to contact the VR program in your state to ask for information about eligibility and application procedures.

WHAT TYPES OF SERVICES MIGHT BE PROVIDED BY MY STATE'S VOCATIONAL REHABILITATION PROGRAM?

The state's VR services might include the following:

- A thorough rehabilitation evaluation to determine extent of disability and need for treatment to correct or reduce the disability
- Vocational guidance and counseling
- Medical appliances and prosthetic devices, if needed, to increase your ability to work
- Vocational training to prepare you for gainful employment
- Provision of occupational equipment and tools
- Job placement and follow-up
- Post-employment services

Keep in mind that, although these programs are mandated by federal law, they tend to vary considerably from state to state.

RECOMMENDED READINGS

Bishop M, Frain M, Rumrill P, Rymond C. The relationship of self-management and disease-modifying therapy use to employment status among adults with multiple sclerosis. *Journal of Vocational Rehabilitation.* 2009;31:119–128.

Fraser R. Employment strategies and community resources. In: *The MS Workbook: Living Fully with Multiple Sclerosis.* Oakland, CA: New Harbinger Publications; 2006:95–104.

Johnson K. Disclosure to employer and using job accommodations. In: *The MS Workbook: Living Fully with Multiple Sclerosis.* Oakland, CA: New Harbinger Publications; 2006:105–116.

Kraft G, Kennedy P, Lowenstein N, et al. Staying connected: The use of computer-related accessible technology among people with multiple sclerosis. *International Journal of MS Care.* 2009;11(suppl 1):1–13.

McCabe M, DiBattista J. Role of health, relationships, work and coping on adjustment among people with multiple sclerosis: a longitudinal investigation. *Psychology, Health, and Medicine.* 2004;9:431–439.

Miller A, Dishon S. Health-related quality of life in multiple sclerosis: The impact of disability, gender, and employment status. *Quality of Life Research: An International Journal of Quality of Life Aspects of Treatment, Care & Rehabilitation.* 2006;15:259–271.

Neath J, Roessler R, McMahon B, Rumrill P. Patterns in perceived employment discrimination for adults with multiple sclerosis. *Work: A Journal of Prevention, Assessment, and Rehabilitation.* 2007;29:255–274.

Roessler R, Neath J, Rumrill P, Nissen S. The employment discrimination experiences of Americans with multiple sclerosis: survey findings and implications for rehabilitation counseling practice. *Journal of Rehabilitation.* 2011;77:20–30.

Roessler R, Rumrill P, Fitzgerald S. Predictors of employment status for people with multiple sclerosis. *Rehabilitation Counseling Bulletin.* 2004;47:96–103.

Roessler R, Turner R, Robertson J, Rumrill P. Gender and perceived illness severity: differential indicators of employment concerns for adults with multiple sclerosis? *Rehabilitation Counseling Bulletin.* 2005;48:66–74.

Rumrill P. Challenges and opportunities related to the employment of people with multiple sclerosis. *Journal of Vocational Rehabilitation.* 2009;31:83–92.

Rumrill P, Hennessey M, Nissen S. *Employment Issues and Multiple Sclerosis.* 2nd ed. New York, NY: Demos Medical Publishing, 2008.

Rumrill P, Roessler R, Fitzgerald S. Vocational rehabilitation-related predictors of quality of life among people with multiple sclerosis. *Journal of Vocational Rehabilitation.* 2004;20:155–163.

Rumrill P, Roessler R, McMahon B. Multiple sclerosis and workplace discrimination: The national EEOC ADA research project. *Journal of Vocational Rehabilitation.* 2005;23:179–187.

Rumrill P, Roessler R, Vierstra C. Workplace barriers and job satisfaction among employed people with multiple sclerosis: an empirical rationale for early intervention. *Journal of Vocational Rehabilitation.* 2004;20:177–183.

Rumrill P, Tabor T, Hennessey M, Minton D. Issues in employment and career development for people with multiple sclerosis: meeting the needs of an emerging vocational rehabilitation clientele. *Journal of Vocational Rehabilitation.* 2000;14:109–117.

Unger D, Rumrill P, Roessler R. A comparative analysis of employment discrimination complaints filed by people with multiple sclerosis and individuals with other disabilities. *Journal of Vocational Rehabilitation.* 2004;20:165–170.

Selected publications available from the National Multiple Sclerosis Society, 1-800-344-3867, or online at http://www.nationalMSsociety.org/Brochures:
- *Disclosure: The Basic Facts*
- *"But You Look So Good"*
- *ADA and People with MS*
- *The Win-Win Approach to Reasonable Accommodations: Enhancing Productivity on Your Job*
- *Information for Employers*
- *Should I Work? Information for Employees*
- *A Place in the Workforce*
- *Focus on Employment*
- *Know Your Rights: A Legal Guide for People Living with MS*
- *Solving Cognitive Problems*

RECOMMENDED RESOURCES

U.S. Department of Labor Office of Disability Employment
200 Constitution Ave, NW
Washington, DC 20210
1-866-633-7365 (voice) (TTY 1-877-889-5627)
http://www.dol.gov/odep:

- *Americans with Disabilities Act, A Summary*
- *Employer Incentives When Hiring People with Disabilities*
- *Ready, Willing and Available*

U.S. Equal Employment Opportunity Commission
131 M St, NE
Washington, DC 20507
1-800-669-4000 (Voice) (TTY 1-800-669-6820)
http://www.eeoc.gov:

- *The Americans with Disabilities Act: Your Employment Rights as an Individual with a Disability*
- *The Americans with Disabilities Act: Your Responsibilities As an Employer*
- *ADA: Questions and Answers*
- *Facts About the American Disability Act*
- *Facts About the Disability-Related Tax Provisions*

National Multiple Sclerosis Society
733 Third Ave
New York, NY 10017
1-800-344-4867
http://www.nationalMSsociety.org

- Career Crossroads: Employment and MS manuals (in-person or self-study) and DVD
- MS in the Workplace: A Guide for Employers DVD
- Self-Advocacy for Employment materials available on http://www.nationalMSsociety.org

Multiple Sclerosis Society of Canada
175 Bloor St East, Ste 700
North Tower
Toronto, Ontario M4W 3R8
1-800-268-7582
http://www.mssociety.ca

Multiple Sclerosis Foundation
6520 North Andrews Ave
Fort Lauderdale, FL 33309
1-888-MSFOCUS
http://www.msfocus.org

The Job Accommodation Network
West Virginia University
P.O. Box 6080
Morgantown, WV 26506-6080
1-800-526-7234 voice, 1-877-781-9403 TTY
http://askJAN.org
http://askjan.org/cgi-win/TypeQuery.exe?902 for full list of state Vocational Rehabilitation
Agencies

ADA National Network (Disability and Business Technical Assistance Center/DBTAC)
1-800-949-4232
http://www.adata.org

National Organization on Disability
1625 K St, NW Ste 850
Washington, DC 20006
1-202-293-5960 (voice)
http://www.nod.org

American Association of People with Disabilities
1629 K St, NW Ste 950
Washington, DC 20006
1-800-840-8844
http://www.aapd.com

Paralyzed Veterans of America
801 18th St, NW
Washington, DC 20006
1-800-424-8200
http://www.pva.org

Operation Job Match
1800 M St, NW Ste 750 South
Washington, DC 20036
1-202-887-0136
http://www.OperationJobMatch.org

National Business and Disability Council
201 I.V. Willets
Road Albertson, NY 11507-1595
1-516-465-1515
http://www.nbdc.com

Virginia Commonwealth University Rehabilitation Research and Training Center
1314 West Main St
P.O. Box 842011
Richmond, VA 23284-2011
1-804-828-1851
http://www.worksupport.com

University of Washington MS Rehabilitation Research and Training Center
Department of Rehabilitation Medicine, University of Washington
Box 356490
Seattle, WA 98195
1-888-634-6778
http://msrrtc.washington.edu/

Rehabilitation Engineering and Assistive Technology Society of North America
1700 North Moore St
Arlington, VA 22209
1-703-524-6686
http://www.resna.org

Social Security Administration
1-800-722-1213 (Voice), 1-800-325-0778 (TTY)
http://www.socialsecurity.gov

- Disability Benefits (publication 05-10029)
- Working While Disabled—How We Can Help (publication 05-10095)
- Red Book: A Summary Guide to Employment Support for Individuals with Disabilities (publication 64-030)
- Your Ticket to Work (publication 05-10061)

Managing the Insurance Maze

*Kimberly Calder, MPS**

Obtaining insurance can be a complex and stressful process, particularly for people who are dealing with the added uncertainties of multiple sclerosis (MS). But the effort you make to examine your insurance needs and explore the available options is well worth your while, because insurance can provide vitally important financial protection for you and your family. The aim of this chapter is to simplify that process for you.

Although there are many types of insurance, the four that are usually most important to people affected by MS or other disabling conditions are health (including hospitalization and major medical coverage), disability, long-term care, and life insurance. Although this chapter addresses all of these, particular emphasis is given to health insurance. This should not be surprising in view of the lifelong, unpredictable, and varying medical and allied health needs that confront many people with MS. Disability insurance—whether government or private—is also extremely important, since it provides income to replace the wages lost when one must leave the workforce because of a disability. Long-term care insurance (LTCI), which covers an array of home, community, and nursing home services, can be an important resource for some people with MS, although the insurance coverage must usually be secured prior to the MS diagnosis. Life insurance can also be challenging to obtain once a diagnosis of MS is established, despite the fact that MS is not considered a fatal disease.

HEALTH INSURANCE

In March 2010, the Patient Protection and Affordable Care Act (ACA) was signed into federal law. This comprehensive legislation outlines major reforms to the health insurance system through changes in federal and state laws and regulations that take effect over a 10-year implementation timeline. At this writing, the ACA is the subject

*With grateful acknowledgment of materials from earlier editions written by Robert Enteen, PhD, and Dorothy Northrop, MSW, ACSW.

of numerous legal challenges, and will likely be reviewed by the U.S. Supreme Court. Additional changes to the law, delayed implementation, and/or its replacement are all possible and hard to predict. It is especially important for people with MS, family members, and others reading this chapter to be aware of these possibilities, and to seek reliable and verifiable advice before making assumptions about their health insurance, or making major changes to it.

The federal government's comprehensive Web site (http://www.healthcare.gov) is a reliable and detailed resource for anyone seeking information on health coverage in their state. In addition, the National Multiple Sclerosis Society offers information and assistance on insurance issues over the phone (1-800-344-4567) and on their Web site at http://www.nationalmssociety.org/insurance.

Editor's Note: As mentioned, the ACA is facing numerous legal challenges that may not be resolved for several years. In reading this book, you will find that two authors—each an expert in her field—have approached the new law a bit differently. In this chapter, the author has incorporated the provisions of the law into the questions and answers. In Chapter 23 on effective life planning, the author has addressed insurance and related issues as though most of the law's provisions will not take place for several years, if ever. This difference in approach highlights the complexities of the current health care environment.

The following commonly asked questions and answers provide a basic overview of insurance.

Because the health insurance arena is complex and constantly evolving, and insurance planning is such a central component of financial and "life" planning, you are urged to use this chapter as a starting point and general guide rather than as a complete and sufficient source of advice on making insurance decisions. At the end of the chapter is a list of resources you can turn to for additional, comprehensive information and advice.

WHAT ARE THE MOST IMPORTANT THINGS TO KNOW ABOUT HEALTH INSURANCE?

You do not need to become an expert on health insurance in order to get and keep health coverage, or even to get the greatest value from your plan. However, it is important to have a basic understanding of a few critical concepts and terms, including (1) how fee-for-service health coverage differs from managed care plans; (2) how your choice of health plan can be limited by the type(s) for which you are eligible; (3) what the major types of health insurance are and what they cover; and (4) how you can get the most from your health plan once you have enrolled. Equally important is knowing where to go for clarification and assistance. This chapter will provide the basic information you need as well as a list of important resources.

HOW DOES FEE-FOR-SERVICE HEALTH INSURANCE DIFFER FROM "MANAGED" CARE?

For most of the 20th century, the majority of health insurance plans were organized as indemnity or fee-for-service contracts. Policyholders used the health services of their choice, paid the health care providers' bill(s), and were reimbursed for them to the extent the services were covered under the terms of the contract.

Fee-for-service plans have become much less common in recent years as the cost-containment strategies of managed care have been incorporated into both employer-based health plans and public insurance programs. However, traditional Medicare still operates as a fee-for-service option and some job-based health plans still provide a fee-for-service option for those who are eligible for their group health plan benefits.

Many other job-based health plans operate as a hybrid of fee-for-service and managed care, so it is important to understand how and where these concepts apply to you. Many people still prefer fee-for-service health insurance because they value the ability to choose their own health care providers. The exact amount you will be reimbursed through a fee-for-service plan is typically a percentage of the providers' total charge, which should be described in your health plan guide or "Summary of Benefits."

In contrast to fee-for-service plans, managed care plans contract with specific doctors, hospitals, pharmacies, and other health care professionals to form a provider "network" for plan members. In health maintenance organizations (HMOs), the original and most restrictive form of managed care, plan enrollees are only covered for health services furnished by "in-network" providers. Because of these limitations in coverage, HMOs generally charge policyholders less in premiums and out-of-pocket costs than fee-for-service plans. The simplicity of managed care plans also appeals to many people; members pay little to no direct fees to health care providers and therefore do not have to file claims for reimbursement. Some HMOs have no annual deductible and little or no out-of-pocket costs for covered services.

Numerous variations of the strict HMO model have evolved in recent years as Americans have responded to these coverage restrictions by demanding more flexible health plans. Preferred provider organizations (PPOs)—which are a hybrid of fee-for-service and HMO plans—are now the most common form of job-based group health plan arrangement. PPO members can choose at any time to use an "out-of-network" provider on a fee-for-service basis, or pay less out-of-pocket by choosing an "in-network" provider. However, the relative freedom to choose either in-network or out-of-network providers makes plans with this flexibility more costly than HMOs, and enrollees pay a higher premium. Point-of-service (POS) health plans are another type of managed care that operates on a basis similar to PPO plans, and is more common in certain geographic areas.

HOW DO I DETERMINE MY HEALTH COVERAGE ELIGIBILITY?
Health coverage in the United States is constantly evolving. The way health plans function is a reflection of federal and/or state laws as well as each plan's rules of operation. In the past, these laws, regulations, and rules have primarily governed eligibility criteria. However, they are now undergoing significant but gradual liberalization as a result of the ACA. Because eligibility for coverage continues to play such a critical role in access to coverage and health care, some basic explanation about eligibility for each major type of coverage is presented here. Describing eligibility for health insurance by distinguishing between government insurance programs and private health plans makes these concepts easier to understand.

Government Insurance Programs

The chief types of government health insurance are Medicare, Medicaid, VA (veterans) benefits, TRICARE, the Federal Employee Health Benefits Program (FEHB), and state or local government employee insurance programs. Millions of Americans are eligible for government insurance program(s) when one or more of the following scenarios applies to them: (1) They are now, or were formerly, employed by a government agency or program, including the uniformed services; (2) They meet the legally defined criteria for a benefit "entitlement" program; or (3) They are the family member of a living or deceased person who is/was eligible for these insurance programs.

- *Medicare.* Medicare is a federal health insurance entitlement program, which means that anyone who meets the eligibility criteria for Medicare is legally entitled to enroll in the program. It is the chief source of coverage for people aged 65 and older. People younger than 65 years with disabilities, including MS, also qualify for Medicare benefits if they meet the Social Security Administration's disability criteria and receive Social Security Disability Insurance (SSDI) benefits (see Chapter 20 for a discussion of SSDI eligibility). This Medicare coverage does not begin immediately upon disability determination however. Once a person has qualified for disability benefits, a 24-month waiting period is required before Medicare coverage begins.

- Medicare's traditional coverage is fairly comprehensive, providing both hospital (Part A) and medical (Part B) protection. Medicare Part C, referred to as "Medicare Advantage," is the managed care option of Medicare. In fact, Medicare Advantage offers Medicare beneficiaries a number of options for accessing all of their Medicare-covered benefits—and sometimes additional benefits such as eyeglasses or prescription drug benefits. These options are available through a choice of plans approved by Medicare for sale by managed care companies. Medicare Part D is Medicare's prescription drug program, which is sold and administered through private health plans approved by Medicare. Part D plans are only necessary for Medicare-eligible individuals who want prescription drug coverage and do not have it from some other source, such as an employer or retiree health plan. Because Medicare beneficiaries have important decisions to make about organizing their Medicare benefits, including prescription drug coverage, it is strongly recommended that individuals and families seek thorough and reliable information to ensure that they are making informed choices regarding Medicare benefits, enrollment procedures, and their rights as Medicare beneficiaries.

- *Medicaid.* Medicaid is a medical assistance entitlement program for certain individuals and families with low incomes and assets. A joint program of federal and state government, it offers comprehensive hospital and medical protection. Medicaid, unlike Medicare, also provides coverage for an array of long-term care services, including nursing home stays. Because the funding for Medicaid comes primarily from the states, benefits vary from one state to another. Far fewer people with MS are eligible for Medicaid than Medicare because their family incomes are usually too high to meet the Medicaid requirements.

- Full implementation of the ACA will make all legal U.S. residents with incomes at or below 133% of the federal poverty level eligible for Medicaid regardless of their assets or state of residence. It will also expand and standardize Medicaid eligibility in every state and assure that all Medicaid enrollees have access to the same comprehensive set of "essential benefits" outlined in the federal law.

- *State Child Health Insurance Programs* (S-CHIPs). Every state has now adopted legislation providing program eligibility for children from households with incomes too high for Medicaid, but too low to purchase insurance on their own. Like Medicaid, S-CHIP benefits can vary from state to state, often using the same health providers as the state's Medicaid program. Check http://www.health-care.gov or contact your state health or social services department for eligibility information. Eligibility rules for each state's S-CHIP program are not due to change under the Affordable Care Act.

- *Veterans' Benefits.* The U.S. Department of Veterans Affairs (VA) offers comprehensive VA health care to veterans with "service-connected" disabilities and to disabled veterans whose disabilities are not service-connected who meet certain eligibility criteria. Of particular relevance to readers of this book, onset of MS in a veteran may be considered service connected under specified conditions (referred to as the "7-year rule"). VA benefits are not scheduled to change as a result of the ACA.

- *TRICARE.* TRICARE is the Department of Defense's managed care health benefit program for all seven uniformed services: the Air Force, Army, Navy, Marine Corps, Coast Guard, Public Health Service, and the National Oceanic and Atmospheric Administration. Any active duty members and their families, Reserve Component members on duty for over 30 days on Federal orders, retirees and their families, and survivors of all uniformed services who are not eligible for Medicare are eligible for TRICARE. TRICARE offers three plans: TRICARE Prime (military treatment facilities are the primary source of health care), TRICARE Extra (a preferred provider option), and TRICARE Standard (a fee-for-service option).

- *Federal Employee Health Benefits Program.* The FEHB program provides a choice of health plans for federal civilian employees. It includes a federal government contribution toward the cost of premiums. FEHB coverage is available immediately from the date of enrollment, without a medical examination or restrictions due to the subscriber's age or physical condition. If certain conditions are met, the FEHB offers continued protection for the subscriber and eligible family members after the subscriber's retirement from federal service, and for eligible family members after the enrollee's death.

- *State and Local Government Employee Programs.* In general, state and municipal governments offer health benefit plans to their employees and eligible family members. Although the choice of options is typically not as broad as the FEHB program offerings, it is common for employees and their families to have a choice of two or more options.

Private Health Insurance

For the purposes of this discussion, the term "private health insurance" refers to any health insurance coverage that is not provided by the federal or state governments. Many people in the United States are eligible for private health insurance as a benefit of their employment, or as a dependent of an employee whose employer chooses to extend eligibility to dependents. The chief types of private health insurance include group coverage provided by an employer, union, or membership organization; individual (or individual and family) plans; high-risk pools; and Medicare supplemental (or "Medigap") insurance.

- *Group health plans.* Many employers choose to offer group coverage to their employees, and often to the employees' families as well. Significantly, the ACA does not compel employers to provide health insurance to their employees. Instead, it provides strong tax incentives for all employers to offer coverage to their employees, as well as penalties for large employers that do not. Many unions and trade associations also offer group coverage to their individual members and their dependents. In the past, membership organizations, professional societies, and fraternal organizations sometimes offered group health plan membership, but these plans are extremely rare now.

  An important concept to understand regarding group coverage is that the plan can be either "fully insured" or "self-insured." "Fully insured" means that the group sponsor (typically an employer or union) purchases an insurance policy from an insurance company and in exchange for payment (premiums), the insurance company assumes the risk of all group enrollees and pays for their covered health care. Fully insured health plans are regulated by the state's Department of Insurance and therefore subject to all health insurance laws in the state where the master contract or policy was purchased.

  In a "self-insured" plan, the group sponsor (employer or union) acts as the insurance company, collecting the premiums, accepting the risk of all those covered by the group, and paying benefits directly or through contractual arrangement with a "third party administrator." These self-insured plans operate through guidance provided by the Federal Department of Labor and historically have not been subject to state insurance regulation. This may change as the ACA is implemented.

  Because it is not always clear whether one's employer health plan is fully insured or self-insured, it is a good idea to ask. This is important information to know, particularly if a serious dispute over your legal rights as a plan member arises, and you need to know who regulates your health plan.

  Eligible employees and their dependents are often given a choice of different health plans in which they can enroll, including an assortment of HMO and PPO plans with different cost-sharing arrangements. With few exceptions, employers pay the majority of the group plan's premiums and individual members pay a portion, typically through a deduction from their paycheck. Some employers choose to extend eligibility for group health benefits to their retirees and retirees' dependents, although most employers do not.

  In general, group health insurance is less costly than individual or individual and family coverage because the insurer can "share" or "spread" the risk of paying out money for services across a number of enrollees. Whereas some enrollees will prove to be relatively heavy users of care, and may cost more than the premiums paid by them or on their behalf, others will use little or no care, and therefore will be less costly enrollees. In contrast, in individual or individual and family plans (see next section), there is less opportunity for the insurer to spread that risk. Therefore, higher premiums are usually charged.

- *Individual and family plans.* Individual and family plans, as the names suggest, are purchased by individuals to cover themselves, or themselves and their family members. Many people, including those who are self-employed and others who are not eligible for group health coverage, need to purchase individual coverage. However, many seeking this coverage have been disappointed and frustrated by their inability to find an insurer or managed care company willing to accept their application, or offer affordable coverage. At the time the ACA was enacted in 2010, health insurance and managed care companies were within their legal rights in most states to reject applications from individuals and families they considered to be a poor risk, such as those with a preexisting condition. The ACA promises to prohibit health insurers from denying applications for coverage based on preexisting conditions. The ACA also seeks to ensure that coverage will be affordable through tax credits and various risk adjustment mechanisms and that basic standards of comprehensive coverage be defined.

- *Medicare supplement (or "Medigap") plans.* Traditional Medicare pays a large part of the health care costs of its beneficiaries, but the insured individual remains responsible for Medicare deductibles and coinsurance, and for services and excess provider charges not covered under Medicare. These additional costs can be substantial. In response to these unpaid costs and the demand for additional insurance coverage for them, many private insurers offer Medicare supplement (also called "Medigap") plans to supplement Medicare services and to cover costs not covered by traditional Medicare.

  Initially, there was a bewildering array of Medigap plans on the market. The confusion surrounding these plans was compounded by questionable marketing practices, such as companies selling several overlapping plans to the same individual. To address these problems, the National Association of Insurance Commissioners standardized Medigap plans and labeled them Plan A, B, C, and so on—with lower premiums for less extensive coverage toward the beginning of the alphabet and higher premiums for more extensive coverage as they move up the alphabet. Each plan level is consistent across the country, so a Plan B purchased in New York, for example, is identical to Plan B in any other state.

  Although this standardization has improved the situation, problems remain. Medigap plans are not always available for purchase by disabled Medicare beneficiaries younger than 65 years who receive their Medicare benefit through SSDI. Because state laws continue to have jurisdiction over the Medigap marketplace, access to Medigap plans varies considerably from state to state. Although any Medigap carrier operating in a state must offer at least Medigap Plan A, it is not compelled to offer other Medigap options in the same state—and the timing of an application for Medigap coverage can be critical; Medigap carriers are free to turn down the application of anyone based on a preexisting condition if that application is received after the individual's first 6 months of Medicare eligibility. Medigap will not be substantially altered by the ACA.

- *High-risk pools.* Beginning in the 1980s, many states created "high-risk pools" to provide protection for state residents who were otherwise uninsurable due to a preexisting condition. The pools offered guaranteed availability of health insurance to individuals regardless of their health status, which in time led to sharp escalations in their premiums, stricter eligibility rules, reductions in benefits, and, in some states, waiting lists for enrollment. With passage of the ACA, however, the ability of insurers to deny applications based on preexisting condition is expected to be phased out. This process began in 2010 (the year of enactment) and is scheduled for completion by 2014 when all uninsured persons will be eligible for individual coverage regardless of any preexisting condition. Existing high-risk pools will continue providing coverage until that time. In the mean time, additional and temporary high-risk pools for previously uninsured individuals denied insurance due to a preexisting condition have also been established pursuant to the ACA and will remain in operation until 2014 as well.

- *COBRA.* Health benefit provisions in the Consolidated Omnibus Budget Reconciliation Act of 1985 (COBRA) are designed in part to ensure that people who lose employment-related group health insurance benefits due to a "qualifying event" can continue to buy the group coverage for themselves and their families for limited periods of time. COBRA qualifying events are a change or termination of a job; separation or divorce; retirement, death, disability, or Medicare enrollment of a working spouse; or loss of status as a "dependent child."

  - The law generally covers group health plans maintained by employers or unions with 20 or more employees. It applies to plans in the private sector as well as those sponsored by state and local governments. COBRA does not apply to plans sponsored by the federal government and certain church-related organizations, although comparable programs exist for those individuals and families.

  - Many states also have "mini-COBRA" laws that provide continuation protection for those employed in businesses with less than 20 employees. Their protections, however, are often not as generous as the federal legislation.

  - If the employee has worked for a company subject to the federal COBRA law, and leaves work for almost any reason other than "gross misconduct," that individual will be able to maintain the same coverage for 18 months (or more under certain circumstances), at only 2 percent above the group premium. His or her dependents who were also group plan enrollees can maintain their coverage through COBRA for up to 36 months. However, when COBRA rights are used (or "elected"), the employer no longer contributes financially toward the premium, and the full cost of coverage is the responsibility of the employee. If an employed person leaves work, and is certified by the Social Security Administration as being disabled within the first 60 days of COBRA coverage, then the group coverage can be extended for a total of 29 months, at which point the individual would become eligible for Medicare. However, there may be an increase of as much as 50 percent in premiums from months 19 to 29.

  - For companies that are not subject to COBRA, a standard conversion to another health plan may be offered. This coverage will generally be less comprehensive than in the employer group plan and will likely cost more than the premium charged within the group.

  - Health plans subject to COBRA must inform plan members of their COBRA rights, both when they first enroll in the plan and when they leave the job or go through any other qualifying event. Enrollees with dependents in a group plan are obligated to notify the plan administrator of any changes in the dependents' status.

The basic COBRA provisions described were not impacted by the ACA, although less costly alternatives to electing COBRA may be possible in the future.

WHAT IS A "PREEXISTING CONDITION," AND WHAT IMPLICATIONS DOES IT HAVE FOR ACCESS TO INSURANCE?

In the past, insurers applied different standards in their definition of a *preexisting condition,* which could be excluded from coverage of private (nongovernment) health plans. Finally, in 1996, the Health Insurance Portability and Accountability Act (HIPAA) established one nationwide definition of a *preexisting* condition as "any physical or mental condition for which medical advice, diagnosis, care, or treatment was recommended or received within a six-month period prior to the enrollment date" in a health plan. Since most people with MS who enroll in a health plan are likely to have received health care (including taking prescription drugs) during the previous 6 months, MS is considered a preexisting condition. This is an important concept to be aware of because group health plans have the right to exclude or limit their coverage of preexisting conditions for certain individuals on a time-limited basis until the provision of the ACA that prohibits this practice is fully implemented.

Since HIPAA was enacted, group health plans have been prohibited from denying enrollment to any individual who would otherwise be eligible for group health benefits on the basis of his or her health status. However, if a new group health plan member has been uninsured for 62 days or more prior to enrolling in the new group, the plan may exclude from coverage any costs associated with the person's preexisting condition for 12 months or longer. For this reason, it is especially important for people with preexisting conditions to stay insured through COBRA or other means when they change jobs or experience any other interruption in their group health coverage.

As of 2010, group health plans are prohibited from imposing this "preexisting condition exclusion period" on children up to age 19, but may continue to do so for new group plan enrollees aged 19 and older. This change is the first step toward phasing out preexisting condition exclusion periods altogether through the ACA.

HOW MUCH HEALTH INSURANCE DO I AND MY FAMILY NEED?

Ideally, everyone should have sufficient health insurance to prevent them and their dependents from financial devastation in the event of a serious condition, accident, or unanticipated need. One of the goals of the ACA is to define the "essential" health benefits that would meet that need for most working age people and their dependents. As a requirement of the ACA, health plans available for purchase by individuals and small employer groups as of 2014 must provide these "essential benefits." Significantly, the ACA only broadly outlines the essential benefits package and promises further definition in regulations to be issued at a later date. Congress signaled its intention with regard to the scope of the essential benefits by stating that they should be "like a typical employer plan." Proponents of the ACA believe that defining an essential benefits package for people who buy their own coverage, who enroll in Medicaid, or are insured through a small employer group, will set a national standard of comprehensiveness for all health plans and reduce the likelihood of problems related to underinsurance. Until that time, however, individuals and families living with MS are encouraged to carefully consider their health insurance needs depending on their individual circumstances. See Table 21-1 to help you lay out the differences between private health plans.

At the very least, your health insurance should cover (1) standard risks of illness and injury for yourself and your family, and (2) special needs, if any member of your family has a condition, such as MS, which may require special, major, costly, and/or continuing or long-term medical attention. Although the ACA will require that health plan options be presented in standardized and simple language, allowing for "apples-to-apples" comparison among shoppers, there will still be choices to make. Remember that you and your dependents may be eligible for different types of coverage at different times, and that overlapping sources of coverage may also be an option.

TABLE 21-1. Plan comparison grid.

Benefit	Plan 1	Plan 2	Plan 3
Coverage of general medical and preventive care needs for you/your family			
Coverage of special medical needs (e.g., MS-related) for you/your family [list specific services/rates here]			
Coverage limitations/exclusions			
Preexisting condition waiting period (no. of days)			
Choice of providers (yes, no)			
Access to MS specialist neurologist			
Prescription drug coverage			
• Formulary tiers			
Costs			
• Premiums			
• Individual and family deductibles			
• Coinsurance or copays			
• Formulary copays			
• Out-of-pocket maximum			
• Cost for seeing out-of-network providers [for managed care plans only]			
Is the premium rate guaranteed?			
Is there a policy renewal guarantee?			
Yearly/lifetime maximums on coverage			
Company reputation/financial rating			

MS, multiple sclerosis.

Especially if you and/or a family member are living with MS or other condition and are preparing to make decisions about your health coverage, you will want to consider the following:

- Any significant medical condition that you or your family members have (or are at significant risk for in the future)
- Your/their past health care use due to the condition(s)
- The prognosis—that is, the likely future course of the condition and consequent likely future use of services, including prescription drugs

With regard to future service needs and use, the best source of advice is your (or your family member's) primary care physician. (For people with MS, a neurologist may serve as the primary care physician and, if so, he or she should be consulted about likely future medical needs.)

If you determine that certain types of services are likely to be especially important to you or your family member (e.g., physical therapy, psychotherapy, inpatient rehabilitation, nursing care), you should seek out plans that provide appropriate levels of coverage for these needs, without imposing problematic limitations on use of relevant services.

HOW CAN I KNOW WHAT I AM ELIGIBLE FOR? CAN I BE ELIGIBLE AND COVERED BY MORE THAN ONE TYPE OF PLAN AT ANY ONE TIME?

Many individuals and families find that they are eligible for different types of coverage at different times, and need help exploring the pros and cons of overlapping or coordinating their coverage. For example, one family member may be eligible for both Medicare and VA benefits, while others in the same household are eligible for employer-based coverage. To determine what you and your dependents may be eligible for, consider the following questions as a first step:

- Are you employed? If so, are you eligible for coverage under your employer's plan? Is your spouse employed and does his/her employer provide health coverage to dependents? If yes, you may want to enroll in both plans if the benefits of coordinating your coverage seem to outweigh the costs of contributing toward the premium for both. One plan will be your primary payer and the other will provide secondary coverage.
- Are you or your spouse starting a new job, or considering a new job with an employer that offers health coverage to employees and dependents? If yes, enroll as soon as possible to keep your portion of the premium (typically deducted from your paycheck) as low as possible. Late enrollment for group health benefits often results in a premium penalty.
- Does your employer provide health coverage to your spouse and children? If not, look into options for private, individual coverage for the nonworking spouse and children, as well as your State Child Health Insurance Program (S-CHIP). Check http://www.healthcare.gov for eligibility and price information in your state.
- Have you left employment due to a disability or some other reason? If so, make sure you understand your rights to continuation of coverage under COBRA (or comparable program for smaller group plans).
- Do you have a plan in mind for coverage once you have exhausted your COBRA coverage? Check http://www.healthcare.gov or your state department of insurance

to check any/all possibilities. This is especially important for people leaving a job due to a disability.

- If you have established eligibility for SSDI (see Chapter 20), are you aware that after 24 months on SSDI, you automatically become eligible for Medicare?
- If you are leaving SSDI and returning to work, are you aware that you may be able to continue or repurchase your Medicare coverage? Call 1-800-MEDICARE to review your eligibility and enrollment details.
- Are you in danger of losing your group coverage because your working spouse is retiring or going on Medicare before you? Review your options online at http://www.healthcare.gov and plan ahead.
- Is your family's combined income (and until 2014, your assets) low enough that you might qualify for your state's Medicaid program? The formula excludes such items as the value of your house or your first car. If your income is too high for Medicaid, do you qualify for another state health insurance program or tax credits to help you pay for private coverage?
- Are your medical monthly expenses so high that if you deducted them from your monthly income you would qualify for your state's medically needy program (a program in some states extending Medicaid eligibility to individuals with extraordinary health care costs)? Contact your state Medicaid authority to learn more.
- Are you on active duty or a veteran? Are you the family member of an active duty, retired, or deceased veteran? If so, have you checked with the U.S. Department of Veterans Affairs or TRICARE?
- Have you researched http://www.healthcare.gov thoroughly to determine whether you are eligible for your state "high-risk pool" or Pre-Existing Condition Insurance Plan?
- Have you contacted your state insurance department to determine whether "special," or "recently enacted" programs are available for state residents that could provide access to certain services or programs, including those for people with MS or other disabling conditions?
- If you are younger than 26 years and were formerly covered by a parent's employer plan, are you aware that you may now reenroll and remain covered under that plan until your 26th birthday unless you are or become eligible for your own employer-based group plan?
- If you are a student, does your college or university offer a plan you can afford and for which you are eligible? Are you aware that student plans must provide the same "consumer protections" as other group plans subject to the Affordable Care Act?
- Have you contacted the National Multiple Sclerosis Society Chapter (800-344-4867) and/or the manufacturer of any specific drug(s), equipment, or supplies, for assistance in securing something for which you have no coverage?
- Have you reached the lifetime limit on your private health plan? If so, are you aware that the ACA includes a provision allowing you to reenroll in that plan?

DO I NEED TO TELL AN INSURANCE COMPANY THAT I HAVE MS WHEN I APPLY TO JOIN THEIR PLAN?
Yes. But remember that the health care reform law (ACA) will soon prohibit health insurers from denying you coverage or charging you more because of your MS or any

other preexisting condition. These protections went into effect in 2010 for children up to age 19 and will apply to everyone after January 2014. Nonetheless, you are legally obligated to provide honest and complete information in response to anything asked of you by an insurance broker or agent, or on an application form for health or any other kind of insurance. Although the health care reform law put an end to policy "rescissions," your health insurance may still be cancelled for nonpayment or "misrepresentation of material fact." If asked, make sure you accurately answer questions about your health, age, smoking history, and even possible health problems not yet fully diagnosed.

ARE MS TREATMENTS COVERED BY HEALTH INSURANCE?

By the year 2010, when the ACA was enacted and began its slow phase-in, health plans varied significantly in terms of what they covered. Even health plans that covered all medically necessary physicians' services may have restricted coverage to in-network providers only. Other common coverage limitations included restrictions on the number of covered mental health visits, magnetic resonance imaging, or hours of rehabilitation within a calendar year. However, in general, most services (with some exceptions) considered medically necessary to treat MS have been covered by standard group health plans. Exceptions, or "excluded benefits" which should be listed as such in your plan materials or "summary of benefits," are standard as well.

Some common exceptions to group health plans have included neuropsychological evaluations to test for possible cognitive impairments, wheelchairs, or other types of durable medical equipment, as well as home care and rehabilitation therapy (including physical, cognitive, and speech therapy). At this writing (early 2011), health plans that include prescription drug coverage will generally include all of the FDA-approved MS disease-modifying drugs, although the amount you will have to pay out-of-pocket for your prescription can be prohibitively expensive for some people. There are other types of services and care that can be necessary for people with MS that will not be covered by standard health insurance plans, including home and automobile modifications, and long-term care. Working with a trusted advisor on a personal financial plan to include these possible needs is recommended for anyone living with a potentially disabling condition like MS.

HOW DO I GET THE BEST VALUE OUT OF MY HEALTH COVERAGE?

Fortunately, more attention has been put on the value of health insurance coverage as scrutiny over the rising cost of health insurance and care has increased. Although there are no simple solutions to the challenge of making health care and coverage affordable for everyone, there are some strategies that can help. Consider the following:

- Pay attention to deadlines. Enroll in any health insurance plan on time to avoid a premium penalty or limitation of coverage. This is especially important for new Medicare beneficiaries considering enrollment in a Medigap policy, as well as those newly eligible for group health, disability, or LTCI benefits.

- Make use of in-network health care providers as much as possible. If given the choice between different types of health plans in which you can enroll, select a PPO or POS plan that will cover your use of in-network *and* out-of-network health care providers. As a cost-saving measure to you, use the in-network providers whenever possible, and plan on spending more for out-of-network providers on occasion, when it really matters to you.

- Get to know your health coverage well enough to know where the cost savings to you can be found, including the use of mail order pharmacies for your maintenance prescription drug needs; the most up-to-date listing of in-network providers; covered prescription drugs at the lowest cost to you; allowable limits on covered services such as mental health or home care visits; avoiding penalties for not getting a prior authorization for certain services; and using "wellness" incentives such as low or no-cost annual physicals, cancer screenings, or gym memberships.

- Use your right to appeal coverage denials or limitations by your health plan to the full extent possible, starting with an "internal appeal" or review of the initial coverage determination by your health plan. If your internal appeal is upheld and you still believe it to be improper, pursue it further through your right to an "external review." Contact your plan administrator, state department of insurance, or the National MS Society for information about how to pursue an effective appeal, and do so before time runs out.

- Always ask your doctor if a prescribed drug is available in generic form and, if yes, ask if there is any reason it would not be recommended for you.

- Familiarize yourself with the cost of your prescription drugs and do comparison shopping between pharmacies. The "Prescription Price Checker" in the Pharmacy section of the Web site http://www.drugstore.com is one point of reference.

- Talk to your health care providers about their charges, and find out from your health plan how much will be covered by the plans and how much you will have to pay. Review your "Explanation of Benefits" (details of the charges, amounts covered, and payment due provided by your health plan) for accuracy, as mistakes are common. Question the discounted amount and how much in addition to it you will be asked to pay. Arrange to pay off any medical debt by telling health care providers how much you can pay each month. Most health care providers will allow you to pay off your debt over time, as long as you honor your obligation to them. You will not be bothered by collection agencies if you pay some portion of your balance due on a scheduled basis.

- Avoid harm to your credit history, if at all possible, by staying out of medical debt. Avoid interest or financing charges by paying for uncovered health services with a check or cash instead of a credit card.

- Make the best use of a flexible spending account (if available) to pay for uncovered medical needs in pretax earnings throughout the year.

HOW DOES THE AMERICANS WITH DISABILITIES ACT DEAL WITH THE INSURANCE QUESTIONS OF SOMEONE WITH CHRONIC ILLNESS AND/OR DISABILITY?
In June 1993, the U.S. Equal Employment Opportunity Commission ruled that under the Americans with Disabilities Act (ADA): (1) employers cannot refuse

to hire people with disabilities due to concern over the effects on the employer's health insurance costs, and (2) employees with disabilities must generally be given "equal access" to any employer health insurance. In other words, the ADA prohibits employers from limiting benefits that single out a particular disability, a discrete group of disabilities, or disability in general. In addition, the ADA requires that these rules apply both to employers that buy commercial insurance and to self-insured employers (even though this group is free from certain other insurance laws and regulations). Moreover, the burden is on the challenged employer, rather than the employee, to prove that differential treatment of an employee with a disability was not "subterfuge."

WHAT IS LONG-TERM CARE INSURANCE, AND WILL I BE ELIGIBLE FOR IT NOW THAT I HAVE MS?

Long-term care includes a wide range of medical, social, and support services. These services are designed for elderly people, the chronically ill, or people with disabilities who live in the community or in extended-care facilities and need ongoing or periodic assistance to compensate for lost functional abilities. Long-term care services are generally categorized as in-home assistance, community care, or residential care. In evaluating a person's dependence on others for assistance with everyday activities, insurance companies usually divide personal functioning into two categories: ***activities of daily living*** (ADLs) such as feeding, bathing, dressing, toileting, bowel and bladder continence, and getting into and out of a chair; and *instrumental activities of daily living*, including household and community activities such as meal preparation, doing laundry, grocery shopping, managing money, making telephone calls, doing light work, getting around outside, and going places that are beyond walking distance.

Most standard health insurance plans of the sort described earlier cover only very limited or no long-term care services. Many private insurance companies, however, market LTCI policies that cover at least some of these services, although they are free to turn down individual applicants considered poor risks. The ACA includes provisions for a voluntary LTCI program for eligible workers known as the CLASS Act. Meanwhile, government programs such as Medicaid (and Medicare for certain very specific situations) cover some or many such services to certain eligible individuals.

The purpose of private LTCI is to protect against catastrophic costs associated with expensive services over a long period. In view of the risk to insurers, these policies are often costly. Information and advice for consumers about LTCI are available from the following:

● Your state insurance department (generally located in the state's capital city—see the state government section of the local phone book)
● National Association of Insurance Commissioners—http://www.naic.org
● American Association of Retired Persons—http://www.aarp.org

Experience suggests that insurers are not likely to offer LTCI to people with MS once the diagnosis has been established. Some may do so on a case-by-case basis and, if so, will favor individuals (1) who currently exhibit no significantly disabling MS symptoms—who have no ADL deficiencies and function independently,

(2) whose "recent" medical records are free from evidence of recurrent need to treat MS-generated symptoms, and (3) who are in good general health.

Some employers offer LTCI to their employees as part of the benefits package, although a health questionnaire may be used resulting in a denial of coverage for a person with a diagnosis of MS. Just as with group health benefits, an offer for LTCI enrollment should be pursued by interested employees as soon as possible to avoid additional premiums or medical underwriting. Consultation with specialized brokers who focus on "impaired risk" insurance coverage may be helpful.

WHAT IS DISABILITY INSURANCE, AND AM I ELIGIBLE FOR IT NOW THAT I HAVE MS?

Disability insurance is more aptly called "disability income insurance." It is a form of health insurance that provides periodic payments to replace regular income when one cannot work as a result of illness, injury, or disease. Employers often offer group disability coverage to eligible employees, and some states mandate that employers provide "short-term disability insurance." Generally, a minimum number of days when you are unable to work is required before your "sick pay" ends and your disability insurance begins. "Short-term disability insurance" typically provides partial coverage (e.g., 60 percent) of your lost earnings for a period of time, usually 3 to 6 months. If your inability to work extends beyond that period, and you continue to be eligible, you begin to receive "long-term disability benefits."

Both private (including employer-provided) and government forms of disability insurance exist. The most common and important form of government disability insurance for people with MS is SSDI, as described in Chapter 20. A person may be found eligible for SSDI if he or she has worked and paid social security taxes (FICA) for at least 10 years (five of which must be in the 10 years prior to leaving the workforce), and meets the listing of impairments criteria as established by the Social Security Administration.

If you are employed by a company that has a group disability insurance plan for its employees, you should be eligible for this coverage. If you have the opportunity to purchase disability insurance through your employer or any other source, you should try to do so. You may automatically be entitled to the basic amount of disability insurance that is offered to members of certain groups, regardless of your MS diagnosis or other medical history. Your MS diagnosis would prevent you from buying coverage over and above this basic amount, but you would still be assured of some basic coverage. It is certainly in your best interest to obtain disability coverage while you are actively working; it is virtually impossible to obtain disability coverage once a person leaves work due to disability.

HOW WILL THE FACT THAT I HAVE MS AFFECT MY ABILITY TO OBTAIN LIFE INSURANCE?

Life insurance is protection against a future (perhaps very distant) eventuality. For those who want to obtain life insurance, there are companies that will sell it to you. You must shop around to find them since many will refuse coverage for a person with MS even though MS is not considered a fatal disease. Working with an insurance broker who is aware of your MS diagnosis may be easier than researching your options on your own. Often the amounts of life coverage they will sell to you are less than standard, and you may be charged higher premiums than the general population.

RECOMMENDED READINGS

Cooper L. *Insurance Solutions: Plan Well, Live Better.* New York: Demos Medical Publishing, 2003. (This book uses a workbook approach to look at various insurance options including life, disability, health, and long-term care.)

Kalb R, Holland N, Giesser B. *Multiple Sclerosis for Dummies.* Hoboken, NJ: Wiley, 2007.

Northrop DE, Cooper S, Calder K. *Health Insurance Resources: A Guide for People with Chronic Disease and Disability.* 2nd ed. New York: Demos Medical Publishing, 2006. (This resource guide was developed to assist people with disabilities and chronic health conditions, as well as health care professionals, understand the health care system and maximize rights and entitlements within that system.)

RECOMMENDED RESOURCES

GOVERNMENT AGENCIES AND PRIVATE ORGANIZATIONS

A variety of organizations and government agencies can provide you with useful information and advice, generally at no cost. Your state's insurance department, listed in the blue pages of your phone book, offers information and assistance about virtually any insurance matter. By 2014, state health insurance exchanges will be available to help individuals and small businesses research, compare and enroll in private health plans. Exchange services will be available in every state to provide a Web site and easy to understand information to state residents at no cost. Until that time, the federal government's interactive Web site, http://www.healthcare.gov, will provide information about health coverage and Medicaid for individuals in every state. Other useful government agencies include your state office on aging, the agency on developmental disabilities, health department, social services department (Medicaid), workers' compensation agencies, and veterans' affairs agencies. Although the names of these departments and agencies may differ somewhat from state to state, they can generally be located by calling telephone information in your state's capital city. The Appendices in Northrop's book, Health Insurance Resources (cited previously), provide numerous listings and Web sites.

American Association of Retired Persons (Web site: http://www.aarp.org) offers information on all types of insurance through online and print publications, reports, and advocacy.

Center for Medicare and Medicaid Services (Web site: http://www.Medicare.gov or 1-800-MEDICARE) provides information about Medicare, Medicaid, and the State Children's Health Insurance Program (S-CHIP).

Families USA (Web site: http://www.familiesusa.org) provides information and advocacy on public and private health insurance and insurance reforms.

National Association of Insurance Commissioners (Web site: http://www.naic.org) provides consumer alerts and helpful manuals on various types of insurance at no cost.

Thinking Proactively About
Long-Term Care

Debra Frankel, MS, OTR

It is not possible to predict what the future holds for any one individual with multiple sclerosis (MS). While for many the disease remains mild, others will experience more severe problems and disability. Remaining optimistic about the future is important, but it is also helpful to think ahead about the different possibilities that may be in store.

This chapter answers questions about long-term care options. The phrase *long-term care* refers to all the services that people with an illness or disability might need to help them perform their activities of daily life, such as dressing, showering, preparing meals, managing their home and finances, and engaging in their communities. Long-term care encompasses a wide range of services, including housekeeping, personal assistance, adult day health care, respite care, support for caregivers, community housing options, and nursing home care. This chapter addresses questions about these services and programs, describing what they are, how much they cost, and how to determine when and if you might need them. The chapter also identifies challenges related to coping with the complex feelings that may accompany the decision to use these services and programs.

It is unlikely that you will need to use many of the programs and services described here. However, planning and preparing for an unpredictable future is generally a better strategy than waiting until you are in the midst of a crisis to make difficult decisions. Planning ahead can give you the comfort and security of knowing that you have this information, in the event you ever need to use it.

MY HUSBAND'S MS IS GETTING MUCH WORSE, AND WE'RE HAVING A HARD TIME MANAGING WITHOUT HELP. I FEEL GUILTY ABOUT NOT BEING ABLE TO DO IT ALL, AND MY HUSBAND FEELS LIKE HE'S A BURDEN TO THE FAMILY. EVERY TIME I BRING IT UP, IT TURNS INTO AN ARGUMENT. WHAT CAN WE DO?
Facing up to difficult realities and planning for an unknown future are stressful for every member of the family. Family members may feel overwhelmed with added responsibilities, scared about an unpredictable future, guilty about not being able to manage it all, and angry about the changes MS has forced upon them. The person

with MS may feel discouraged about needing to ask for help, ashamed of becoming more dependent, and guilty or angry about the changes MS has imposed on the family. Sometimes these strong feelings interfere with a family's ability to talk calmly about these matters. At a time when family members may need to make important decisions about the future, their feelings can become barriers to honest and effective communication.

Sometimes, just giving family members a chance to air their feelings and voice their points of view in a planned family meeting is the best way to address these issues. It often works best to lay some ground rules, such as no interrupting, taking turns speaking, agreeing to disagree on some topics, and recognizing that this is a hard conversation for everyone to have.

Some families enlist the services of a care manager or case coordinator to help them focus on the decisions at hand and identify available resources. In addition, talking to a social worker or family therapist may promote healthy communication and mutual understanding, helping to separate the emotions from the objective realities that need to be addressed.

Acknowledging to one another that talking about these harsh realities is unpleasant and often frightening, but deciding that you are in it together, can be the beginning of more open communication.

WHAT IS A CARE MANAGER?

Care managers (also called care coordinators or case managers) are health professionals who specialize in providing information, referral, advocacy, and coordination of health and social services to individuals who need assistance with personal care and health care. They usually have a background in social work, nursing, counseling, gerontology, or another health care field. A care manager can provide a range of personalized services to the individual and his or her family, including the following:

- Helping to identify needs
- Arranging for home care or other long-term services (e.g., adult day health care, nursing home care)
- Providing crisis intervention
- Offering counseling and support
- Reviewing financial and insurance questions
- Acting as a liaison to family members who are far away

The care manager may charge a flat fee or hourly rate. When hiring, ask for the person's credentials, obtain and check references, and develop or obtain a written agreement or contract regarding fees and work to be performed. Be sure to clarify whether expenses (e.g., phone charges, mileage) are included in the fee or will be charged separately. The services of a care coordinator or case manager are generally not covered by insurance, although it is always best to check with your specific insurance carrier. The benefits gained from hiring someone to help you and your family navigate through the complex system of long-term services may be well worth the cost.

Contact the National Multiple Sclerosis Society (800-344-4867) for a referral to a care manager, and to see if they can help with the costs of these services. Many local chapters contract with local care managers to provide these services to persons with MS in the chapter area. Also, the National Association of Professional Geriatric Care Managers (520-881-8008 or http://www.caremanager.org) can provide information and help you locate a care manager in your area.

HOME CARE

MY WIFE NEEDS MORE HELP NOW, AND I HAVE TO BE AT WORK ALL DAY. WHAT KINDS OF IN-HOME SERVICES ARE AVAILABLE?

Home care services include the following:

- Housekeeping—basic homemaking tasks, light cleaning, errands, light chores, laundry, and cooking
- Personal care—assistance with dressing, bathing, grooming, transfers, exercise, and toileting
- Nursing care—assistance with medications, catheter care, and other medical procedures
- Rehabilitation services—occupational therapy, physical therapy, speech therapy, and social work
- Companionship—conversation, supervision, company, and entertainment

WHO PROVIDES HOME CARE SERVICES?

The two primary options available when hiring help at home are (1) using a home health care agency or (2) finding and hiring someone on your own. There are benefits and drawbacks to both options.

Professional home health care agencies select, train, insure, and supervise their staff of homemakers, home health aides, nurses, therapists, and social workers. The agency manages record keeping, scheduling, coordinating, and insurance billing— all of which can lift a burden from an already overwhelmed family. Agency rates vary, however, and home care through an agency can be costly. Also, the agency's scheduling practices may not offer you flexibility in terms of the helpers' available hours.

Hiring privately offers you greater control. You can decide who comes to your home, and you are the one to negotiate their schedules, salaries, and responsibilities. In most cases, this option is less costly because the arrangements are made without the involvement of a third party. Although it is unlikely that an insurance company will pay for someone you hire on your own, Medicaid (in certain states) will pay for personal care assistants hired independently through independent living or personal assistance programs.

When hiring someone privately, it is useful to explore local colleges and churches, or put a notice in your local paper. Word of mouth is often the best method of identifying potential helpers. You might even be able to recruit a personal assistant through a local community service program, a retired senior volunteer program, or through your church or synagogue. However you decide to recruit candidates, it is critical to screen each person carefully and obtain personal references.

WHO PAYS FOR HOME HEALTH CARE?

Medicare, Medicaid, and private insurance cover some home-based services. However, there are usually strict eligibility criteria and limitations on coverage.

- Medicare will pay for personal care or homemaker services if there is also a need for short-term skilled care (e.g., nursing or rehabilitation services following a hospital discharge). Medicare does not cover ongoing care.
- Medicaid—for which eligibility is largely determined by income—covers home care services for eligible individuals. Because Medicaid is a state-administered program, quite a bit of variability exists from state to state. However, most states have developed Medicaid programs that support and encourage people with disabilities on Medicaid to live in the community. These programs offer a wider range of home- and community-based services, including personal care assistance and case management. Many state Medicaid personal care assistance programs allow you to hire helpers on your own and receive Medicaid funds to pay them. Check with your chapter of the National Multiple Sclerosis Society (800-344-4867) or your local public health department to find out what types of home- and community-based services are offered by Medicaid in your state.
- Private insurance and health maintenance organizations (HMOs) may cover some home care services through an agency—usually for a limited period. They, like Medicare, may require that you need a skilled service along with personal care or homemaker services.
- If you are a veteran, you might also want to check with the Office of Veterans' Affairs to see if you are covered for home health care.
- Many long-term care insurance policies also provide some coverage of home health services. Each policy is different, so check your policy document or call your insurance agent for details.
- Some people older than 60 years might find that their local Council on Aging offers assistance with home care.

If you are paying privately for agency assistance, some home health agencies offer a sliding fee scale, allowing individuals to pay according to their ability to do so. Since the cost of hiring a helper privately will come out of your own pocket, you are well advised to comply with Social Security regulations in hiring household help. The Social Security Administration can explain your responsibilities when paying assistants in your home.

The cost of not asking for help can be very high for you and your family. The stress of too much responsibility and the consequences of unattended needs can be overwhelming. Do not wait for a crisis to begin using helpers at home.

I FEEL UNCOMFORTABLE HAVING STRANGERS COME INTO MY HOUSE. WHAT CAN I DO TO FEEL MORE SECURE ABOUT THAT?

A home health agency usually conducts a careful screening and interview process with its potential employees. The agency provides training and supervision of its employees, so you can generally feel confident about the helpers you have hired from a home health agency. If you feel uncomfortable about the behavior of anyone coming to your home from an agency, alert the agency immediately. When hiring on your own, remember that you are in charge.

- Prepare a written job description that clearly outlines your needs and expectations.
- Conduct a lengthy interview and invite a family member or friend to be present during the interview to offer another impression.
- Require three references whom you can contact personally.
- Conduct a criminal background check on a potential employee. Check with your state government as to whether they have a Criminal History Systems Board that enables you to conduct a Criminal Offender Record Information check.
- Trust your instincts when hiring. If someone makes you uncomfortable, do not hire that individual, even if he or she "looks good on paper."
- Once you have decided to hire a particular individual, establish a trial period during which you and the employee will have an opportunity to evaluate how things are going. At the end of the trial period, you have the option to terminate the person's employment if you are dissatisfied with his or her behavior, manner of speaking to you, job performance, or if something just does not feel right.

Other ways to protect yourself include the following:

- Keeping track of how much cash you have in the house, and putting it in a safe place.
- Keeping checkbooks, credit cards, and other valuables safely out of view.
- Keeping track of your medication supply.
- Discussing finances only with family and trusted friends.
- Requiring receipts for any shopping done on your behalf.
- Asking friends or relatives to stop by periodically when your helper is on duty.

I'VE BEEN DEPENDING ON MY CHILDREN TO HELP ME GET UP AND DRESSED IN THE MORNINGS. SOMETIMES I THINK IT'S GOOD FOR THEM TO LEARN HOW TO HANDLE THIS KIND OF RESPONSIBILITY, BUT AT OTHER TIMES I WONDER IF IT WILL BE HARMFUL FOR THEM. IS IT ALL RIGHT FOR KIDS TO HELP OUT AT HOME?

Children of parents with MS may have extra responsibilities around the house. Such tasks as doing laundry, taking out the trash, cleaning up, and preparing meals can help youngsters learn valuable life skills. As long as youngsters have time to enjoy their own age-appropriate activities, these extra responsibilities are not harmful to them (even though they may complain from time to time). However, children should not be involved in the personal care of a parent. It is inappropriate to ask a child to assist a parent with toileting, showering, dressing, and other personal activities. Wherever possible, arrange for assistance from adult family members, friends, and home health agencies for this type of care. You can contact your local chapter of the National Multiple Sclerosis Society for help in finding personal care assistance.

MY MOTHER COMES TO MY HOUSE EVERY DAY TO COOK AND CLEAN AND HELP ME OUT. I NEED HER HELP, AND I APPRECIATE IT, BUT I WOULD LIKE TO GIVE HER A MUCH-NEEDED BREAK. DO YOU HAVE ANY IDEAS?

Respite care is a service that provides family caregivers a break from their caregiving responsibilities. Respite care might involve hiring a personal care assistant or home health aide to fill in at home and provide caregiving and/or companionship for a set number of hours each week, or weeks each year. Resources and/or funding for respite care may be available from your local National Multiple Sclerosis Society chapter.

Some families are able to make arrangements with friends to stay with the person with MS for an evening, afternoon, or weekend, so that the family caregiver can have a break and the individual with MS a change of routine. Respite can also be provided by having the person with MS admitted to a nursing facility for a few days or weeks so that round-the-clock care is available while family caregivers are away or taking a break.

Caregiving, while satisfying and rewarding for most people, can also be exhausting and time-consuming. A planned respite provides an essential, refreshing break from routine for everyone.

ADULT DAY CARE

SINCE LEAVING WORK BECAUSE OF MY DISABILITY, I SEEM TO BE SPENDING ALL MY TIME AT HOME ALONE. GETTING OUT HAS JUST BECOME TOO TIRING AND DIFFICULT. MY DOCTOR SUGGESTED I TRY AN ADULT DAY CARE PROGRAM TO GET OUT OF THE HOUSE MORE REGULARLY AND INTERACT WITH OTHERS. WHAT IS ADULT DAY CARE?

Adult day centers provide a planned, daytime program that includes a variety of health, social, and support services in a supervised setting. This is a community-based service designed to meet the needs of people who, due to a disability or illness, may need personal assistance, health monitoring, opportunities to socialize, and/or supervision. Specific services might include social activities, meals, rehabilitation therapies, nursing care, personal care, and counseling. Most adult day health programs are geared to elders, although some serve a more heterogeneous population—and some programs are specifically targeted to young and middle-aged adults with disabilities.

HOW WILL I KNOW WHAT KIND OF ADULT DAY HEALTH PROGRAM IS RIGHT FOR ME, AND WHO IS GOING TO PAY FOR IT?

Several types of adult day care are available: Social day care offers minimal personal care assistance and emphasizes social activities and mental stimulation. Adult day health care offers moderate personal care assistance, health monitoring, and rehabilitation therapies. Some programs are specifically geared to those with cognitive impairments. A high-quality, adult day health center will do a thorough assessment to determine your needs and interests, and offer you the opportunity to ask questions and observe the program. The staff should also work with you to develop an individualized plan (to be reevaluated periodically) that meets your social, recreational, and health needs. In general, you are looking for a program that:

- Provides a range of services in a safe and secure environment
- Offers a flexible schedule of full- or part-time care
- Has well-trained staff and volunteers and a low staff-to-participant ratio
- Adheres to state and national standards and guidelines

Most adult day programs are targeted to seniors, although some may offer special activities for younger participants. You can often determine whether a program is right for you by asking about the types of activities offered and the age and disability range of the participants. It is also important to check a program's references and talk to two or three participants about their experience. The National Adult Day Services Association (http://www.nadsa.org; 877-745-1440) can provide information about choosing a program.

Fees for adult day care vary, depending on the region of the country and the range of services provided by the center. Daily fees may range from $50 to $200 or more per day. Medicaid provides funding for adult day care, including transportation to and from the program, for eligible individuals. Some private insurance or HMOs may partially cover adult day care or specific services provided as part of a program (e.g., occupational or speech therapy). Medicare may also cover some components of the program (e.g., rehabilitation therapies), but does not cover the cost of the program in full. Some private long-term care insurance policies cover adult day care. Check with your agent or refer to your policy documents. If you do not have coverage and are paying privately, ask the center if they offer a sliding fee scale.

HOUSING OPTIONS

MY HUSBAND AND I HAVE HEARD THAT THERE ARE SOME TYPES OF APARTMENTS WHERE HOUSEKEEPING AND MEALS, AND EVEN SOME PERSONAL CARE SERVICES, ARE INCLUDED IN THE RENT. IS THAT A GOOD CHOICE FOR SOMEONE WITH MS?

You are referring to a housing option called *assisted living*. Assisted living residences combine housing, personalized supportive services, and health care designed to meet the needs (both scheduled and unscheduled) of those who require help with ***activities of daily living (ADLs)***. These programs foster independence and resident choice while providing a safe and supportive environment.

The types of services offered at these programs usually include meals served in a common dining area (apartments may also have their own kitchens or kitchenettes), housekeeping services, transportation, personal care assistance, emergency call systems, medication management, health promotion programs, social activities, and laundry services. Assisted living programs may offer single rooms, studio apartments, or one- or two-bedroom apartments. They may be free-standing or housed with other residential options such as nursing homes or independent living units.

Today, most residents of assisted living facilities are elderly. However, more and more younger, disabled individuals and couples are finding that these programs meet their needs. It is very important to obtain enough information to determine whether assisted living is a good option for you. Many programs have specific admission criteria with regard to the amount of assistance you require with transfers and personal care. Ask about what your options would be if your need for personal assistance increases while you are living there. Determine exactly what services are offered and if they can be supplemented if necessary, and finally, ask about the circumstances under which you might no longer be eligible to live there.

**HOW MUCH DOES ASSISTED LIVING COST, AND HOW CAN WE TELL
IF A FACILITY IS ADEQUATE FOR OUR NEEDS?**

Costs vary with the program and the types of services needed by the residents, so it is important that you fully understand the costs and available services. Monthly fees (including rent and services) range from $1,500 to over $6,000 per month. Some programs charge a basic fee, with additional charges for special services. Most residences offer month-to-month arrangements, although some may require a long-term commitment. You may be required to demonstrate that you have assets to cover the costs for a specific time period.

Regulations and licensing requirements for assisted living programs vary from state to state. Residences must comply with local building codes and fire safety regulations, and some states require that staff be certified and receive special training. When considering a particular program, look into state licensure and certification requirements; staff credentials and ratios of staff to residents; services and activities offered; costs; contracts; accessibility of the physical plant; availability of common areas; security, quality, and size of living space; and menus and special dietary requirements. It is very important to read informational materials and contracts very carefully and be a cautious consumer. Marketing brochures can be misleading or unclear as to costs and availability of services. Contact the Assisted Living Facilities Association at http://www.alfa.org or 703-894-1805 for a directory of facilities in your area.

ARE THERE OTHER HOUSING OPTIONS FOR ME?

Over the past several years, new options for accessible and supported housing have become available for people with disabilities. Some are rental properties that offer rental subsidies, with the resident making his or her own arrangements for personal care assistance. Others combine accessible housing with these supportive services. Contact the National MS Society for information about accessible housing in your area.

**I'M LIVING ALONE AND FEEL LESS SECURE NOW BECAUSE I NEED MORE HELP
THAN I USED TO. DO I HAVE ANY OPTIONS THAT WOULD ALLOW ME TO
FEEL MORE SECURE AND INDEPENDENT?**

An emergency response system (ERS) can offer a sense of safety and security to many people who live by themselves. An ERS usually consists of a call button (worn as a necklace or bracelet) that can be pushed if you fall or need emergency help. Once activated, the system alerts an attendant at the system headquarters who will try to contact you to determine your needs. The attendant will then contact predetermined family members, neighbors, or local fire/emergency services to respond to your call. The call device can be worn in the shower and to bed, and the system is in operation 24 hours a day.

Another option is to find a roommate who, in exchange for rent, can offer some personal care assistance and/or companionship. Other personal care and home care assistance options are described in the answers to previous questions.

Home modifications might also help you feel safer and more independent. Widening doorways, creating an accessible bathroom, building a ramped entrance, or purchasing adaptive equipment can often enable someone to stay at home safely and more independently. A consultation with an ***occupational therapist*** or home modification specialist will help you identify your options.

Other housing opportunities or innovative programs may exist in your community. Such options might include:

- *Congregate housing*, in which several people with disabilities share common space and personal care services while each has a private room and/or bath
- *Cooperatives*, in which people who have similar needs share personal care assistants
- *Adult foster care*, which places a disabled adult with a "foster family" that provides companionship, supervision, and, perhaps, personal care

Check with the National Multiple Sclerosis Society for information about housing and independent living options that may be available in your area.

CAREGIVER ISSUES

I FEEL FULLY CONSUMED BY MY RESPONSIBILITIES AS A CAREGIVER.
I LOVE MY WIFE AND DON'T WANT TO BECOME RESENTFUL OF THE
DEMANDS MS HAS PLACED ON ME. WHAT CAN I DO?
The responsibilities of caregiving may cause family members to neglect their own health and personal needs. It is important for your well-being to be attentive to your personal needs for leisure time, exercise, and the pursuit of personal interests. You deserve to have your own needs met, and a person who is feeling less overwhelmed and frustrated will be more effective and patient as a caregiver.

Try to arrange respite care—that is, time when you are relieved from caregiving responsibilities. You can hire help through a home health agency or see if other family members or friends will agree to stay with your wife while you have time for yourself. Your wife might enjoy the change of company as well! The National Multiple Sclerosis Society can refer you to community agencies and facilities that provide respite care. Some Society chapters are also able to provide funding for respite care.

In addition, you might want to consider joining a caregivers' support group. The sharing of experiences and mutual support provided by these groups can be invaluable. Talking to others in a similar situation (as well as to your health care providers) can also help you learn how to distinguish between real, or immediate, needs and unduly demanding behaviors. This may help you set limits and clarify with your partner the best ways you can provide help and still take care of yourself. Contact the National Multiple Sclerosis Society chapter near you for information about support groups in your area. The Well Spouse Foundation (http://www.wellspouse.org; 800-838-0879) and the National Family Caregiver's Association (http://www.nfcacares.org; 800-896-3650) can also be invaluable sources of support, offering excellent newsletters and resource information.

I RECENTLY FELT SO TIRED AND WORN OUT THAT I SHOUTED AT MY HUSBAND AND PUSHED HIM INTO HIS WHEELCHAIR WHEN I WAS HELPING WITH A TRANSFER. MY LOSS OF CONTROL FRIGHTENED HIM (AND ME), AND I FELT TERRIBLE AFTERWARDS. HOW CAN WE PREVENT THIS FROM HAPPENING AGAIN?

When people are frustrated, overwhelmed, and stretched beyond their emotional and physical capabilities, they may lash out verbally and physically. While care partners can control such impulses most of the time, there are situations in which even the most thoughtful, loving person can lose control. People with MS, who must depend on others, are very vulnerable to abusive treatment or neglect. They too, however, can lose control, lashing out physically or verbally at the people who care for them. When tensions mount, and family members are troubled by their own behavior or the way they are being treated, it is time to seek professional help. If you would be embarrassed or ashamed for someone to see your behavior or overhear the way you speak to your partner, you know it is time to seek help. No one in a family should have to accept abusive treatment. When this situation occurs, it means that the family is in need of additional resources to address relationship issues and conflicts, improve communication, and ease the stresses on the care partnership. Your local chapter of the National Multiple Sclerosis Society can direct you to a counselor who is sensitive to the stresses experienced by those living with chronic illness.

NURSING HOME CARE

WE JUST AREN'T ABLE TO MANAGE ANY MORE AT HOME; MY WIFE NEEDS SOMEONE WITH HER ALMOST ALL THE TIME NOW. HOW DO YOU KNOW WHEN YOU'VE REACHED THE LIMIT OF WHAT YOU CAN DO AT HOME?

The answer to this question will differ for each family, but is usually a function of many factors:

- Number of family members and friends available to help
- Financial resources of the family
- Level of disability and health care needs of the person with MS
- Needs and wishes of the person with MS
- Health status of the caregiver
- Types of support available in the community
- Accessibility and safety of the home

Although it is never an easy conclusion to draw, a skilled nursing facility may be the best option if the resources available to you in your home are insufficient to meet the family's needs.

IS A NURSING HOME THE RIGHT CHOICE FOR SOMEONE WITH SEVERE MS?

When care needs exceed the resources available at home, a nursing home is a reasonable and viable choice. A nursing home can provide the full range of necessary services and may well enhance the quality of life of someone who is unsafe or socially isolated at home.

There are many misconceptions about nursing home care, and most people find that their fears about nursing home life are never realized. In fact, life in a nursing home can offer many benefits, including more opportunities for socializing and recreational activities, peace of mind, safety, security, and 24-hour professional care and supervision. While many people perceive a nursing home as "the end of the road," it can provide those who need it a positive, comfortable, and healthy life. Furthermore, the person living in a nursing home can return home for holidays and special visits, or on a more permanent basis if there is a significant change in his or her condition.

While most nursing homes are geared to the elderly, some facilities have special programs for young and middle-aged residents. Some nursing facilities actually specialize in MS care. Be sure to ask each facility for the age range of its residents. The good news is that there are increasing numbers of innovative models of nursing home care that are more resident-centered—offering small, home-like settings, flexible schedules, and greater resident choice. One excellent example is The Greenhouse model—http://www.thegreenhouseproject.org. The National Multiple Sclerosis Society may be able to refer you to these innovative facilities and to those where the staff have experience caring for people with MS.

WHAT IS THE COST OF NURSING HOME CARE, AND HOW DO PEOPLE PAY FOR IT?
Nursing home care can range from $150 to well over $400 per day, and Medicaid is the most common source of payment.

- To qualify for Medicaid, an individual is required to have very limited assets and income. Your state Division of Medical Assistance can give you information about Medicaid eligibility. To qualify for long-term care Medicaid, you may have to demonstrate the need for skilled nursing care and for help with specific ADLs. These requirements tend to vary from state to state.
- Medicare will cover up to 100 days of skilled nursing or rehabilitation under certain circumstances. You can call the Social Security Administration at 800-772-1213 or visit http://www.medicare.gov for specific information. Medicare may also cover some rehabilitation services for someone who is living in a nursing home over the long term.
- Private long-term health insurance often covers a portion of the daily nursing home rate for a specified period of time, and may cover other services you receive there as well. Be sure to read your policy carefully because there are often caps and limitations on coverage.
- Private health insurance and HMOs generally do not cover the cost of nursing home care. Some services, however, may be covered (e.g., physical therapy or durable medical equipment). Again, it is important to check your policy carefully.

Finances are often the most confusing and misunderstood part of the whole process of finding and entering a nursing home. Be sure to ask questions of the admissions staff when visiting nursing homes. You may also want to consult a lawyer or care manager who can help you understand the complexities of financing long-term care.

MY HUSBAND AND I ARE BEGINNING TO LOOK FOR A NURSING HOME FOR HIM. WHAT SHOULD WE BE LOOKING FOR IN MAKING OUR CHOICE?
Ask for referrals from your physician and other health care providers, friends, the National Multiple Sclerosis Society chapter, and other families with MS. Try to plan ahead and visit as many facilities as possible. You might also want to check the

results of government surveys and report cards conducted by your state (http://www. medicare.gov/Nhcompare/Home.asp). It is important to be an informed (but skeptical) consumer, accepting that even the best facility will not be perfect or ideal. If possible, the person with MS should be involved in visiting and selecting a facility. This involvement can make a critical difference in his or her future adjustment in the new situation. When choosing a nursing home, look for the following:

- Current operating license from the state
- Administrator with a current state license
- Certification from Medicaid and Medicare
- Location that suits the resident and makes it convenient for family and friends to visit
- Clean, accessible, bright, and roomy bedrooms and living areas
- Common space for activities and entertaining
- Inviting dining area
- Appetizing food
- Physician who visits the facility regularly and is also available for emergencies
- Residents who are well groomed and dressed appropriately
- Staff who are friendly, skilled, caring, and accommodating
- Adequate staffing (staffing will vary depending on the shift and the level of care required by residents on a particular floor or unit. The ratio can range from four to ten residents for each nursing assistant. Talk to the staff at the facility as well as to other residents and their families about their feelings regarding staffing patterns)
- Active resident council, or other ways in which residents can participate in the life of the home
- Residents' Bill of Rights
- Privacy
- Appropriate range of activities, trips, and social events
- Availability of rehabilitation activities
- Ability to bring personal belongings
- Volunteer program
- Generous visiting policy
- Security and safety
- Experience with MS

Once your husband has moved into the nursing home, visit during different shifts, make unannounced visits, and ask him about the quality of care he is receiving. Even after your husband has moved into a facility, it is possible to make a change or transfer if either or both of you are dissatisfied with the care. A nursing home checklist is available from the Centers for Medicare and Medicaid Services and can be obtained by calling 800-638-6833 or visiting their Web site at http://www. medicare.gov.

MY MOTHER-IN-LAW CANNOT UNDERSTAND HOW WE COULD HAVE COME TO THE DECISION TO HAVE MY WIFE LIVE IN A NURSING HOME. SHE IS MAKING ME FEEL SO GUILTY! HOW DO WE HANDLE IT WHEN FAMILY MEMBERS DISAGREE ABOUT SUCH IMPORTANT DECISIONS?
Decisions like these are often complicated by intense feelings, and harsh realities are obscured by our wishes that things were different. Try to sit down together as a family

and talk honestly about the situation. Talk about the resources you have used, the solutions you have tried, and the thought processes that went into making this decision. Do your best to give a clear picture of the situation—the personal care that is needed, your safety concerns, the impact of caregiving on other family members, the financial factors, and the medical issues. This will help distinguish the objective reality from the sadness, frustration, and anger that family members may be feeling. If communication breaks down, consider seeing a family therapist who can facilitate a reasoned, calm discussion. While family members may not ultimately agree, they might become more sensitive to your point of view and understand the decision you have reached.

MY WIFE WILL SOON BE MOVING INTO A NURSING HOME. ARE THERE ANY STRATEGIES WE CAN USE TO MAKE THE TRANSITION A SMOOTH ONE?

For the person entering a nursing home, as well as family members, the days before and after the move can be filled with anxiety. As with every transition, there will be fears and doubts. With care and understanding, planning and help, the uncertainties of adjusting to nursing home life can be minimized.

If possible, arrange for several visits to the facility prior to moving day. On the day of the move, you and other family members can help your wife set up her room. It helps to bring along personal possessions to create a welcoming space. You can also begin to help your wife learn her way around. You and other family members and friends might plan on staying for the first meal or activity and meeting other residents and staff.

Anger and depression are not uncommon reactions to moving into a nursing home. Your wife may withdraw initially, or seem angry or bitter. You may find yourself the target of these angry feelings, even if you and she made this decision together. It will be important to share your feelings with one another, tap into social and mental health services that are available to you both, and enlist religious or spiritual supports to help ease the transition.

Your wife's adjustment can also be helped along by frequent visits from you and other family members and friends, invitations to join family gatherings outside the nursing home, and reassurances that family relationships will remain caring and strong in spite of the change in living arrangements. Your own adjustment is important as well. Do not hesitate to seek the support of family, friends, your clergyman, or a counselor.

It is important to keep in mind that caring and caregiving do not end because your loved one is no longer living with you. You may find yourself more relaxed and more emotionally available to your wife once you feel less overwhelmed and frustrated with providing the physical care yourself. Some couples report an improvement in their relationship as the stresses of caregiving and fears about safety are removed. Be prepared to get involved in the life of the nursing home. Your involvement and visibility in the home will keep you aware of the quality of ongoing care, help you identify and solve problems before they grow, and help you create a new kind of relationship with your spouse.

MY WIFE AND I HAVE DONE A LOT OF TALKING ABOUT THIS DECISION, BUT NOW THAT IT'S DECIDED, I FEEL GUILTY AND UNSURE. I EVEN FEEL EMBARRASSED TO TELL OUR FRIENDS. IS THIS REALLY THE RIGHT THING?

You and your family may have second thoughts as the move gets closer. Remind yourself that you have carefully thought about this decision, reviewed the options, and debated the pros and cons before arriving at your decision. Review the benefits of the move—the increased security, professional care, and companionship of others. As with all major life transitions, you can expect this decision to be accompanied by anxieties and doubts. With the support of nursing home staff, family, and friends, however, these problems can be minimized.

You may feel that some family members or friends are being judgmental, but this may just be a reflection of your ambivalence and guilt, rather than reality. You need not feel compelled to defend your decision to anyone outside your family, because they have not walked in your shoes. Try to focus on the benefits of the move, and avoid the people in your life who cannot be supportive and helpful to you during this difficult transition.

RECOMMENDED READINGS

Meyer MM, Derr P. *The Comfort of Home: Multiple Sclerosis Edition: An Illustrated Step-by-Step Guide for Multiple Sclerosis Caregivers.* Portland, OR: Care Trust Publications, LLC, 2006.

Miller D, Crawford P. The caregiving relationship. In: Kalb R, ed. *Multiple Sclerosis: A Guide for Families.* 3rd ed. New York: Demos Medical Publishing, 2006.

Mintz SG. *Love, Honor, and Value: A Family Caregiver Speaks Out About the Choices & Challenges of Caregiving.* Herndon, VA: Capital Books, National Caregivers Association (800-896-3650; http://www.nfcacares.org), 2002.

Selected publications available from the National Multiple Sclerosis Society (800-FIGHT-MS; 800-344-4867) or online at http://www.nationalmssociety.org/multimedia-library/brochures/managing-major-changes/index.aspx

- *A Guide for Caregivers*
- *Hiring Help at Home: The Basic Facts*
- *At Home with MS: Adapting Your Environment*
- *Managing Progressive MS*
- *Plaintalk: A Booklet About MS for Families*
- *So You Have Progressive MS?*

RECOMMENDED RESOURCES

Assisted Living Facilities Association
(http://www.alfa.org; 703-894-1805)

Centers for Medicare and Medicaid (800-MEDICARE 800-633-4227;
Web site: http://www.cms.gov)

National Association for Home Care (Tel: 202-547-7424;
Web site: http://www.nahc.org)

National Association of Professional Geriatric Care Managers
(Tel: 520-881-8008; Web site: http://www.caremanager.org)

National Council on Aging
(Tel: 202-479-1200; Web site: http://www.ncoa.org)

National Family Caregivers Association
(Tel: 800-896-3650; Web site: http://www.nfcacares.org)

Social Security Administration (800-772-1213;
Web site: http://www.medicare.gov)

Well Spouse Foundation
(Tel: 800-838-0879; Web site: http://www.well-spouse.org)

RECOMMENDED WEB SITES

Family Caregiving Organization (http://www.familycaregiving101.org). Two leaders in the movement to better understand and assist family caregivers—The National Family Caregivers Association and the National Alliance for Caregiving—have joined together to recognize, support, and advise this vital group of Americans.

Medicare (http://www.medicare.gov/nhcompare). A federal Web site for comparing nursing home quality data and finding state inspection agencies.

Johnson & Johnson (http://www.strengthforcaring.com). A Web site supported by Johnson & Johnson that makes it possible for caregivers to connect and chat with one another.

Effective Life Planning Begins Now

Laura Cooper, Esq

The purpose of this chapter is to highlight some of the ways in which individuals with multiple sclerosis (MS) and their family members can take action and problem-solve now, in an effort to safeguard the family's financial well-being in the future. Of all the topics in this book, life planning may be the one that people are most reluctant to explore. The questions touch on topics relating to severe or incapacitating disability, long-term care, making provisions for financial security, and self-determination in regard to medical decisions and treatment. Although many people with MS will never have to deal with some of the questions raised here, there is no way to predict exactly who will be confronted with severe disability and who will not. Therefore, while many prefer the strategy of waiting and hoping for the best, a more prudent approach is to plan for the worst while hoping for the best. This chapter is designed to illustrate ways to safeguard the future for yourself and your family in the event that your MS becomes severely disabling. Having engaged in this type of long-range thinking and planning, you can feel more secure no matter what the future brings.

The legal and financial questions raised here are meant to provide you with some basic information about very complicated issues. In-depth answers are necessarily more complex than a single chapter could cover, particularly given that the level of complexity required for thorough insurance planning has increased significantly since the passage of federal health care legislation. In addition, the circumstances of each family are unique, and the laws governing many of these issues also differ from state to state, and from country to country.

As of the printing of this book, significant uncertainty has arisen in the United States due to the status of the federal health reform law known as the "Patient Protection and Affordable Care Act." It is impossible at this time to determine whether that legislation will ultimately survive judicial scrutiny; for that reason, this chapter is written under the assumption that most provisions of the federal law will not take effect, at least for the next several years. If that law is ultimately enforced, much of what is written here about health planning and long-term care planning will need to be revisited. Therefore, this chapter is written in the expectation that federal health reform will *not* apply. For example, federal health reform includes two forms of coverage for long-term care that are significant—including a voluntary program of long-term care insurance open to all employees regardless of diagnosis, and strengthened support for home and community-based services in existing Medicaid programs. In its absence, this chapter is designed to help you identify questions you might want to raise with an attorney, certified financial planner, life planner, or specialized postdiagnosis insurance planner who is familiar with the laws where you live.

The term "partner" is used throughout this chapter to refer to spouses, unmarried partners of the opposite sex, and married or unmarried same-sex partners. However, it is important to keep in mind that the legal status of unmarried partners can vary significantly from state to state. Unmarried partners, whether same-sex or opposite-sex, need to consult legal and financial experts about their rights within the state in which they live.

IF I NEED HELP PUTTING TOGETHER A WORKABLE FINANCIAL STRATEGY WITH LIMITED RESOURCES, WOULD A FINANCIAL PLANNER BE HELPFUL?

The simplest answer to this question is that some financial planners would be very helpful while others would not. It is very important to work with planning professionals who have the experience and expertise necessary to construct a rational and workable financial plan in the face of potentially life-altering disability or illness. Very few professionals are by temperament or training prepared to undertake the mammoth and complex task of creating a workable plan under these circumstances. It is therefore critical to begin thinking early on about the types of advisors you may need to assist you throughout your life, and to forge solid working relationships with them as soon as possible. For example, as state law becomes more complex and care costs increase, an elder lawyer may be an invaluable advisor in setting up a Medicaid-qualified Special Needs Trust that may become useful if you or your family member requires care over an extended period of time.

In beginning your search for advisors, it is important to understand that labels can be deceiving. For example, most financial planners are not really *financial* planners in the true sense; they are better understood as *wealth* planners whose expertise is *not* designed for middle-class clients with limited resources. Thus, most "financial planners" are not experts in assisting average or middle-class people in making sound financial decisions that would use their resources most effectively. For example, the typical financial planner's advice would be to have sufficient savings (or other liquid assets) available to cover about 6 months' of expenses in case of unemployment or other career-interrupting disability. However, such advice is totally inadequate for anyone who might have to survive the lengthy waiting period for a Social Security Disability claim (see Chapters 20 and 21).

The mislabeling of financial planners is particularly critical to keep in mind when an individual is trying to construct a sound financial plan in the face of a progressive illness or disability. Standard planning strategies are inadequate in this situation because individuals who mistakenly rely on "traditional wisdom" are likely to face serious—but often avoidable—financial disasters. For example, most financial planners encourage their clients to rely heavily on employer-sponsored insurance benefits. However, these benefits may not be sufficient for someone who is forced to leave the workforce because of illness or disability, especially when loss of employment translates into loss of insurance coverage upon the expiration of COBRA (*Consolidated Omnibus Budget*

Reconciliation Act) benefits and Health Insurance Portability and Accountability Act benefits (see Chapter 21 for more information about health insurance coverage).

As a consequence, *it is critical that you exercise great caution about selecting financial "experts" or advice and screen for specific expertise in the area of disability planning.* Some key points:

- A well-versed financial advisor assisting an individual with a potentially career-shortening disability will focus on your financial plan to address your total long-term needs, paying particular attention to ensuring insurance coverage in the event that you lose your employer-sponsored insurance plan. If the advice offered is simplistic, or relies solely on "traditional" insurance or savings strategies, that advice is likely not designed to assist people who have potentially career-shortening illnesses to reach specific financial objectives.

- Look for an expert who understands *how* to obtain insurance after diagnosis, including health, life, and disability coverage; also look for an expert who knows how to integrate these products into an overall, effective risk-management portfolio. Under some circumstances, it may be important to consciously take into account the rules for specific government benefits, such as long-term care; a good advisor will know how to integrate these considerations into your overall plan.

- Look for an expert who will make appropriate referrals to assist you in constructing an effective "life circumstances plan" to maximize your long-term independence, and therefore also help you defer or reduce the need for long-term care.

IS THERE ANYTHING ABOUT MY RECORDKEEPING THAT I NEED TO CHANGE NOW THAT I HAVE BEEN DIAGNOSED WITH A SERIOUS ILLNESS?

One of the things that you should begin to do right away is establish and maintain a file with all your current medical records, including copies of objective findings and examinations that establish your diagnosis and show the details of your illness or disability. Do not assume that your providers will keep a thorough record for you. These same records may be necessary to justify any expensive or controversial treatments you might receive later, as well as to ensure ongoing availability of information—which increases the likelihood that you can establish continuity of care for yourself even if you find that you are shuffled around to many different medical providers. As medical privacy laws expand, and providers become more reluctant to maintain records—especially for inactive patients—you may find it difficult to go back and accumulate your medical records should the need arise. It is much easier to maintain a file with information as it accumulates. As part of that file, you should obtain a standard medical records release form. Keep copies of it in the file so that one is available each time you need to obtain a copy of a medical record for your own file.

I HAVE HAD A DIFFICULT TIME FINDING PROFESSIONALS WHO KNOW MUCH ABOUT FINANCIAL PLANNING FOR A NONELDERLY, DISABLED PERSON. WHAT TYPES OF PROFESSIONALS COULD HELP ME WITH PLANNING FOR A DISABILITY BEFORE I AM ELDERLY?

Planning to meet financial goals following pre–retirement-age disability is a fundamentally different task than the traditional "wealth planning" process that is the primary focus of certified financial planners. In fact, most financial planners may neglect to take into account (1) the realities of the costs of disability, (2) the ever-changing nature of insurance coverage, and (3) the steps necessary to ensure eligibility for government entitlement program when all private resources have been exhausted.

For legal matters, younger people with disabilities and the elderly often have similar needs. Therefore, one type of attorney who may be helpful in disability-related planning is one who specializes in "elder law" (see Recommended Resources). The National Multiple Sclerosis Society (800-344-4867) can help you locate a qualified professional in your area to help you with life planning.

MY HUSBAND HAS RECENTLY BEEN DIAGNOSED WITH MS. HE IS THE PRIMARY BREADWINNER RIGHT NOW WHILE I AM HOME WITH OUR YOUNG CHILDREN. SHOULD WE BE DOING ANY KIND OF SPECIAL PLANNING, FINANCIAL OR OTHERWISE, NOW THAT HE HAS MS?

You and your husband should begin immediately to create a financial plan that includes insurance and other protection planning, as well as a comprehensive estate plan that also includes the *advance directives* discussed later. Financial planning is the methodical process of assessing your total assets and liabilities, as well as future income potential and anticipated expenses, and then using that information to determine your best options for meeting future needs and wants. Planning should be done as soon as possible and then revised periodically as new circumstances dictate.

The planning process may include the assessment of myriad financial options, including insurance plans, annuities, pensions, home equity, and availability of government benefits. The difficulty will be finding qualified planners who have sufficient expertise in disability issues to construct a thorough plan. The National MS Society can help you identify a certified financial planner or lawyer who can help you sort through the options and identify the possible legal and tax consequences of various choices and choice combinations. If your husband is the primary breadwinner, you will need to pay special attention to his disability, life, health, and long-term care insurance issues so that your income stream will be protected if his disease progresses and he becomes unable to work. You might also want to begin thinking about the type of employment you would seek in the event that you need to provide additional income for the family. If you would need further training in a particular area in order to become employable, you might want to think about taking some courses now. Then, in the event that your husband becomes unable to continue working, you would feel less financially vulnerable and more prepared to take on the breadwinner role.

SAVING FOR THE FUTURE WAS HARD ENOUGH BEFORE I GOT MS. HOW CAN MY PARTNER AND I PLAN FOR OUR FINANCIAL FUTURE NOW THAT I HAVE SUCH AN UNPREDICTABLE ILLNESS?

Your first priority should be to increase the rate of retirement savings as much as you possibly can, since MS may shorten the time you have before retirement. If there is any danger that your own income stream will be insufficient to fund your financial needs, you should also make sure that your financial plan includes consideration of the potential future need for government benefits, as described later.

Next, it is important for you to safeguard yourself and your family from the potential extraordinary costs of the unpredictable illness. When you are planning for such risk, the sensible approach is to assume that the worst will happen, and assess what your needs would be if the worst were to occur. You should never plan for the best; such a strategy is doomed to fail in all but the most ideal and infrequent circumstances. By planning for the worst, even though the best is what you hope for, you will feel pleasantly surprised and adequately prepared if less than the worst comes your way.

Consider, for example, the following grim scenario. If you, as your family's primary breadwinner, become disabled, the continuation of your family's entire health insurance package might be jeopardized if it is based on your employment. In addition, you would need to provide income replacement for any time that you were not working, including finding income supplements for added expenses attributable to any disability you might experience. You might find it difficult or impossible to increase your life insurance to provide financial security for your family members in the event of your death. And, even upon returning to work (assuming that you were able to do so, and that you could obtain adequate health insurance coverage from your employer following a period of disability), you might find that you were no longer as productive as you were before your disability occurred, and therefore could not earn as much money. You might even lose your job altogether. All of these possibilities are frightening, to say the least. If you planned for all of them, you might be able to preserve whatever lifestyle you had before your disability occurred. If you adequately planned for none or only part of them, and you experienced a significant disability for a substantial period of time, your family's quality of life would no doubt be negatively affected.

The ultimate question in this circumstance is how can a person deal with the financial risks attributable to ill health but still maintain adequate income and savings? The answer to this question lies mostly in devising a strategy of protection planning for the risk of ill health. The object of this kind of protection planning is to find ways to lessen the risks—to make yourself and your loved ones as "bullet-proof" as possible—given whatever unpleasant surprises your MS or other health conditions might bring your way. Your best strategy is to devise an insurance package that covers your family's five separate elements of health risk:

(1) major medical coverage for any preexisting conditions, such as the MS, that may be excluded from your primary policy;
(2) major medical coverage for all other conditions;
(3) hospitalization for the excluded health condition(s);
(4) hospitalization for all other conditions; and
(5) some provisions for long-term services.

You should also make special efforts to obtain adequate life and disability insurance that is not contingent upon your or someone else's employment or any other circumstance over which you have no control. Refer to Chapter 21 for a discussion of available insurance options. Once your savings rate is on target, and your assets are protected from depletion with sufficient insurance, you are well on your way to financial security despite the potential intrusion of disability.

I HAVE PROGRESSIVE MS AND SEEM TO BE SLOWLY GETTING MORE DISABLED. MY PARTNER AND I WANT TO PROTECT THE MONEY WE HAVE SAVED TOWARD OUR CHILDREN'S EDUCATIONS AND OUR OWN RETIREMENT BUT WE BOTH KNOW THAT MY MEDICAL EXPENSES MAY GROW CONSIDERABLY IF MY MS GETS MUCH WORSE. ARE THERE ANY STRATEGIES TO DEAL WITH THIS?

The most important strategy is to maintain a "stop-loss" in insurance coverage. This refers to the maximum out-of-pocket expense you will have to absorb before you are completely insured for the medical costs. There are two basic elements to this strategy. The first is to obtain adequate basic major medical and hospitalization coverage that has a built-in "stop-loss" provision that limits your maximum out-of-pocket expenses in any calendar year. The second element is to obtain a good "catastrophic" or "excess" major medical policy. These policies are usually available to members of large organizational groups, and your diagnosis will not necessarily exclude you from eligibility for these group policies. Although you will be excluded from some, others will only impose a waiting period (perhaps a year or two) before you can claim benefits for your preexisting condition. The benefit of such a policy is that it will provide an additional measure of protection by enlarging the scope of expenses that may be covered for your illness. For example, many of these policies expressly provide for at least some custodial (as opposed to skilled nursing) home health care, a benefit that is specifically excluded in most major medical policies. In addition, these policies are relatively inexpensive, so their expense is usually manageable in addition to your usual major medical coverage.

Another strategy you might consider if you find that you are spending a significant amount of time in the hospital is to collect multiple hospital indemnity insurance policies. These policies will pay you a specific indemnity—or dollar amount—for every day that you are in the hospital. These can be real money makers if you are hospitalized with any frequency due to your MS or related conditions. In addition, many of these policies can be obtained without preexisting condition exclusions (usually only with waiting periods). These policies can be obtained from many organizational groups, and they are fairly inexpensive. Unless you find yourself having more than sporadic, brief hospitalizations, you might only want to carry a single good policy of this type to help pay for the deductibles and copayments you may have when you are hospitalized. Keep information on other available indemnity policies for which you qualify in a file. Then, if your amount of hospitalization increases to a point that justifies the cost of multiple premiums, you can sign up for additional policies.

THE MEDICAL EXPENSES RELATED TO MY PARTNER'S MS ARE ALREADY PRETTY HIGH. IF HE SHOULD NEED NURSING CARE IN THE FUTURE, WE WOULD BE UNABLE TO AFFORD IT. WE EARN SALARIES, BUT NOWHERE NEAR ENOUGH TO COVER NURSING CARE IN ADDITION TO OUR LIVING EXPENSES. ARE THERE ANY WAYS TO HANDLE THIS PROBLEM?

The first step in assessing what money is available for long-term care is to identify all your joint income and assets. Once you have a complete picture of income and assets, you will want to take steps to protect as many of those assets as possible against the expense of long-term care or other extraordinary costs. For example, you want to make sure that you have adequate insurance to protect against catastrophic losses, that you make careful investments, and that you protect your credit rating. If regular in-home or outside care does become necessary, try to determine which of the necessary services might be at least partially covered by government programs or private insurance, and which are available at low cost. You should also engage in "life circumstances planning" to try to establish a "life circumstance" that could defer or reduce the need for assistance to begin with. For example, if you lived in a barrier-free home on an accessible transportation line and assisted your partner in acquiring independent living skills that would help him maneuver independently in and through your community, much of the help you are currently considering might not be needed. Life circumstances planning could therefore eliminate the need for care that might otherwise be necessary.

It is also important to think about your natural support groups, and how much informal care those relationships could be relied on to provide. Similarly, if your care is not critically tied to your current residence, you could consider relocating to a lower cost-of-living location, a place where lower wages purchase better care, or a place where state or local laws or programs could help to obtain more complete or better care. Any of those strategies could increase the residual income you have available for care, reduce your overall cost of care, and thereby enhance your overall quality of care arrangement for a substantially lower cost. Finally, extended family members should begin to think about their financial contributions. While there may be no immediate need for money or assistance from relatives, planning for possible long-term care expenses will allow you to determine when financial or other assistance from relatives might be required. The earlier the possibility is discussed, the easier it will be for people to plan and provide for it.

If you do not have enough resources to pay for long-term services, you will need to try to create a source of money to cover the costs. For example, people with a significant amount of "whole life" insurance, or a home with a significant amount of equity in it, have possible avenues for raising cash. The whole life insurance policy may have a high enough cash value to provide you with a lump sum of cash via a policy loan that does not have to be repaid until the death of the insured person. You would probably, however, be required to make annual interest-only payments on the loan. You would have to read your insurance policy to determine the exact loan provisions that would apply to you. You might also be able to convert home equity into cash while continuing to live in the home. The mechanism for doing this is called a *reverse mortgage*, which is basically a loan against the value of a home that does not require repayment until the borrower sells or otherwise (permanently) leaves the home. For information about reverse mortgages, contact the National Center for Home Equity Conversion (see Recommended Resources).

If you find that you still cannot obtain the resources necessary to pay for your partner's long-term care, your only realistic, available option is for your partner to become eligible for Medicaid, the state health care program for low-income individuals (see Chapter 21). The amount of your joint income and assets, in conjunction with the requirements of your state Medicaid program, will determine whether Medicaid would provide care at home or would only cover your partner's care in a residential nursing facility. Since at-home care is more expensive than residential nursing care in many states, Medicaid may balk at paying for a person to receive nursing care at home if the family's assets or income are above a certain level. However, in recent years, and in light of the Supreme Court's *Olmstead Decision* (1999), most states have developed plans to offer care in the least restrictive environment possible; you should advocate for in-home care if your partner qualifies for Medicaid and explore all your legal rights in that regard before you allow the state to force your partner into a nursing home.

I NEED TO APPLY FOR MEDICAID IF MY WIFE AND I ARE GOING TO BE ABLE TO PAY FOR MY NURSING-HOME CARE. HOW DO I GO ABOUT BECOMING ELIGIBLE FOR MEDICAID COVERAGE?

You must be very careful when trying to make your income and assets low enough to qualify for Medicaid coverage (see Chapter 21). Medicaid rules severely restrict protective transfers of income and assets. In other words, the rules prohibit you from reducing your assets simply by taking them out of your own name and "giving" them to children or other relatives. These issues keep evolving, and vary from state to state. To understand how complex these issues are, it helps to understand the basic rules—which may not even apply in your own state. The transfer of any assets out of a person's name during the 30-month period prior to entering a nursing facility or applying for Medicaid is generally considered a nonvalid transfer and will delay eligibility for Medicaid.

There are, however, certain exceptions to this 30-month rule. Medicaid rules allow a couple to change the title on their home when one partner enters a nursing facility and permit the at-home spouse to keep some assets and income. The family may also keep a low-value car and some personal belongings. In addition, there are certain individuals to whom a person is permitted to transfer anything at any time, including a minor child who is blind or disabled. The person applying for Medicaid may transfer any assets to his or her at-home spouse as long as the spouse does not transfer it to anyone else within 30 months for less than its true value. A couple is also permitted to invest liquid assets in their home by paying off an outstanding mortgage, making home improvements, or buying a new home for more money than the present home is worth. Of course, an additional benefit of paying off the mortgage or increasing the value of the home is to make more equity available in case a reverse mortgage might be useful at a later time. Whatever you do, however, must result in a home in which the at-home spouse actually resides.

In addition to reducing your assets to qualify for Medicaid, it will be necessary to deal with your various income sources. If your well spouse has enough independent income (from employment, for example), and if you receive your care in a skilled nursing facility, you may be able to set up an *income-cap trust* (also known as a *Miller trust*) for any personal income you personally receive over the Medicaid qualifying amount. The essential problem here is that all of one spouse's income and assets are deemed to be available to the other spouse if they are living together (but not if they are divorced). Also, the rules involving these trusts have been in a great deal of flux, and an elder-care lawyer should be consulted before you consider setting up such a trust.

If you move into a nursing facility for more than a month, most states have income eligibility limits that use a "name-on-the-check" rule. (Since individual states may have their own versions of this rule that place other restrictions or limits on exempt income, you should check with your state Medicaid agency for more specific information.) Essentially, after the first month in the nursing facility, any income that is received in your wife's name is generally not counted toward the state's maximum income limit for your own Medicaid eligibility. Therefore, the only income that remains at issue after your first month in the facility is income received in your name. If that income is still too high for you to be eligible for Medicaid, it may be possible to set up a trust to divert that income so that you can still become eligible for Medicaid.

The main function of an income-cap trust is to change the way that Medicaid measures your available income. In this type of trust, any income over the Medicaid limit is sheltered for special needs. The money in trust cannot be used for basic support or for services that are covered by Medicaid. The trust will have a "trustee" who administers any income of yours that goes into the trust, and the trustee can use the funds only to pay for items or services, not covered by Medicaid, which would provide you with some benefit. Money in the trust cannot be used for your wife, and the state will be entitled to the proceeds of the trust after your death (up to the total amount already spent by Medicaid on your care). It is important to keep in mind that each state's Medicaid agency may impose different requirements on the trust. If you are considering an income-cap trust, you should contact your state Medicaid agency for information about the specific requirements for this type of trust, and consult with an elder-law attorney familiar with your state's laws.

If, after examining your income and assets, you and your spouse determine that Medicaid would be your only option to pay for nursing care, you should start as quickly as possible to arrange the "ownership" of your funds so that you will be immediately eligible for Medicaid when the time comes. This not only includes transferring assets in acceptable ways (taking into account the ineligibility period or transfer restrictions), but also arranging your income sources, to the extent possible, so that income is in the proper spouse's name. While it is not usually possible to put your own pension or Social Security checks in your spouse's name, it may be possible to put other sources of income, such as investments, in your spouse's name.

If you desire to have your nursing care at home rather than in a nursing facility, and you are not able to make yourself eligible under your state's income limitations, a last resort may be to obtain a divorce that divides your income and assets in such a way that you are left with transferable assets and no disqualifying income sources. While this may be a distressing option to consider, it might make it possible for you to live together and yet redistribute your assets to make yourself eligible for Medicaid. Since some state Medicaid programs do not recognize divorce settlements for Medicaid-qualification purposes, be sure to consult your state Medicaid agency about its restrictions.

MY SAME-SEX PARTNER AND I ARE NOT ELIGIBLE FOR SPOUSE OR DOMESTIC PARTNER BENEFITS IN OUR STATE. WHAT CONSIDERATIONS DO WE NEED TO TAKE TO AVOID LEGAL PITFALLS IN OUR PLANNING, GIVEN THE NATURE OF OUR LEGAL RELATIONSHIP?

Although the term "partner" has been used throughout this text to include same-sex partners as well as opposite-sex partners, not all same-sex partners enjoy the same legal status as opposite-sex spouses in all locations. Because laws vary from state to state, and in some cases location to location, you should consult with relevant planning professionals to obtain accurate and thorough information for your specific area. For example, planning issues and considerations will be dependent on what provisions are contained within your own state law. However, federal law still clearly distinguishes between same-sex and opposite-sex legal partners in that it only recognizes the latter. Thus, even though same-sex partners may be eligible for some insurance benefits based on local law, such partners will not be eligible for spousal treatment under federal government programs (including Medicare and Medicaid), and explicit consideration of such limitations may need to become part of the overall planning paradigm for same-sex couples. Similarly, even if your state provides same-sex partner legal recognition, you will nevertheless need to complete a set of powers of attorney and advance directives to enable your partner to make medical decisions for you—just as you would be well advised to do if you were a member of an opposite-sex partnership.

WHAT IS THE DIFFERENCE BETWEEN A LIVING WILL AND A HEALTH CARE PROXY, AND WHY DO I NEED TO HAVE ONE OR BOTH OF THEM?

Every competent person has the right to accept or refuse medical care. Unfortunately, illness or injury can intrude on the decision-making process, limiting a person's ability to communicate or carry out his or her wishes when the time for a decision arrives. What actually happens is that although the person retains the right to make a decision, the legal ability to exercise the right may be lost due to the incapacity to make such decisions. When an individual is judged legally incompetent (through unconsciousness or severe *cognitive impairment*, for example), health care providers do not need to abide by the person's choices if those choices conflict with medical judgments. If, however, personal choices about medical treatment have been made in advance and incorporated into a legally enforceable advance directive, the legal ability to make decisions is protected even after the person becomes incapacitated. Health care providers can then be directed by the wishes that the person made clear in advance, even if those wishes conflict with medical judgments.

Advance medical directives take the form of written documents in which competent persons state their medical decisions for the future. This can be accomplished in two ways: (1) via a *living will*, in which you outline specific instructions for your health care providers; or (2) by a *health care proxy* (also known as a *power of attorney for health care decision making*), in which you designate another person, who knows and would be sympathetic to your desires, to make medical decisions for you in the event that you become too incapacitated to make them for yourself.

Although the living will and health care proxy are both known as advance directives, they differ in the type of directive that is involved. A living will establishes certain treatment guidelines that are to be followed in the future (e.g., an instruction that no "extraordinary measures" are to be used to prolong life in the event of permanent unconsciousness). A health care proxy does not establish treatment guidelines directly. Instead, it appoints a trusted individual to act as your agent and make any necessary decisions in the event that you cannot act for yourself. A health care proxy can incorporate provisions of a living will by requiring that the health care proxy follow any directives that you have included in your living will. Because it is almost impossible to predict all the circumstances that might arise during an illness, it would be difficult for you to include an exhaustive list of advance directives in a living will. Hence, a health care proxy is necessary, in addition to a living will, if you wish to preserve completely the right to self-determination; any decision that is not determined by the directives in your living will would then be made by the person you have entrusted to speak for you. Consequently, a good set of advance directives will include both a living will and a health care proxy, or a single document incorporating both items.

Advance medical directives are recommended for all adults, with or without *chronic* illness or disability. In fact, new federal privacy rules make it more critical than ever before for all competent adults to execute advance directives, since even spouses and other close relatives may now be denied access by health providers to private medical information without explicit written permission. For that reason, regardless of your formal marital or family status, you should make certain that you execute and maintain advance directives empowering a trusted individual to act on your behalf.

Many hospitals now routinely ask any person being admitted whether he or she has made an advance directive. Once you have written your directives, be sure to give copies to your health care providers and close family members so that they can be informed of your wishes. At least one online repository for advance directives has been established in Montana. You may want to explore the option of storing these documents online so that they could be made available to health providers over the Internet no matter when or where you may need them, without losing your ability to modify them as you choose.

IF MY PARTNER DOES NOT EXECUTE AN ADVANCE DIRECTIVE, HOW WILL MEDICAL DECISIONS BE MADE FOR HIM IF HE BECOMES UNABLE TO MAKE THOSE DECISIONS FOR HIMSELF?

Once it has been determined that an incapacitated person cannot make decisions and has not left specific directives, family members are usually considered to be the appropriate decision makers. In theory, most courts agree that even in the absence of a proxy, family members are the appropriate decision makers. In practice, however, health care providers are not required to follow the family's decisions (to withhold or remove life support, for example) if the providers question the good faith or the medical advisability of those decisions. Therefore, appointing a proxy would provide a safeguard in the event that health care providers hesitate to follow the requests of the incapacitated person as understood or interpreted by family members. Since proxies are considered to directly exercise the wishes of the incapacitated person, health care providers cannot disregard any proxy decisions that conform to the terms of the advance directive.

It is precisely because of this issue that an important legal distinction must be made between a *proxy* and a *surrogate*. A proxy is named in the advance directive and is therefore chosen directly by the incapacitated individual. A surrogate is someone who is legally appointed by the court and is not, therefore, considered to be directly exercising the wishes of the incapacitated person. For example, if no valid health care proxy exists, a surrogate may be appointed to make the incapacitated person's decisions. This surrogate may be empowered to make these decisions in one of two ways: (1) by virtue of a legal relationship (e.g., spouse, parent, or adult child) that automatically gives the person the authority to make surrogate decisions, or (2) by court appointment as a guardian.

The extent to which you can enforce decisions concerning your partner's future care will depend on whether you are acting as his proxy or as his surrogate. If your partner named you as his proxy, you are acting for him and have the same authority as if he were making his own decisions. If you were named his surrogate decision maker by some other process of law, your decisions will only be honored if you are thought to be acting in good faith, and if his health care providers think your decisions are medically advisable.

MY PARTNER HAS EXPERIENCED SIGNIFICANT COGNITIVE CHANGES AS A RESULT OF HER MS. HER MEMORY, JUDGMENT, AND DECISION-MAKING ABILITIES ARE SEVERELY IMPAIRED. HOW CAN WE MAKE SURE THAT SHE WILL GET PROPER CARE IF I DIE BEFORE SHE DOES?

Assuming that your partner executed a health care proxy naming you as her proxy prior to her severe cognitive impairment, and also designated your successor, this successor could take over if you were to die or become legally incapacitated and unable to make decisions for her. However, if your partner executed a proxy without designating your successor, your death would leave her in the same position as if she had not designated a proxy at all. If your partner did not execute a health care proxy, the court will generally appoint surrogate (substitute) decision makers according to a hierarchy established by state law, with close relatives being given priority over more distant relatives. Thus, if no valid proxy exists, a legal spouse would probably be appointed her surrogate decision maker and then replaced by another surrogate if that spouse became incapacitated or died.

A surrogate chosen by the court does not have the power to delegate his or her surrogate decision-making authority to other persons. Therefore, if you acquired your ability to make medical decisions for your partner as a court-appointed surrogate, rather than as her designated proxy, the court will simply appoint another surrogate in the event that you die or become incapacitated. As a surrogate, you cannot control in any legal or formal way who this successor will be. However, there are steps that you can take to try to assist the court to make an appropriate decision in such a matter. The best strategy is to define her wishes, as you understand them, in a *values history form*. The purpose of such a form is to assist you in describing your partner's feelings and preferences concerning her health as you understand them. Values history forms are usually available from elder-law attorneys.

In addition to making decisions about your partner's medical care, you will also want to try to ensure that sufficient resources will be available after your death (or during your life if you are also incapacitated and are using substantial resources for your own care) to provide for that care. The best way to do this is to develop plans to increase, protect, and preserve your assets.

OUR 46-YEAR-OLD DAUGHTER HAS PROGRESSIVE MS. SHE IS FAIRLY WELL AT PRESENT, BUT WE WOULD LIKE TO MAKE FINANCIAL PROVISIONS FOR HER IN OUR ESTATE PLANNING. WHAT IS THE BEST WAY FOR US TO DO THIS?

Your best strategy will be to develop a cohesive estate plan in which you accomplish the following: (1) determine who will get your property when you die, (2) set up procedures to make sure that your property passes to others free from probate or with the lowest possible probate fees, (3) set up ways to pass your property to others while reducing or avoiding taxes, and (4) set up a mechanism to manage property you are leaving to others who might be unable to manage it themselves, including your disabled daughter.

In general, the method you choose to distribute your assets will involve either a *will*, a *trust*, or both. In using estate planning tools to protect your daughter, it would be advisable to consult an experienced attorney; the law is quite complex and mistakes in planning could have unfortunate consequences. For example, a problem that is commonly overlooked in estate planning is the effect that inheritances or gifts can have on a person's eligibility for public benefits such as Medicaid. Under certain circumstances, it might be preferable to limit or eliminate the transfer of assets to your daughter so that she is not put in the position of missing out on valuable (government) social services.

A written will generally serves as the cornerstone of your financial estate plan. A will is a binding legal document that determines how your estate should be distributed after you die. In addition to distributing property, wills may be used to handle certain personal affairs such as ensuring that your disabled daughter is cared for properly in the event that she becomes legally incompetent. Parents and guardians may use wills to name their successors. Such designations, depending on the state in which they are made, may be legally binding or of invaluable assistance to a court in any necessary guardianship proceedings. These designees are known either as *successor* or *testamentary guardians*.

A trust is a binding legal arrangement in which a person transfers assets to another person, known as a *trustee*, who manages it for the named beneficiary. This arrangement may be made as part of a will, in which case it is called a *testamentary trust*, or it may become effective during your lifetime, in which case it is called a *living trust*. In addition, a living trust may be changeable during your lifetime (*revocable*) or it may be fixed (*irrevocable*). A trust can be used to select a trustee who will look out for the financial and personal interests of your daughter without the need for a guardian, and it may result in substantial tax savings. The disadvantages of a trust may include complexity, cost, and the possibility that changing circumstances will leave the trustee without the most appropriate options. Although trusts may come in many forms, the most important for this purpose include:

- *Contingent testamentary trusts*—proceeds of an estate go first to the surviving spouse and then are held in trust for your daughter after the spouse's death
- *Living trust with a pour-over provision*—allows property to be added to the trust for your daughter after your death

- *Discretionary trust*—carefully defines the amount and kind of discretion that the trustee will have in distributing or withholding benefits
- *Sprinkling trust*—allows you to instruct the trustee, in the event that the trust has more than one beneficiary, to distribute the benefits unequally according to the unique needs of each of those beneficiaries
- *Life insurance trust*—ensures that the benefits of a life insurance policy will be managed properly

It is advisable to consult with an estate planning attorney to make sure, given your financial and social circumstances, that the best strategies are used to ensure that your daughter will be protected both financially and socially once you pass away. In many states, experts in estate planning are available for families with children who have disabilities. You can obtain current information about such experts by contacting the National Information Center for Children and Youth with Disabilities.

Although this chapter comes at the end of the book, its more suitable placement might well be at the very beginning. Effective planning means looking ahead in an effort to make the future as workable and predictable as it can possibly be in the face of life's uncertainties. MS only adds to those uncertainties. Every chapter in this book is designed to help you familiarize yourself and your family members with the possibilities inherent in living with this type of unpredictable chronic illness. While many people will never experience much of what is described in these pages, being educated about the disease and the resources that are available to help you will enable you to feel more prepared to deal with whatever the future brings.

RECOMMENDED READINGS
....

Cooper L. *Insurance Solutions: Plan Well, Live Better. A Workbook for People with Chronic Illness or Disability.* New York: Demos Medical Publishing, 2000.

Northrop D. Life planning: Financial and legal considerations. In: Kalb R, ed. *Multiple Sclerosis: A Guide for Families.* 3rd ed. New York: Demos Medical Publishing, 2006.

Northrop D, Cooper S, Calder K. *Health Insurance Resources: A Guide for People with Chronic Disease and Disability.* 2nd ed. New York: Demos Medical Publishing, 2007.

Selected publications available from the National Multiple Sclerosis Society (800-FIGHT-MS; 800-344-4867):
- National Endowment for Financial Education: *Adapting: Financial Planning for a Life with Multiple Sclerosis,* 2004.

RECOMMENDED RESOURCES—FEDERAL HEALTH CARE REFORM
....

Health Reform Source: an online timeline for changes, published by the Kaiser Family Foundation at http://kff.org/healthreform/8060.cfm

Health Reform GPS: a joint project of George Washington University's Hirsh Health Law and Policy Program and the Robert Wood Johnson Foundation, providing an overview of health reform at http://healthreformgps.org

Helpful Federal Web sites:
http://healthcare.gov
http://cms.gov
http://medicare.gov

RECOMMENDED RESOURCES—GENERAL

American Association of Retired Persons (AARP) (Tel: 202-434-2277; Web site: http://www. aarp.org). Disseminates valuable information on all types of insurance.

Center for Medicare Advocacy (Tel: 860-456-7790; Web site: http://www.medicareadvocacy. org). Provides assistance to people with disabilities (and their advocates) in areas of Medicare, educational materials, home care, and referrals.

Center for the Study of Services, The Consumer Guide to Health Plans, 733 15th Street NW, Suite 820, Washington, DC 20005 (Tel: 800-475-7283; Web site: http://www.cssresearch. org). Ranks managed care plans and publishes its findings.

Consumer Federation of American (CFA), 1424 16th Street NW, Washington, DC 20036 (Tel: 202-387-6121 or 212-387-0087; Web site: http://www.consumerfed.org). This insurance consumer advocacy group publishes a useful life insurance guide called *Taking a Bite Out of Insurance.*

Medicare Rights Center: a national, nonprofit consumer service organization that works to ensure access to affordable health care for older adults and people with disabilities at http://medicarerights.org.

National Academy of Elder Law Attorneys, Inc., 1604 N. Country Club Road, Tucson, AZ 85716 (Tel: 602-881-4005; Web site: http://www.naela.com). If you send them a stamped, self-addressed, legal-sized envelope, they will send you a brochure entitled "Questions and Answers When Looking for an Elder Law Attorney."

National Association of Personal Financial Advisors—NAPFA (Tel: 800-366- 2732; Web site: http://www.napfa.org). They will send you names of association members in your area.

National Center for Home Equity Conversion, Reverse Mortgage Locator, National Center for Home Equity Conversion, 7373 147th St, Ste 115, Apple Valley, MN 66124 (Tel: 612-953-4474; Web site: http://www.reverse.org).

National Committee for Quality Assurance (NCQA) (Tel: 800-839-6487; Web site: http://www.ncqa.org). Collects information on managed care plans, including HMOs and rates them on factors such as physician credentials and subscriber turnover, publishes its findings, and accredits the plans. The accreditation report is provided free-of-charge upon request, or can be accessed via the NCQA Web site.

National Information Center for Children and Youth with Disabilities, P.O. Box 1492, Washington, DC 20013 (Tel: 800-695-0285; 202-884-8200; Web site: http://www. nichcy.org).

People's Medical Society (Tel: 610-770-1670; Web site: http://www.peoplesmed.org). Publishes useful information about health insurance.

Appendix A: Glossary

Activities of daily living (ADLs): Activities of daily living include any daily activity a person performs for self-care (feeding, grooming, bathing, dressing), work, homemaking, and leisure. The ability to perform ADLs is often used as a measure of ability/disability in MS.

Acute: Having rapid onset, usually with recovery; not chronic or long lasting.

Acute attack: *See* Exacerbation.

ADLs: *See* Activities of daily living.

Advance (medical) directive: Advance directives preserve the person's right to accept or reject a course of medical treatment even after the person becomes mentally or physically incapacitated to the point of being unable to communicate those wishes. Advance directives come in two basic forms: (1) a living will, in which the person outlines specific treatment guidelines that are to be followed by health care providers; (2) a health care proxy (also called a power of attorney for health care decision making), in which the person designates a trusted individual to make medical decisions in the event that he or she becomes too incapacitated to make such decisions. Advance directive requirements vary greatly from one state to another and should therefore be drawn up in consultation with an attorney who is familiar with the laws of the particular state.

Afferent pupillary defect: An abnormal reflex response to light that is a sign of nerve fiber damage due to optic neuritis. A pupil normally gets smaller when a light is shined either into that eye (direct response) or the other eye (indirect response). In an afferent pupillary defect (also called Marcus Gunn pupil), there is a relative decrease in the direct response. This is most clearly demonstrated by the "swinging flashlight test." When the flashlight is shined first in the abnormal eye, then in the healthy eye, and then again in the eye with the pupillary defect, the affected pupil becomes larger rather than smaller.

AFO: *See* Ankle-foot orthosis.

Ankle-foot orthosis (AFO): An ankle-foot orthosis is a brace, usually plastic, that is worn on the lower leg and foot to support the ankle and correct foot drop. By holding the foot and ankle in the correct position, the AFO promotes correct heel-toe walking. *See* Foot drop.

Antibody: Protein produced by certain cells of the immune system in response to bacteria, viruses, and other types of foreign antigens. *See* Antigen.

Anticholinergic: Refers to the action of certain medications commonly used in the management of neurogenic bladder dysfunction. These medications inhibit the transmission of parasympathetic nerve impulses and thereby reduce spasms of smooth muscle in the bladder.

Antigen: Any substance that triggers the immune system to produce an antibody; generally refers to infectious or toxic substances. *See* Antibody.

Aspiration: Inhalation of food particles or fluids into the lungs.

Aspiration pneumonia: Inflammation of the lungs due to aspiration.

Assistive devices: Any tools that are designed, fabricated, and/or adapted to assist a person in performing a particular task, for example, cane, walker, shower chair.

Assistive technology: A term used to describe all of the tools, products, and devices, from the simplest to the most complex, which can make a particular function easier or possible to perform.

Ataxia: The incoordination and unsteadiness that result from the brain's failure to regulate the body's posture and the strength and direction of limb movements. Ataxia is most often caused by disease activity in the cerebellum.

Atrophy: A wasting away or decrease in size of a cell, tissue, or organ of the body because of disease or lack of use. *See* Brain atrophy.

Attack: *See* Relapse.

Autoimmune disease: A process in which the body's immune system causes illness by mistakenly attacking healthy cells, organs, or tissues in the body that are essential for good health. Multiple sclerosis is believed to be an autoimmune disease, along with systemic lupus erythematosus, rheumatoid arthritis, scleroderma, and many others. The precise origin and pathophysiologic processes of these diseases are unknown.

Autonomic nervous system: The part of the nervous system that regulates involuntary vital functions, including the activity of the cardiac (heart) muscle, smooth muscles (e.g., of the gut), and glands. The autonomic nervous system has two divisions: the sympathetic nervous system accelerates heart rate, constricts blood vessels, and raises blood pressure; the parasympathetic nervous system slows heart rate, increases intestinal and gland activity, and relaxes sphincter muscles.

Axon: The extension or prolongation of a nerve cell (neuron) that conducts impulses to other nerve cells or muscles. Axons are generally smaller than 1 micron (1 micron = 1/1,000,000 of a meter) in diameter, but can be as much as a half meter in length.

Axonal damage: Injury to the axon in the nervous system, generally as a consequence of trauma or disease. This damage may involve temporary, reversible effects or permanent severing of the axon. Axonal damage usually results in short-term changes in nervous system activity, or permanent inability of nerve fibers to send their signals from one part of the nervous system to another or from nerve fibers to muscles. The damage can thus result in a variety of symptoms relating to sensory or motor function.

B cell: A type of lymphocyte (white blood cell) manufactured in the bone marrow that makes antibodies.

Babinski reflex: A neurologic sign in MS in which stroking the outside sole of the foot with a pointed object causes an upward (extensor) movement of the big toe rather than the normal (flexor) bunching and downward movement of the toes. This abnormal response indicates damage to the motor pathways in the brain and spinal cord. *See* Sign.

Black hole: A plaque (lesion) appearing on magnetic resonance imaging (MRI) as a dull spot that may indicate an area of permanent axonal injury or tissue loss. *See* Axonal damage.

Bell's palsy: A paralysis of the facial nerve (usually on one side of the face), which can occur as a consequence of MS, viral infection, or other infections. It has acute onset and can be transient or permanent.

Blinding: An attempt to eliminate bias in the interpretation of clinical trial outcomes. It indicates that at least one party involved in the clinical trial is unaware of which patients are receiving the experimental treatment and which are receiving the control substance. Trials may be either single-blind (patients do not know which treatment they are receiving) or double-blind (neither the examining physicians nor the patients know which treatment each patient is receiving).

Blood-brain barrier: A semipermeable cell layer around blood vessels in the brain and spinal cord that prevents large molecules, immune cells, and potentially damaging substances and disease-causing organisms (e.g., viruses) from passing out of the blood stream into the central nervous system (brain and spinal cord). A break in the blood-brain barrier may underlie the disease process in MS.

Brain atrophy: A loss or shrinkage of brain tissue that occurs in MS as a result of damage to axons. Loss of myelin and changes in brain fluids probably contribute as well. *See* Axon, Axonal damage, Myelin.

Brainstem: The part of the central nervous system that houses the nerve centers of the head as well as the centers for respiration and heart control. It extends from the base of the brain to the spinal cord.

Catheter: A hollow, flexible tube, made of plastic or rubber, which can be inserted through the urinary opening into the bladder to drain excess urine that cannot be excreted normally.

Central nervous system: The part of the nervous system that includes the brain, optic nerves, and spinal cord.

Cerebellum: A part of the brain situated above the brainstem that controls balance and coordination of movement.

Cerebrospinal fluid (CSF): A watery, colorless, clear fluid that bathes and protects the brain and spinal cord. The composition of this fluid can be altered by a variety of diseases. Certain changes in CSF that are characteristic of MS can be detected with a lumbar puncture (spinal tap), a test sometimes used to help make the MS diagnosis. *See* Lumbar puncture.

Cerebrum: The large, upper part of the brain that acts as a master control system and is responsible for initiating thought and motor activity. Its two hemispheres, united by the corpus callosum, form the largest part of the central nervous system.

Cerebral: Pertaining to the cerebrum.

Chronic: Of long duration, not acute; a term often used to describe a disease that shows gradual worsening.

Chronic progressive: A former "catch-all" term for progressive forms of MS. *See* Primary-progressive MS, Secondary-progressive MS, and Progressive-relapsing MS.

Clinical finding: An observation made during a medical examination indicating change or impairment in a physical or mental function.

Clinically isolated syndrome (CIS): A first neurologic episode, lasting at least 24 hours, which is caused by inflammation/demyelination in one or more sites in the central nervous system (CNS). A person with CIS can have a single neurologic sign or symptom—for example, an attack of optic neuritis—that is caused by a single lesion (and referred to as *monofocal*), or more than one sign or symptom—for example, an attack of optic neuritis accompanied by weakness on one side—caused by lesions in more than one place (and referred to as *multifocal*). Individuals who experience a clinically isolated syndrome may or may not go on to develop multiple sclerosis. Studies have shown that when the CIS is accompanied by asymptomatic MRI-detected brain lesions that are consistent with those seen in MS, there is a high risk of a second neurologic event, and therefore a diagnosis of clinically definite MS, within several years. Individuals who experience CIS with no evidence of MRI-detected lesions are at relatively low risk for developing MS over the same time period.

Clinical trial: Rigorously controlled studies designed to provide extensive data that will allow for statistically valid evaluation of the safety and efficacy of a particular treatment. *See* Double-blind clinical study; Placebo.

Cognition: High level functions carried out by the human brain, including comprehension and use of speech, visual perception and construction, calculation ability, attention (information processing), memory, and executive functions such as planning, problem-solving, and self-monitoring.

Cognitive impairment: Changes in cognitive function caused by trauma or disease process. Some degree of cognitive impairment occurs in approximately 50 to 60 percent of people with MS, with memory, information processing, and executive functions being the most commonly affected functions. *See* Cognition.

Cognitive rehabilitation: Techniques designed to improve the functioning of individuals whose cognition is impaired because of physical trauma or disease. Rehabilitation strategies are designed to improve the impaired function via repetitive drills or practice, or to compensate for impaired functions that are not likely to improve. Cognitive rehabilitation is provided by psychologists and neuropsychologists, speech/language pathologists, and occupational therapists. While these three types of specialists use different assessment tools and treatment strategies, they share the common goal of improving the individual's ability to function as independently and safely as possible in the home and work environment.

Combined (bladder) dysfunction: A type of neurogenic bladder dysfunction in MS (also called detrusor-external sphincter dyssynergia—DESD). Simultaneous contractions of the bladder's detrusor muscle and external sphincter cause urine to be trapped in the bladder, resulting in symptoms of urinary urgency, hesitancy, dribbling, and incontinence.

Condom catheter: A tube connected to a thin, flexible sheath that is worn over the penis to allow drainage of urine into a collection system; can be used to manage male urinary incontinence.

Constipation: A condition in which bowel movements happen less frequently than is normal for the particular individual, or the stool is small, hard, and difficult or painful to pass.

Contraction: A shortening of muscle fibers that results in the movement of a joint.

Contracture: A permanent shortening of the muscles and tendons adjacent to a joint, which can result from severe, untreated spasticity and interferes with normal movement around the affected joint. If left untreated, the affected joint can become frozen in a flexed (bent) position. *See* Spasticity.

Controlled clinical trials: A clinical trial that compares the outcome of a group of randomly assigned patients who receive the experimental treatment to the outcome of a group of randomly assigned patients who receive a standard treatment or inactive placebo.

Coordination: An organized working together of muscles and groups of muscles aimed at bringing about a purposeful movement such as walking or standing.

Corpus callosum: The broad band of nerve fiber tissue that connects the two cerebral hemispheres of the brain.

Cortex: The outer layer of brain tissue.

Corticosteroid: Any of the natural or synthetic hormones associated with the adrenal cortex (which influences or controls many body processes). Corticosteroids include glucocorticoids, which have an anti-inflammatory and immunosuppressive role in the treatment of MS exacerbations. *See* Glucocorticoids; Immunosuppression; Exacerbation.

Cortisone: A glucocorticoid steroid hormone, produced by the adrenal glands or synthetically, which has anti-inflammatory and immune-system–suppressing properties. Prednisone and prednisolone belong to this group of substances.

Cranial nerves: Nerves that carry sensory, motor, or parasympathetic fibers to the face and neck. Included among this group of twelve nerves are the optic nerve (vision), trigeminal nerve (sensation along the face), vagus nerve (pharynx and vocal cords). Evaluation of cranial nerve function is part of the standard neurologic exam.

Cystoscopy: A diagnostic procedure in which a special viewing device called a cystoscope is inserted into the urethra (a tubular structure that drains urine from the bladder) to examine the inside of the urinary bladder.

Cystostomy: A surgically created opening through the lower abdomen into the urinary bladder. A plastic tube inserted into the opening drains urine from the bladder into a plastic collection bag. This relatively simple procedure is done when a person requires an indwelling catheter to drain urine from the bladder but passage through the urethral opening is not desirable for reasons such as uncontrollable frequency or incontinence. *See* Indwelling catheter.

Cytokines: Messenger chemicals produced by various cells, particularly those of the immune system, to influence the activity of other cells.

Deep tendon reflexes: The involuntary jerks that are normally produced at certain spots on a limb when the tendons are tapped with a hammer. Reflexes are tested as part of the standard neurologic examination.

Dementia: A generally profound and progressive loss of intellectual function, sometimes associated with personality change, which results from loss of brain substance and is sufficient to interfere with a person's normal functional activities.

Demyelination: A loss of myelin in the white matter of the central nervous system (brain, spinal cord, optic nerves).

DESD: *See* Detrusor-external sphincter dyssynergia.

Detrusor muscle: A muscle of the urinary bladder that contracts and causes the bladder to empty.

Detrusor-external sphincter dyssynergia (DESD): *See* Combined (bladder) dysfunction.

Diplopia: Double vision, or the simultaneous awareness of two images of the same object that results from a failure of the two eyes to work in a coordinated fashion. Covering one eye will erase one of the images.

Disablement: As defined by the World Health Organization, a disability (resulting from an impairment) is a restriction or lack of ability to perform an activity in the manner or within the range considered normal for a human being.

Double-blind clinical study: A study in which none of the participants, including experimental subjects, examining doctors, attending nurses, or any other research staff, know who is taking the test drug and who is taking a control or placebo agent. The purpose of this research design is to avoid inadvertent bias of the test results. In all studies, procedures are designed to "break the blind" if medical circumstances require it.

Dysarthria: Poorly articulated speech resulting from dysfunction of the muscles controlling speech, usually caused by damage to the central nervous system or a peripheral motor nerve. The content and meaning of the spoken words remain normal.

Dysesthesia: Distorted or unpleasant sensations experienced by a person when the skin is touched, which are typically caused by abnormalities in the sensory pathways in the brain and spinal cord.

Dysphagia: Difficulty in swallowing. It is a neurologic or neuromuscular symptom that may result in aspiration (whereby food or saliva enters the airway), slow swallowing (possibly resulting in inadequate nutrition), or both.

Dysphonia: Disorders of voice quality (including poor pitch control, hoarseness, breathiness, and hypernasality) caused by spasticity, weakness, and incoordination of muscles in the mouth and throat.

EAE: *See* Experimental allergic encephalomyelitis.

EEG: *See* Electroencephalography.

Electroencephalography (EEG): A diagnostic procedure that records, via electrodes attached to various areas of the person's head, electrical activity generated by brain cells.

Electromyography (EMG): Electromyography is a diagnostic procedure that records muscle electrical potentials through a needle or small plate electrodes. The test can also measure the ability of peripheral nerves to conduct impulses.

EMG: *See* Electromyography.

Enhancement: *See* Gadolinium-enhancing lesion.

Epidemiology: The study of the pattern of disease occurrence in human populations and of the factors that influence these patterns (i.e., risk factors).

Erectile dysfunction: The inability to attain or retain a rigid penile erection.

Etiology: The study of all factors that may be involved in the development of a disease, including the patient's susceptibility, the nature of the disease-causing agent, and the way in which the person's body is invaded by the agent.

Euphoria: Unrealistic cheerfulness and optimism, accompanied by a lessening of critical faculties; generally considered to be a result of damage to the brain.

Evoked potentials (EPs): EPs are recordings of the nervous system's electrical response to the stimulation of specific sensory pathways (e.g., visual, auditory, general sensory). In tests of evoked potentials, a person's recorded responses are displayed on an oscilloscope and analyzed on a computer that allows comparison with normal response times. Demyelination results in a slowing of response time. EPs can demonstrate lesions along specific nerve pathways whether or not the lesions are producing symptoms, thus making this test useful in confirming the diagnosis of MS. Visual evoked potentials are considered the most useful in MS. *See* Visual evoked potential.

Exacerbation: *See* Relapse.

Expanded Disability Status Scale (EDSS): A part of the Minimal Record of Disability that summarizes the neurologic examination and provides a measure of overall disability. The EDSS is a 20-point scale, ranging from 0 (normal examination) to 10 (death due to MS) by half-points. A person with a score of 4.5 can walk three blocks without stopping; a score of 6.0 means that a cane or a leg brace is needed to walk one block; a score over 7.5 indicates that a person cannot take more than a few steps, even with crutches or help from another person. The EDSS is used for many reasons, including deciding future medical treatment, establishing rehabilitation goals, choosing subjects for participation in clinical trials, and measuring treatment outcomes. This is currently the most widely used scale in clinical trials.

Experimental allergic encephalomyelitis (EAE): Experimental allergic encephalomyelitis is an autoimmune disease resembling MS that has been induced in some genetically susceptible research animals. Before testing on humans, a potential treatment for MS may first be tested on laboratory animals with EAE to determine the treatment's efficacy and safety.

Extensor spasm: A symptom of spasticity in which the legs straighten suddenly into a stiff, extended position. These spasms, which typically last for several minutes, occur most commonly in bed at night or on rising from bed.

Failure to empty (bladder): A type of neurogenic bladder dysfunction in MS resulting from demyelination in the voiding reflex center of the spinal cord. The bladder tends to overfill and become flaccid, resulting in symptoms of urinary urgency, hesitancy, dribbling, and incontinence.

Failure to store (bladder): A type of neurogenic bladder dysfunction in MS resulting from demyelination of the pathways between the spinal cord and brain. Typically seen in a small, spastic bladder, storage failure can cause symptoms of urinary urgency, frequency, incontinence, and nocturia.

FDA: *See* Food and Drug Administration.

Finger-to-nose test: As a test of dysmetria and intention tremor, the person is asked, with eyes closed, to bring an outstretched index finger in repeatedly to touch the tip of his or her nose. This test is part of the standard neurologic examination.

Flaccid: A decrease in muscle tone resulting in weakened muscles and therefore loose, "floppy" limbs.

Flexor spasm: Involuntary, sometimes painful contractions of the flexor muscles, which pull the legs upward into a clenched position. These spasms, which last two to three seconds, are symptoms of spasticity. They often occur during sleep, but can also occur when the person is in a seated position.

Foley catheter: *See* Indwelling catheter.

Food and Drug Administration (FDA): The U.S. federal agency that is responsible for enforcing governmental regulations pertaining to the manufacture and sale of food, drugs, and cosmetics. Its role is to prevent the sale of impure or dangerous substances. Any new drug that is proposed for the treatment of MS in the United States must be approved by the FDA.

Foot drop: A condition of weakness in the muscles of the foot and ankle, caused by poor nerve conduction, which interferes with a person's ability to flex the ankle and walk with a normal heel-toe pattern. The toes touch the ground before the heel, causing the person to trip or lose balance.

Frontal lobes: The largest lobes of the brain. The anterior (front) part of each of the cerebral hemispheres that make up the cerebrum. The back part of the frontal lobe is the motor cortex, which controls voluntary movement; the area of the frontal lobe that is further forward is concerned with learning, behavior, judgment, and personality.

Functional magnetic resonance imaging (fMRI): A relatively new MRI technique that studies brain function. Using fMRI technology, scientists can determine which part of the brain is active during a given task by tracking blood oxygen levels. Brain regions that are active require more oxygen. Oxygen is delivered by increasing the blood flow to these active brain regions. In MS, researchers are using fMRI to look at how the brain compensates for damage in one area by recruiting other areas of the brain to help perform a task.

Gadolinium: A chemical compound that can be administered to a person during magnetic resonance imaging to help distinguish between new lesions and old lesions.

Gadolinium-enhancing lesion: A lesion appearing on magnetic resonance imagery, following injection of the chemical compound gadolinium, which reveals a breakdown in the blood-brain barrier. This breakdown of the blood-brain barrier indicates either a newly active lesion or the reactivation of an old one. *See* Gadolinium.

Gastrocolic reflex: A mass peristaltic (coordinated, rhythmic) smooth muscle contraction that acts to force food through the digestive tract movement of the colon that often occurs 15 to 30 minutes after ingesting a meal.

Gastrostomy: *See* Percutaneous endoscopic gastrostomy.

Glucocorticoid hormones: Steroid hormones that are produced by the adrenal glands in response to stimulation by adrenocorticotropic hormone (ACTH) from the pituitary. These hormones, which can also be manufactured synthetically (prednisone, prednisolone, methylprednisolone, betamethasone, dexamethasone), serve both an immunosuppressive and an anti-inflammatory role in the treatment of MS exacerbations: they damage or destroy certain types of T-lymphocytes that are involved in the overactive immune response, and interfere with the release of certain inflammation-producing enzymes.

Health care proxy: *See* Advance (medical) directive.

Heel-knee-shin test: A test of coordination in which the person is asked, with eyes closed, to place one heel on the opposite knee and slide it up and down the shin. This test is part of the standard neurological exam.

Helper T-lymphocytes: White blood cells that are a major contributor to the immune system's inflammatory response against myelin.

Hemiparesis: Weakness of one side of the body, including one arm and one leg.

Hemiplegia: Paralysis of one side of the body, including one arm and one leg.

Immune system: A complex network of glands, tissues, circulating cells, and processes that protect the body by identifying abnormal or foreign substances and neutralizing them.

Immune-mediated disease: A disease in which components of the immune system—T cells, antibodies, and others—are responsible for the disease either directly (as occurs in autoimmunity) or indirectly (e.g., when damage to the body occurs secondary to an immune assault on a foreign antigen such as a bacteria or virus).

Immunoglobulin: *See* Antibody.

Immunology: The science that concerns the body's mechanisms for protecting itself from abnormal or foreign substances.

Immunosuppression: In MS, a form of treatment that slows or inhibits the body's natural immune responses, including those directed against the body's own tissues. Examples of immunosuppressive treatments in MS include mitoxantrone, cyclosporine, methotrexate, and azathioprine.

Impairment: Any loss or abnormality of psychological, physiological, or anatomical structure or function. It represents a deviation from the person's usual biomedical state. An impairment is thus any loss of function directly resulting from injury or disease.

Incidence: The number of new cases of a disease in a specified population over a defined period of time. The incidence of MS in the United States is approximately 10,000 newly diagnosed people per year.

Incontinence: Also called spontaneous voiding; the inability to control passage of urine or bowel movements.

Indwelling catheter: A type of catheter that remains in the bladder on a temporary or permanent basis. It is used only when intermittent catheterization is not possible or is medically contraindicated. The most common type of indwelling catheter is a Foley catheter, which consists of a flexible rubber tube that is inserted into the bladder to allow the urine to flow into an external drainage bag. A small balloon, inflated after insertion, holds the Foley catheter in place. *See* Catheter.

Inflammation: A tissue's immunologic response to injury, characterized by mobilization of white blood cells and antibodies, swelling, and fluid accumulation.

Intention tremor: Rhythmic shaking that occurs in the course of a purposeful movement, such as reaching to pick something up or bringing an outstretched finger in to touch one's nose.

Interferon: A group of immune system proteins, produced and released by cells infected by a virus, which inhibit viral multiplication and modify the body's immune response. Four interferon beta medications have been approved by the U.S. Food and Drug Administration (FDA) for treating relapsing forms of MS: IFN beta-1β (Betaseron and Extavia); IFN beta-1α (Avonex and Rebif).

Intermittent self-catheterization (ISC): A procedure in which the person periodically inserts a catheter into the urinary opening to drain urine from the bladder. ISC is used in the management of bladder dysfunction to drain urine that remains after voiding, prevent bladder distention, prevent kidney damage, and restore bladder function.

Internuclear ophthalmoplegia: A disturbance of coordinated eye movements in which the eye turned outward to look toward the side develops nystagmus (rapid, involuntary movements) while the other eye simultaneously fails to turn completely inward. This neurologic sign, of which the person is usually unaware, can be detected during the neurologic examination.

Intrathecal space: The space surrounding the brain and spinal cord that contains cerebrospinal fluid.

Intravenous: Within a vein; often used in the context of an injection into a vein of medication dissolved in a liquid.

Lesion: *See* Plaque.

Lhermitte's sign: An abnormal sensation of electricity or "pins and needles" going down the spine into the arms and legs that occurs when the neck is bent forward so that the chin touches the chest.

Living will: *See* Advance (medical) directive.

Lofstrand crutch: A type of crutch with an attached holder for the forearm that provides extra support.

Lumbar puncture: A diagnostic procedure that uses a hollow needle to penetrate the spinal canal at the level of third-fourth or fourth-fifth lumbar vertebrae to remove cerebrospinal fluid for analysis. This procedure is used to examine the cerebrospinal fluid for changes in composition that are characteristic of MS (e.g., elevated white cell count, elevated protein content, the presence of oligoclonal bands). *See* Oligoclonal bands.

Lymphocyte: A type of white blood cell that is part of the immune system. Lymphocytes can be subdivided into two main groups: B lymphocytes, which originate in the bone marrow and produce antibodies, and T lymphocytes, which are produced in the bone marrow and mature in the thymus. Helper T lymphocytes heighten the production of antibodies by B lymphocytes; suppressor T lymphocytes suppress B-lymphocyte activity and seem to be in short supply during an MS exacerbation.

Macrophage: A white blood cell with scavenger characteristics that has the ability to ingest and destroy foreign substances such as bacteria and cell debris.

Magnetic resonance imaging (MRI): A diagnostic procedure that produces visual images of different body parts without the use of X rays. Nuclei of atoms are influenced by a high frequency electromagnetic impulse inside a strong magnetic field. The nuclei then give off resonating signals that can produce pictures of parts of the body. An important diagnostic tool in MS, MRI makes it possible to visualize and count lesions in the white matter of the brain and spinal cord.

Marcus Gunn pupil: *See* Afferent pupillary defect.

Minimal record of disability (MRD): A standardized method for quantifying the clinical status of a person with MS. The MRD is made up of five parts: demographic information; the Neurological Functional Systems (developed by John Kurtzke), which assign scores to clinical findings for each of the various neurologic systems in the brain and spinal cord (pyramidal, cerebellar, brainstem, sensory, visual, mental, bowel, and bladder); the Expanded Disability Status Scale (developed by John Kurtzke), which gives a single composite score for the person's disease; the Incapacity Status Scale, which is an inventory of functional disabilities relating to activities of daily living; the Environmental Status Scale, which provides an assessment of social handicap resulting from chronic illness. The MRD has two main functions: to assist doctors and other professionals in planning and coordinating the care of persons with MS, and to provide a standardized means of recording repeated clinical evaluations of individuals for research purposes. *See* Expanded Disability Status Scale (EDSS).

Monoclonal antibody: Antibodies are proteins that are generated by the immune system, specifically the white blood cells. They circulate in the blood and attach to foreign proteins called antigens in order to destroy or neutralize them. Monoclonal antibodies are laboratory produced, customized proteins, made from a single cell or its clones, which are designed to locate and bind to specific target molecules. Producing man made proteins is an intricate process that involves placing cells in large stainless steel vats filled with nutrients to produce the specified protein. It is extensively tested to ensure purity before it is ready for patient use. *See* Antibody.

Motor point block: *See* Nerve block.

MRI: *See* Magnetic resonance imaging.

Multiple sclerosis functional composite (MSFC): A three-part, standardized, quantitative assessment instrument for use in clinical trials in MS, that was developed by the Task Force on Clinical Outcomes Assessment appointed by the National MS Society's Advisory Committee on Clinical Trials of New Agents in Multiple Sclerosis. The three components of the MSFC measure leg function/ambulation (Timed 25-Foot Walk), arm/hand function (9-Hole Peg Test), and cognitive function (Paced Auditory Serial Addition Test [PASAT]).

Muscle tone: A characteristic of a muscle brought about by the constant flow of nerve stimuli to that muscle, which describes its resistance to stretching. Abnormal muscle tone can be defined as hypertonus (increased muscle tone, as in spasticity); hypotonus (reduced muscle tone); flaccid (paralysis); atony (loss of muscle tone). Muscle tone is evaluated as part of the standard neurologic examination in MS.

Myelin: A soft, white coating of nerve fibers in the central nervous system, composed of lipids (fats) and protein. Myelin serves as insulation and as an aid to efficient nerve fiber conduction. When myelin is damaged in MS, nerve fiber conduction is faulty or absent. Impaired bodily functions or altered sensations associated with those demyelinated nerve fibers are identified as symptoms of MS in various parts of the body.

Myelin basic protein: One of several proteins associated with the myelin of the central nervous system, which may be found in higher than normal concentrations in the cerebrospinal fluid of individuals with MS and other diseases that damage myelin.

Nerve: A bundle of nerve fibers (axons). The fibers are either afferent (leading toward the brain and serving in the perception of sensory stimuli of the skin, joints, muscles, and inner organs) or efferent (leading away from the brain and mediating contractions of muscles or organs).

Nerve block: A procedure used to relieve otherwise intractable spasticity, including painful flexor spasms. An injection of phenol into the affected nerve interferes with the function of that nerve for up to 3 months, potentially increasing a person's comfort and mobility.

Nervous system: Includes all of the neural structures in the body: the central nervous system consists of the brain, spinal cord, and optic nerves; the peripheral nervous system consists of the nerve roots, nerve plexi, and nerves throughout the body.

Neurogenic: Related to activity of the nervous system, as in "neurogenic bladder."

Neurogenic bladder: Bladder dysfunction associated with neurologic malfunction in the spinal cord and characterized by a failure to empty, failure to store, or a combination of the two. Symptoms that result from these three types of dysfunction include urinary urgency, frequency, hesitancy, nocturia, and incontinence.

Neurologist: Physician who specializes in the diagnosis and treatment of conditions related to the nervous system.

Neurology: Study of the central, peripheral, and autonomic nervous system.

Neuron: The basic nerve cell of the nervous system. A neuron consists of a nucleus within a cell body and one or more processes (extensions) called dendrites and axons.

Neuropsychologist: A psychologist with specialized training in the evaluation of cognitive functions. Neuropsychologists use a battery of standardized tests to assess specific cognitive functions and identify areas of cognitive impairment. They also provide remediation for individuals with MS-related cognitive impairment. *See* Cognition and Cognitive impairment.

Nocturia: The need to urinate during the night.

Nystagmus: Rapid, involuntary movements of the eyes in the horizontal or, occasionally, the vertical direction.

Occupational therapist (OT): Occupational therapists assess functioning in activities of everyday living, including dressing, bathing, grooming, meal preparation, writing, and driving, which are essential for independent living. In making treatment recommendations, the OT addresses (1) fatigue management, (2) upper body strength, movement, and coordination, (3) adaptations to the home and work environment, including both structural changes and specialized equipment for particular activities, and (4) compensatory strategies for impairments in thinking, sensation, or vision.

Oligoclonal bands: A diagnostic sign indicating abnormal levels of certain antibodies in the cerebrospinal fluid; seen in approximately 90 percent of people with multiple sclerosis, but not specific to MS.

Oligodendrocyte: A type of cell in the central nervous system that is responsible for making and supporting myelin.

Olmstead decision: The Supreme Court decision in Olmstead v L.C. (1999) is an interpretation of Title II of the Americans with Disabilities Act (ADA) that affirms the right of people with disabilities to receive services in the most integrated setting appropriate to their needs. The decision recognizes that unnecessary segregation of persons in long-term care facilities constitutes discrimination under the ADA.

Open-label study: Unblinded study in which both the participants and the investigators know which mediation or intervention is being used. Open-label studies are generally small, preliminary investigations done to evaluate the potential safety and efficacy of a treatment before moving on to larger-scale, controlled clinical trials. *See* Controlled study; Double-blind clinical study.

Ophthalmoscope: An instrument designed for examination of the interior of the eye.

Optic atrophy: A wasting of the optic disc that results from partial or complete degeneration of optic nerve fibers and is associated with a loss of visual acuity.

Optic disc: The small blind spot on the surface of the retina where cells of the retina converge to form the optic nerve; the only part of the retina that is insensitive to light.

Optic neuritis: Inflammation or demyelination of the optic (visual) nerve with transient or permanent impairment of vision and occasionally pain.

Orthotic: Also called orthosis; a mechanical appliance such as a leg brace or splint that is specially designed to control, correct, or compensate for impaired limb function.

Orthotist: A person skilled in making mechanical appliances (orthotics) such as leg braces or splints that help to support limb function. *See* Orthotic.

Oscillopsia: Continuous, involuntary, and chaotic eye movements that result in a visual disturbance in which objects appear to be jumping or bouncing.

Osteopenia: Bone mineral density (BMD) that is lower than normal peak BMD but not low enough to be classified as osteoporosis. *See* Osteoporosis.

Osteoporosis: A gradual loss of bone mineral density (BMD). This bone disease is most common in post-menopausal women but can occur in any person as a result of severely impaired mobility and lack of weight-bearing exercise, corticosteroid use, or inadequate levels of vitamin D, among other factors.

Paralysis: Inability to move a part of the body.

Paraparesis: A weakness but not total paralysis of the lower extremities (legs).

Paraplegia: Paralysis of both lower extremities (legs).

Paresis: Partial or incomplete paralysis of a part of the body.

Paresthesia: A spontaneously occurring sensation of burning, prickling, tingling, or creeping on the skin that may or may not be associated with any physical findings on neurologic examination.

Paroxysmal spasm: A sudden, uncontrolled limb contraction that occurs intermittently, lasts for a few moments, and then subsides.

Paroxysmal symptom: Any one of several symptoms that have sudden onset, apparently in response to some kind of movement or sensory stimulation, last for a few moments, and then subside. Paroxysmal symptoms tend to occur frequently in those individuals who have them, and follow a similar pattern from one episode to the next. Examples of paroxysmal symptoms include acute episodes of trigeminal neuralgia (sharp facial pain), tonic seizures (intense spasm of limb or limbs on one side of the body), dysarthria (slurred speech often accompanied by loss of balance and coordination), and various paresthesias (sensory disturbances ranging from tingling to severe pain).

PEG: *See* Percutaneous endoscopic gastrostomy.

Percutaneous endoscopic gastrostomy (PEG): A PEG is a tube inserted into the stomach through the abdominal wall to provide food or other nutrients when eating by mouth is not possible. The tube is inserted in a bedside procedure using an endoscope to guide the tube through a small abdominal incision. An endoscope is a lighted instrument that allows the doctor to see inside the stomach.

Periventricular region: The area surrounding the four fluid-filled cavities within the brain. MS plaques are commonly found within this region.

Physiatrist: Physicians who specialize in physical medicine and rehabilitation, including the diagnosis and management of musculoskeletal injuries and pain syndromes, electrodiagnostic medicine (e.g., electromyography), and rehabilitation of severe impairments, including those caused by neurologic disease or injury. *See* Electromyography (EMG).

Physical therapist (PT): Physical therapists are trained to evaluate and improve movement and function of the body, with particular attention to physical mobility, balance, posture, fatigue, and pain. The physical therapy program typically involves (1) educating the person with MS about the physical problems caused by the disease, (2) designing an individualized exercise program to address the problems, and (3) enhancing mobility and energy conservation through the use of a variety of mobility aids and adaptive equipment.

Placebo: An inactive, nondrug compound that is designed to look just like the test drug. It is administered to control group subjects in double-blind clinical trials (in which neither the researchers nor the subjects know who is getting the drug and who is getting the placebo) as a means of assessing the benefits and liabilities of the test drug taken by experimental group subjects.

Placebo effect: An apparently beneficial result of therapy that occurs because of the patient's expectation that the therapy will help.

Plantar reflex: A reflex response obtained by drawing a pointed object along the outer border of the sole of the foot from the heel to the little toe. The normal flexor response is a bunching and downward movement of the toes. An upward movement of the big toe is called an extensor response, or Babinski reflex, which is a sensitive indicator of disease in the brain or spinal cord. Also called Babinski reflex.

Plaque: An area of inflamed or demyelinated central nervous system tissue (also referred to as a *lesion* or *scar*).

Postvoid residual test (PVR): The PVR test determines how much urine is left in the bladder after an attempt to empty the bladder through urination has been made. It involves passing a catheter into the bladder following urination to drain and measure any urine remaining in the bladder. The PVR is a simple but effective technique for diagnosing bladder dysfunction in MS.

Postural tremor: Rhythmic shaking that occurs when the muscles are tensed to hold an object or stay in a given position.

Pressure sore: An ulcer of the skin—also referred to as a "bed sore"—resulting from pressure and lack of movement such as occurs when a person is limited to bed or requires a wheelchair for mobility. The ulcers occur most frequently in areas where the bone lies directly under the skin, such as elbow, hip, or over the coccyx (tailbone). A pressure sore may become infected and cause general worsening of the person's health.

Prevalence: The number of all new and old cases of a disease in a defined population at a particular point in time. The prevalence of MS in the United States at any given time is about 1/750—approximately 400,000 people.

Primary-progressive MS: A clinical course of MS characterized from the beginning by progressive disease, with no plateaus or remissions, or an occasional plateau and very short-lived, minor improvements.

Prognosis: Prediction of the future course of the disease.

Progressive-relapsing MS: A clinical course of MS that shows disease progression from the beginning, but with clear, acute relapses, with or without full recovery from those relapses along the way.

Pseudobulbar affect: Also called pathological laughing and crying; an involuntary emotional expression disorder in which episodes of laughing and/or crying occur with no apparent precipitating event. The person's actual mood may be unrelated to the emotion being expressed. This condition is thought to be caused by lesions in the limbic system, a group of brain structures involved in emotional feeling and expression.

Pseudoexacerbation: A temporary aggravation of disease symptoms, resulting from an elevation in body temperature or other stressor (e.g., an infection, severe fatigue, constipation) that disappears once the stressor is removed. A pseudoexacerbation involves symptom flare-up rather than new disease activity or progression.

Quad cane: A cane that has a broad base on four short "feet," which provides extra stability.

Quadriplegia: The paralysis of both arms and both legs.

Recent memory: The ability to remember events, conversations, content of reading material or television programs from a short time ago, that is, an hour or two ago or last night. People with MS-related memory impairment typically experience greatest difficulty remembering these types of things in the recent past.

Reflex: An involuntary response of the nervous system to a stimulus, such as the stretch reflex, which is elicited by tapping a tendon with a reflex hammer, resulting in a contraction. Increased, diminished, or absent reflexes can be indicative of neurologic damage, including MS, and are therefore tested as part of the standard neurologic examination.

Rehabilitation: Rehabilitation in MS involves the intermittent or ongoing use of multidisciplinary strategies (e.g., physiatry, physical therapy, occupational therapy, speech therapy) to promote functional independence, prevent unnecessary complications, and enhance overall quality of life. It is an active process directed toward helping the person recover and/or maintain the highest possible level of functioning and realize his or her optimal physical, mental, and social potential given any limitations that exist. Rehabilitation is also an interactive, ongoing process of education and enablement in which people with MS and their care partners are active participants rather than passive recipients.

Relapse: The appearance of new symptoms or the aggravation of old ones, lasting at least 24 hours (synonymous with *attack*, *exacerbation*, or *flare-up*); usually associated with inflammation and demyelination in the brain or spinal cord.

Relapsing-remitting MS: A clinical course of MS that is characterized by clearly defined, acute attacks with full or partial recovery and no disease progression between attacks.

Remission: A lessening in the severity of symptoms or their temporary disappearance during the course of the illness.

Remote memory: The ability to remember people or events from the distant past. People with MS tend to experience few, if any, problems with their remote memory.

Remyelination: The repair of damaged myelin. Myelin repair occurs spontaneously in MS but very slowly. Research is currently underway to find a way to speed the healing process.

Residual urine: Urine that remains in the bladder following urination.

Retrobulbar neuritis: *See* Optic neuritis.

Romberg's sign: The inability to maintain balance in a standing position with feet and legs drawn together and eyes closed.

Scanning speech: Abnormal speech characterized by staccato-like articulation that sounds clipped because the person unintentionally pauses between syllables and skips some of the sounds.

Sclerosis: Hardening of tissue. In MS, sclerosis is the scar tissue that forms when myelin around CNS nerve cells is damaged or destroyed.

Scotoma: A gap or blind spot in the visual field.

Secondary-progressive MS: A clinical course of MS that initially is relapsing-remitting and then becomes progressive at a variable rate, possibly with an occasional relapse and minor remission.

Sensory: Related to bodily sensations such as pain, smell, taste, temperature, vision, hearing, acceleration, and position in space.

Sign: An objective physical problem or abnormality identified by the physician during the neurologic examination. Neurologic signs may differ significantly from the symptoms reported by the patient because they are identifiable only with specific tests and may cause no overt symptoms. Common neurologic signs in multiple sclerosis include altered eye movements and other changes in the appearance or function of the visual system; altered reflexes; weakness; spasticity; circumscribed sensory changes.

Spasticity: Involuntary muscle stiffness and/or spasms resulting from increased muscle tone. Spasticity is a common symptom of MS. *See* Muscle tone.

Speech/language pathologist: Speech/language pathologists specialize in the diagnosis and treatment of speech and swallowing disorders. A person with MS may be referred to a speech/language pathologist for help with either one or both of these problems. Because of their expertise with speech and language difficulties, these specialists also provide cognitive remediation for individuals with cognitive impairment.

Sphincter: A circular band of muscle fibers that tightens or closes a natural opening of the body, such as the external anal sphincter, which closes the anus, and the internal and external urinary sphincters, which close the urinary canal.

Spinal tap: *See* Lumbar puncture.

Spirometer: An instrument used to assess lung function; it measures the volume and flow rate of inhaled and exhaled air.

Spontaneous voiding: *See* Incontinence.

Steroids: *See* ACTH; Corticosteroid; Glucocorticoid hormones.

Straight catheter: A straight but flexible, hollow plastic tube of variable length and diameter, which can be inserted through the urinary opening into the bladder to drain excess urine that cannot be excreted normally. The straight catheter is the type used for intermittent self-catheterization (ISC). *See* Intermittent self-catheterization.

Suppressor T lymphocytes: White blood cells that act as part of the immune system and may be in short supply during an MS exacerbation.

Symptom: A subjectively perceived problem or complaint reported by the patient. In multiple sclerosis, common symptoms include visual problems, fatigue, sensory changes, weakness or paralysis of limbs, tremor, lack of coordination, poor balance, bladder or bowel changes, and psychological changes.

T cell: A lymphocyte (white blood cell) that develops in the bone marrow, matures in the thymus, and works as part of the immune system in the body.

Tandem gait: A test of balance and coordination that involves alternately placing the heel of one foot directly against the toes of the other foot. This test is part of the standard neurological exam.

Titubation: A form of tremor, resulting from demyelination in the cerebellum, which manifests itself primarily in the head and neck.

Transcutaneous electric nerve stimulation (TENS): TENS is a nonaddictive and non-invasive method of pain control that applies electric impulses to nerve endings via electrodes that are attached to a stimulator by flexible wires and placed on the skin. The electric impulses block the transmission of pain signals to the brain.

Trigeminal neuralgia: Lightning-like, acute pain in the face caused by demyelination of nerve fibers at the site where the sensory (trigeminal) nerve root for that part of the face enters the brainstem.

Twins-dizygotic: Also known as fraternal twins, two babies that come from separate, simultaneously-fertilized eggs. If one dizygotic twin develops MS, the other has the same genetic risk for MS (approximately 2–5 in 100 or 3 percent) as any other sibling or first-degree relative.

Twins-monozygotic: Also known as identical twins, two babies that come from single fertilized egg and share identical genetic makeup. If one monozygotic twin develops MS, the other has a 25-to-30 percent risk of developing the disease, indicating that factors other than genetic makeup contribute to the etiology of MS.

Urethra: Duct or tube that drains the urinary bladder.

Urinalysis: Screening test to determine whether urinary tract infection, bladder stones, or other abnormality is, or may be, present.

Urinary frequency: Feeling the urge to urinate even when urination has occurred very recently.

Urinary hesitancy: The inability to void urine spontaneously even though the urge to do so is present.

Urinary incontinence: *See* Incontinence.

Urinary sphincter: The muscle closing the urethra, which in a state of flaccid paralysis causes urinary incontinence and in a state of spastic paralysis results in an inability to urinate.

Urinary urgency: The inability to postpone urination once the need to void has been felt.

Urine culture and sensitivity (C&S): A diagnostic procedure to test for urinary tract infection and identify the appropriate treatment. Bacteria from a midstream urine sample are allowed to grow for 3 days in a laboratory medium and then tested for sensitivity to a variety of antibiotics.

Urologist: A physician who specializes in the branch of medicine (urology) concerned with the anatomy, physiology, disorders, and care of the male and female urinary tract, as well as the male genital tract.

Urology: A medical specialty that deals with disturbances of the urinary (male and female) and reproductive (male) organs.

Vertigo: A dizzying sensation of the environment spinning, often accompanied by nausea and vomiting.

Vibration sense: The ability to feel vibrations against various parts of the body. Vibration sense is tested (with a tuning fork) as part of the sensory portion of the neurologic examination.

Videofluoroscopy: A radiographic study of a person's swallowing mechanism that is recorded on videotape. Videofluoroscopy shows the physiology of the pharynx, the location of the swallowing difficulty, and confirms whether or not food particles or fluids are being aspirated into the airway.

Visual acuity: Clarity of vision. Acuity is measured as a fraction of normal vision. 20/20 vision indicates an eye that sees at 20 feet what a normal eye should see at 20 feet; 20/400 vision indicates an eye that sees at 20 feet what a normal eye sees at 400 feet.

Visual evoked potential: A test in which the brain's electrical activity in response to visual stimuli (e.g., a flashing checker-board) is recorded by an electroencephalograph and analyzed by computer. Demyelination results in a slowing of response time. Because this test is able to confirm the presence of a suspected brain lesion (area of demyelination) as well as identify the presence of an unsuspected lesion that has produced no symptoms, it is extremely useful in diagnosing MS. VEPs are abnormal in approximately 90 percent of people with MS.

Vocational rehabilitation (VR): Vocational rehabilitation is a program of services designed to enable people with disabilities to become or remain employed. Originally mandated by the Rehabilitation Act of 1973, VR programs are carried out by individually created state agencies. To be eligible for VR, a person must have a physical or mental disability that results in a substantial handicap to employment. VR programs typically involve evaluation of the disability and need for adaptive equipment or mobility aids, vocational guidance, training, job-placement, and follow-up.

White matter: The part of the brain that contains myelinated nerve fibers and appears white, in contrast to the cortex of the brain, which contains nerve cell bodies and appears gray.

Appendix B: Medications Commonly Used in MS

BRAND NAME	GENERIC NAME	USAGE IN MS
No brand name formulation[1]	Mineral oil	Constipation
No brand name formulation	Papaverine	Erectile dysfunction
Amitiza	Lubiprostone	Constipation
Ampyra	Dalfampridine	Walking
Antivert	Meclizine	Nausea; vomiting; dizziness
Atarax	Hydroxyzine	Itching
Avonex	Interferon beta-1α	Disease-modifying agent
Bactrim	Sulfamethoxazole + Trimethoprim Combination	Urinary tract infections
Betaseron	Interferon beta-1β	Disease-modifying agent
Botox	OnabotulinumtoxinA	Bladder dysfunction
Caverject	Alprostadil (also called prostaglandin E1)	Erectile dysfunction
Cialis	Tadalafil	Erectile dysfunction
Cipro	Ciprofloxacin	Urinary tract infections
Colace[1]	Docusate	Constipation
Copaxone	Glatiramer acetate	Disease-modifying agent
Cymbalta	Duloxetine Hydrochloride	Depression Neuropathic pain
Dantrium	Dantrolene	Spasticity
DDAVP nasal spray DDAVP tablets	Desmopressin	Bladder dysfunction
Decadron	Dexamethasone	Acute exacerbations
Deltasone	Prednisone	Acute exacerbations
Detrol	Tolterodine	Bladder dysfunction
Dilantin	Phenytoin	Pain (dysesthesias)
Ditropan	Oxybutynin	Bladder dysfunction
Ditropan XL	Oxybutynin chloride (Extended release formula)	Bladder dysfunction
Dulcolax[1]	Bisacodyl	Constipation

Edex	Alprostadil (also called prostaglandin E1)	Erectile dysfunction
Effexor	Venlafaxine	Depression
Elavil	Amitriptyline	Pain (paresthesias)
Enablex	Darifenacin	Bladder dysfunction
Enemeez Mini Enema[1]	Docusate	Constipation
Extavia	Interferon beta-1b	Disease-modifying agent
Fleet Enema[1]	Sodium phosphate	Constipation
Flomax	Tamsulosin	Bladder dysfunction
Gelnique	Oxybutynin gel	Bladder dysfunction
Gilenya	Fingolimod	Disease-modifying agent
Hiprex	Methenamine	Urinary tract infections (preventative)
HP Acthar Gel	Adrenocorticotropic hormone (ACTH)	Acute exacerbations
Hytrin	Terazosin	Bladder dysfunction
Intrathecal Baclofen (ITB)	Baclofen (intrathecal)	Spasticity
Klonopin	Clonazepam	Tremor; pain; spasticity
Laniazid; Nydrazid	Isoniazid	Tremor
Levitra	Vardenafil	Erectile dysfunction
Lioresal	Baclofen	Spasticity
Lyrica	Pregabalin	Pain
Macrodantin	Nitrofurantoin	Urinary tract infections
Metamucil[1]	Psyllium hydrophilic mucilloid	Constipation
Minipress	Prazosin	Bladder dysfunction
MiraLax[1]	Polyethylene glycol	Constipation
Muse	Alprostadil	Erectile dysfunction
Neurontin	Gabapentin	Pain
Nuedexta	dextromethorphan/ quinidine	Pseudobulbar affect
Novantrone	Mitoxantrone	Disease-modifying agent
Nuvigil	Armodafinil	Fatigue
Oxytrol	Oxybutynin (transdermal patch)	Bladder dysfunction
Pamelor	Nortriptyline	Depression
Paxil	Paroxetine	Depression
Phillips' Milk of Magnesia[1]	Magnesium hydroxide	Constipation
Pro-Banthine	Propantheline bromide	Bladder dysfunction
Provigil	Modafinil	Fatigue
Prozac	Fluoxetine	Depression; fatigue
Pyridium	Phenazopyridine	Urinary tract infections (symptom relief)
Rebif	Interferon beta-1α	Disease-modifying agent

Sanctura	Trospium chloride	Bladder dysfunction
Sani-Supp suppository[1]	Glycerin	Constipation
Solu-Medrol	Methylprednisolone	Acute exacerbations
Symmetrel	Amantadine	Fatigue
Tegretol	Carbamazepine	Pain (trigeminal neuralgia)
Tofranil	Imipramine	Bladder dysfunction; pain
Tysabri	Natalizumab	Disease-modifying agent
Valium	Diazepam	Spasticity (muscle spasms)
Vesicare	Solifenacin succinate	Bladder dysfunction
Viagra	Sildenafil	Erectile dysfunction
Wellbutrin	Bupropion	Depression
Zanaflex	Tizanidine	Spasticity
Zoloft	Sertraline	Depression

[1]Available without a prescription.
Detailed medication information is available at www.nationalmssociety.org/meds.

Appendix C: Additional Readings

FROM DEMOS MEDICAL PUBLISHING

Banister KR. *The Personal Care Attendant Guide: The Art of Finding, Keeping, or Being One.* 2007.

Bowling A. *Alternative Medicine and Multiple Sclerosis.* 2nd ed. 2007.

Ettinger AB, Weisbrot DM. *The Essential Patient Handbook: Getting the Health Care You Need—From Doctors Who Know.* 2004.

Farrell P. *It's Not All in Your Head: Anxiety, Depression, Mood Swings and Multiple Sclerosis.* 2010.

Fishman LM, Small E. *Yoga and Multiple Sclerosis: A Journey to Health and Healing.* 2007.

Gingold JN. *Mental Sharpening Stones: Managing the Cognitive Challenges of Multiple Sclerosis.* 2008.

Gingold JN. *Facing the Cognitive Challenges of Multiple Sclerosis* 2nd ed. 2011.

Halper J. *Living with Progressive MS: Overcoming the Challenges.* 2nd ed. 2007.

Harrington C. *Barrier-Free Travel: A Nuts and Bolts Guide for Wheelers and Slow Walkers.* 2nd ed. 2005.

Harrington C. *There Is Room at the Inn: Inns and B&Bs for Wheelers and Slow Walkers.* 2006.

Holland N, Halper J. (eds.). *Multiple Sclerosis: A Self-Care Guide to Wellness.* 2nd ed. 2005.

Holland N, Murray TJ, Reingold SC. *Multiple Sclerosis: A Guide for the Newly Diagnosed.* 3rd ed. 2007.

Kalb RC. (ed.). *Multiple Sclerosis: A Guide for Families.* 3rd ed. 2006.

Karp G. *Life on Wheels: The A to Z Guide to Living Fully with Mobility Issues.* 2008.

LaRocca N, Kalb R. *Multiple Sclerosis: Understanding the Cognitive Challenges.* 2006.

Lowenstein N. *Fighting Fatigue in Multiple Sclerosis: Practical Ways to Create New Habits and Increase Your Energy.* 2009.

Murray TJ. *Multiple Sclerosis: The History of a Disease.* 2005.

Northrop D, Cooper S, Calder K. *Health Insurance Resources: A Guide for People with Chronic Disease and Disability.* 2nd ed. 2007.

Perkins L, Perkins S. *Multiple Sclerosis: Your Legal Rights.* 2nd ed. 1999.

Meyer M, Derr P. *The Comfort of Home: An Illustrated Step-by-Step Guide for Caregivers.* 2nd ed. Demos Medical Publishing, 2002.

Robitaille S. *The Illustrated Guide to Assistive Technology and Devices: Tools and Gadgets for Living Independently.* 2009.

Rogers J. *The Disabled Woman's Guide to Pregnancy and Birth.* 2006.

Rumrill P, Nissen S. *Employment Issues and Multiple Sclerosis.* 2nd ed. 2008.

Saunders C. *What Nurses Know…Multiple Sclerosis.* 2011.

Schapiro RT. *Symptom Management in Multiple Sclerosis.* 5th ed. New York: Demos Medical Publishing. 2007.

Schwarz SP. *300 Tips for Making Life with Multiple Sclerosis Easier.* 2nd ed. New York: Demos Medical Publishing, 2006.

OTHER

Alliance for Technology Access. *Computer Resources for People with Disabilities*. 4th ed. 2004. Available by calling 800-914-3015 or online at http://www.ataccess.org/

Barrett S, Jarvis WT. (eds.). *The Health Robbers: A Close Look at Quackery in America*. Buffalo, NY: Prometheus Books, 1993.

Blackstone M. *The First Year: Multiple Sclerosis: An Essential Guide for the Newly Diagnosed: A Patient Expert Walks You Through Everything You Need to Learn and Do*. New York: Marlowe and Co., 2003.

Burstein E. *Legwork: An Inspiring Journey through a Chronic Illness*. New York: Simon & Schuster, 1994.

Chapman B. *Coping with Vision Loss: Maximizing What You Can See and Do*. Alameda, CA: Hunter House (Tel: 800-265-5592; E-mail: ordering@hunterhouse.com), 2001.

Chatman L, Chatman C. *The Art of Living with Multiple Sclerosis (Six Secrets for Managing MS as a Team)*. Two- Hearts Publishing, 2006.

Cohen MD. *Dirty Details: The Days and Nights of a Well Spouse*. Philadelphia, PA: Temple University Press, 1996.

Cohen R. *Blindsided: Living a Life Above Illness: A Reluctant Memoir*. New York: HarperCollins, 2004.

Cristall B. *Coping When a Parent Has Multiple Sclerosis*. New York: Rosen Publishing (Written for teens), 1992.

Fennell PA. *The Chronic Illness Workbook*. 2nd ed. Spring Harbor Press, 2006.

Foster S, Tyler VE. *Tyler's Honest Herbal: A Sensible Guide to the Use of Herbs and Related Remedies*. 4th ed. New York: Haworth Press, 1999.

Furney K. *When the Diagnosis is Multiple Sclerosis: Help, Hope, and Insights from an Affected Physician*. Westport, CT: Praeger, 2008.

Holland N, Burks J, Schneider D. *Primary Progressive Multiple Sclerosis: What You Need to Know*. New York: Diamedica, 2010.

Garr T. *Speedbumps: Flooring It Through Hollywood*. New York: Hudson Street Press, 2005.

Iezzoni LI. *When Walking Fails*. Berkeley: University of California Press, 2003.

James JL. *One Particular Harbor: The Outrageous True Adventures of One Woman with Multiple Sclerosis Living in the Alaskan Wilderness*. Chicago, IL: Noble Press, 1993.

Kalb R, Holland N, Giesser B. *Multiple Sclerosis for Dummies*. Hoboken NJ: Wiley Publishing, 2007.

Koplowitz A, Celizic M. *The Winning Spirit: Lessons Learned in Readings Last Place*. New York: Doubleday, 1997.

Lander DL. *Fall Down Laughing: How Squiggy Caught Multiple Sclerosis and Didn't Tell Nobody*. New York: Tarcher/Putnam, 2000.

MacFarlane EB, Burstein P. *Legwork: An Inspiring Journey Through a Chronic Illness*. New York: Charles Scribner's Sons, 1994.

Mintz SG. *Love, Honor, &Value: A Family Caregiver Speaks Out About the Choices & Challenges of Caregiving*. Available on the Web site of the National Family Caregivers Association (NFCAcares.org). 2002.

Pitzele SK. *We Are Not Alone: Learning to Live with Chronic Illness*. New York: Workman, 1986.

Pitzele SK. *One More Day: Daily Meditations for the Chronically Ill*. Minneapolis, MN: Hazelden, 1988.

Price J. *Avoiding Attendants from Hell: A Practical Guide to Hiring, Firing, and Keeping Personal Care Attendants*. 2nd ed. Science & Humanities Press (Tel: 636-394-4950; E-mail: banis@banis-associates.com). 2002.

Resources for Rehabilitation. *Resources for People with Disabilities and Chronic Conditions.* 5th ed. Winchester, MA: Resources for Rehabilitation (Tel: 781-368-9094; Web: http://www.rfr.org), 2002.

Resources for Rehabilitation. *A Man's Guide to Coping with Disability.* 3rd ed. Winchester, MA: Resources for Rehabilitation (Tel: 781- 368-9094; Web: http://www.rfr.org), 2003.

Resources for Rehabilitation. *A Woman's Guide to Coping with Disability.* 4th ed. Winchester, MA: Resources for Rehabilitation (Tel: 781- 368-9094; Web: http://www.rfr.org), 2003.

Resources for Rehabilitation. *Living with Low Vision: A Resource Guide for People with Sight Loss.* 6th ed. Winchester, MA: Resources for Rehabilitation (Tel: 781-368-9094; Web: http://www.rfr.org), 2001.

Resources for Rehabilitation. *Making Wise Medical Decisions: How to Get the Information You Need.* 2nd ed. Winchester, MA: Resources for Rehabilitation (Tel: 781-368-9094; Web: http://www.rfr.org), 2001.

Resources for Rehabilitation. *Meeting the Needs of Employees with Disabilities.* 3rd ed. Winchester, MA: Resources for Rehabilitation (Tel: 781- 368-9094; Web: http://www.rfr.org), 1999.

Russell LM, Grant AE, Joseph SM, Fee RW. *Planning for the Future: Providing a Meaningful Life for a Child with a Disability After Your Death.* 2nd ed. Evanston, IL: American Publishing, 1993.

Sherkin-Langer F. *When Mommy Is Sick.* St. Louis: Fern Publications (P.O. Box 16893, St. Louis, MO 63105; Fax: 314-994-0052; Recommended for children ages 2–8), 1995.

Snyder-Grant D. *Just Like Life, Only More So: Other Stories.* Available in paperback (Booklocker.com, P.O. Box 2399, Bangor, ME 04402-2399) or as an e-book (http://www.booklocker.com/books/2544.html).

Spero D. *The Art of Getting Well: A Five-Step Plan for Maximizing Health When You Have a Chronic Illness.* Alameda, CA: Hunter House (Tel: 800-265-5592; E-mail: ordering@hunterhouse.com), 2002.

Stone K. *Awakening to Disability: Nothing About Us Without Us.* Volcano, CA: Volcano Press (P.O. Box 270, Volcano, CA 95689; Tel: 800-879-9636), 1997.

Strong M. *For the Well Spouse of the Chronically Ill.* 3rd rev. Mainstay, NY: Little Brown, 1997.

Webster B. *All of a Piece: A Life with Multiple Sclerosis.* Baltimore, MD: Johns Hopkins, 1989.

Weiner HL. *Curing MS: How Science Is Solving the Mysteries of Multiple Sclerosis.* New York: Crown Publishing, 2004.

Wells SM. *A Delicate Balance: Living Successfully with Chronic Illness.* New York: Plenum Press, 1998.

PUBLICATIONS AVAILABLE FROM THE NATIONAL MULTIPLE SCLEROSIS SOCIETY

Contact the National Multiple Sclerosis Society at 800-344-4867 or online at http://www.nationalmssociety.org/Library.

BOOKLETS

General Information
- *Choosing the Right Health-Care Provider*
- *Genetics: The Basic Facts*
- *The History of Multiple Sclerosis*

- *Research Directions in Multiple Sclerosis*
- *What Everyone Should Know About Multiple Sclerosis*
- *What Is Multiple Sclerosis?*

Information for the Newly Diagnosed
- *Diagnosis: The Basic Facts*
- *Disclosure: The Basic Facts*
- *The Disease Modifying Drugs*
- *Living with MS*
- *Putting the Brakes on MS*

Employment Issues
- *ADA and People with MS*
- *Information for Employers*
- *Should I Work? Information for Employees*
- *A Place in the Workforce*
- *Enhancing Productivity on Your Job: The Win-Win Approach*

Staying Well
- *Acupuncture and MS: The Basic Facts*
- *Clear Thinking About Alternative Therapies*
- *Dental Health: The Basic Facts*
- *Exercise as Part of Everyday Life*
- *Food for Thought: MS and Nutrition*
- *Managing MS Through Rehabilitation*
- *Multiple Sclerosis and Your Emotions*
- *MS and Intimacy*
- *Preventive Care Recommendations for Adults with MS: The Basic Facts*
- *Stretching for People with MS*
- *Stretching with a Helper for People with MS*
- *Taming Stress in Multiple Sclerosis*
- *Vitamins, Minerals, and Herbs in MS: An Introduction*

Managing Specific Issues
- *Bowel Problems: The Basic Facts*
- *Controlling Bladder Problems in Multiple Sclerosis*
- *Controlling Spasticity in MS*
- *Depression and Multiple Sclerosis*
- *Fatigue: What You Should Know*
- *Gait or Walking Problems: The Basic Facts*
- *Hormones: The Basic Facts*
- *MS and the Mind*
- *MS and Pregnancy*
- *Pain: The Basic Facts*
- *Sleep Disorders and MS: The Basic Facts*
- *Solving Cognitive Problems*
- *Speech and Swallowing: The Basic Facts*
- *Tremor: The Basic Facts*
- *Urinary Dysfunction and MS*
- *Vision Problems: The Basic Facts*

Managing Major Changes
- *A Guide for Caregivers*
- *Hiring Help at Home: The Basic Facts*

- *So You Have Progressive MS?*
- *Managing Progressive MS*
- *PLAINTALK: A Booklet about MS for Families*

For Children and Teens
- *Someone You Know Has MS: A Book for Families*
- *When a Parent Has MS: A Teenager's Guide*

Materials Available in Spanish
- *Comparación de los Medicamentos Modificadores de la Enfermedad*
- *Controlando los Problemas de la Vejiga en la Esclerosis Múltiple*
- *Debo Trabajar? Información para Empleados*
- *Diagnóstico: Hechos Básicos sobre Esclerosis Múltiple*
- *Ejercicios Prácticos de Estiramiento para las Personas con Esclerosis Múltiple*
- *Ejercicios Prácticos de Estiramiento con un Ayudante para las Personas con Esclerosis Múltiple*
- *Información para Empleadores*
- *La Fatigua: Lo Que Usted Debe Saber*
- *Lo Que Todo el Mundo Debe Saber Sobre la Esclerosis Múltiple*
- *"¡Pero si te ves tan bien!"*
- *¿ Qué es la Esclerosis Múltiple?*
- *Sobre los Problemas Sexuales Que No Mencionan los Médicos*

OTHER NATIONAL MS SOCIETY PUBLICATIONS
- *Momentum*—a quarterly magazine for people affected by MS, available in hard copy or online http://www.nationalmssociety.org/library.
- *Knowledge Is Power*—a series of articles for individuals newly diagnosed with MS available in hard copy or by email (www.nationalmssociety.org/Knowledge
- *Learn Online Programs*—available at http://www.nationalmssociety.org/MSLearnOnline

CANADIAN MULTIPLE SCLEROSIS SOCIETY PUBLICATION (TEL: 416-922-6065)
- *Coping with Fatigue in MS Takes Understanding and Planning*—Alexander Burnfield, MB, MRC Psych.

UNITED SPINAL ASSOCIATION (FORMERLY EASTERN PARALYZED VETERANS ASSOCIATION) PUBLICATIONS (TEL: 800-444-0120; WEB: HTTP://WWW.UNITEDSPINAL.ORG)
- *Disability Etiquette*—a how-to guide for interacting with someone who has a disability
- *Fire Safety for Wheelchair Users*—fire-prevention tips for private homes and suggestions on how to handle situations before and during a fire
- *Accessible Air Travel*—information for airplane travelers who have a disability
- *Adaptive Automotive Equipment*—information about adaptations for your car that can allow you to keep driving in spite of a disability
- *The Americans with Disabilities Act*—a description of the provisions of this important law

GENERAL PUBLICATIONS
- *International Journal of MS Care*—a quarterly journal published by the Consortium of Multiple Sclerosis Centers at http://www.mscare.org.

- *MS in Focus*—the flagship publication of the Multiple Sclerosis International Federation, available at no charge (http://www.msif.org/applications/people_ profiles/register.rm).
- *New Mobility*—a monthly magazine available from NewMobility.com.
- *Real Living with MS*—a monthly newsletter available from Lippincott, Williams & Wilkins (Tel: 800-638-3030).

Appendix D: Resources

A vast array of resources is available to help you meet the challenges of multiple sclerosis. This list is by no means a complete one. It is designed as a starting point in your efforts to identify the resources you need. Each resource that you investigate will lead you to others and they, in turn, will lead you to even more.

INFORMATION SOURCES

Clearinghouse on Disability Information, Communications and Information Services, Office of Special Education and Rehabilitative Services, U.S. Department of Education. http://www.ed.gov/about/offices/list/osers/codi.html. Created by the Rehabilitation Act of 1973, the Clearinghouse responds to inquiries about federal laws, services, and programs for individuals of all ages with disabilities.

Disabled Rights Advocates (DRA). http://www.dralegal.org. Nonprofit law firm dedicated to securing the civil rights of people with disabilities.

Disability Rights Education and Defense Fund, Inc. (DREDF). http://www.dredf.org. A national law and policy center dedicated to furthering the civil rights of people with disabilities. The Center provides assistance, information, and referrals on disability rights laws; legal representation in cases involving civil rights; and education/training for legislators, policy makers, and law students.

Disaboom. http://www.disaboom.com. Founded by a physician who is also quadriplegic, Disaboom stresses the power of community, advice from medical experts and also from "peers," and comprehensive solutions to the difficulties faced by the more than 100 million adults worldwide living with disabilities.

Easter Seals/March of Dimes National Council. http://www.esmodnc.org. Federation of regional and provincial groups serving individuals with disabilities throughout Canada; operates an information service and publishes a newsletter and a quarterly journal.

Job Accommodation Network (JAN). Tel: 800-526-7234; http://www.jan.wvu.edu. Offers a free consulting service designed to increase the employability of people with disabilities by providing individualized worksite accommodations solutions; technical assistance regarding the ADA and other disability-related legislation; information about self-employment options.

Medline Plus. http://www.medlineplus.gov. A service of the National Library of Medicine and the National Institutes of Health, providing health news, drug information, clinical trials listing, medical encyclopedia, medical dictionary, links to other databases and resources.

National Health Information Center. Tel: 800-336-4797; http://www.health.gov/nhic. Maintains a library and a database of health-related organizations. It also provides referrals related to health issues for consumers and professionals.

President's Committee on Employment of People with Disabilities. http://www.pcepd.gov. Publishes employment-related brochures for individuals with disabilities and their employers, and provides the Job Accommodation Network.

HELPFUL WEB SITES

Many sources of information are available free on the Internet. If you are an experienced "net surfer," switch to your favorite search engine and enter the keywords "MS" or "multiple sclerosis." This will generally give you a listing of dozens of Web sites that pertain to MS. Keep in mind, however, that the Internet is a free and open medium; while many of the Web sites have excellent and useful information, others may contain highly unusual and inaccurate information. Following is a list of some recommended MS sites available through the Web. Each of these will provide links to other sites.

Allsup. http://www.allsup.com. Assists individuals applying for Social Security disability benefits.

Avonex (interferon beta-1α). http://www.avonex.com.

Betaseron (interferon beta-1β). http://www.betaseron.com.

CenterWatch Clinical Trials Listing Service. http://www.centerwatch.com. Ongoing clinical research, including both industry- and government-sponsored trials.

CLAMS—Computer Literate Advocates for Multiple Sclerosis. www.clams.org.

Copaxone (glatiramer acetate). http://www.copaxone.com.

Emerging Therapies Collaborative. http://www.ms-coalition.org/emergingtherapies. A group including all of the organizations in the Multiple Sclerosis Coalition, the American Academy of Neurology, ACTRIMS, and the Multiple Sclerosis VA Centers of Excellence East and West, which was organized to provide organized to provide timely, evidence-based resources regarding the known benefits and risks of newly emerging, FDA-approved medications for multiple sclerosis (MS).

Extavia (interferon beta-1β). http://www.extavia.com.

Gilenya (fingolimod). http://www.gilenya.com.

International Journal of MS Care. http://www.mscare.org. Official peer-reviewed journal of the Consortium of MS Centers, International Organization of Multiple Sclerosis Nurses, International Organization of Multiple Sclerosis Rehabilitation Therapists, and Rehabilitation in Multiple Sclerosis. The journal's mission is to promote multidisciplinary cooperation and communication among MS health care professionals with the goal of maximizing the quality of life of people affected by MS.

Medicare Information. http://www.hcfa.gov/medicare/medicare.htm. Official site for information about Medicare.

Multiple Sclerosis Coalition. http://www.ms-coalition.org. A collaborative network of independent organizations (Accelerated Cure Project, Can Do MS, Consortium of MS Centers, International Organization of MS Nurses, MS Association of American, MS Foundation, National MS Society, and United Spinal) whose mission is to increase opportunities for cooperation and provide greater opportunity to leverage the effective use of resources for the benefit of the MS community.

MS Crossroads. http://www.mscrossroads.org. Comprehensive personal Web site of Aapo Halko, PhD, mathematician with MS in Finland.

Multiple Sclerosis Information Gateway. http://www.ms-gateway.com. Bayer Schering AG, Berlin, Germany. Up-to-date news on multiple sclerosis and health-related topics.

Multiple Sclerosis International Federation/The World of Multiple Sclerosis. http://www.msif.org. Established in 1967 as an international body linking the activities of national MS societies around the world. Provides independent information from MS professionals worldwide in a variety of languages.

Myelin Project. http://www.myelin.org. Established in 1989 with the aim of funding research to find a cure for demyelinating diseases.

National Institute of Neurological Disorders and Stroke (NINDS). http://www.ninds.nih.gov. Created by the U.S. Congress in 1950, NINDS is one of the more than two dozen research institutes and centers that comprise the National Institutes of Health (NIH); conducts and supports research on brain and nervous system disorders.

National Library of Medicine. http://www.nlm.nih.gov. World's largest medical library, located at the National Institutes of Health; collects materials and provides information and research services in all areas of biomedicine and health care.

National Multiple Sclerosis Society. http://www.nationalMSsociety.org. Offering comprehensive information about MS and its treatment, research, strategies to enhance health, wellness and quality of life, a multimedia library, and fundraising and social networking opportunities.

National Organization for Rare Disorders (NORD). http://www.rarediseases.org. A unique federation of voluntary health organizations dedicated to helping people with rare "orphan" diseases and assisting the organizations that serve them.

NARIC—The National Rehabilitation Information Center. http://www.naric.com. Gateway to an abundance of disability- and rehabilitation-oriented information organized in a variety of formats designed to make it easy for users to find and use.

Novantrone (mitoxantrone). http://www.novantrone.com.

Rebif (interferon beta-1α). http://www.rebif.com.

Tysabri (natalizumab). http://www.tysabri.com.

RESOURCE MATERIALS

NARIC—The National Rehabilitation Information Center. http://www.naric.com. Gateway to an abundance of disability- and rehabilitation-oriented information organized in a variety of formats designed to make it easy for users to find and use.

The Complete Directory for People with Chronic Illness (2011–2012 ed.). Grey House Publishing, Inc. Tel: 800-562-2139. http://www.greyhouse.com.

The Complete Directory for People with Disabilities (2011 ed.). Grey House Publishing, Inc. Tel: 800-562-2139. http://www.greyhouse.com.

Complete Drug Reference. (Compiled by United States Pharmacopoeia, published by Consumer Report Books). This comprehensive, readable, and easy-to-use drug reference includes almost every prescription and nonprescription medication available in the United States and Canada. A new edition is published yearly.

Complete Guide to Prescription and Nonprescription Drugs. Written by H. Winter Griffith, MD, and Stephen Moore, published by The Body Press/Perigee 2011.

Exceptional Parent Magazine. A magazine for families and professionals. EP Global Communications, 877-372-7368; http://www.eparent.com This magazine's Resource Guide, which is the largest and most widely referenced directory in the special needs field, includes 10 directories with more than 1,000 resources in the United States and Canada. The directory is useful for adults with disabilities as well.

AGENCIES AND ORGANIZATIONS

Can Do Multiple Sclerosis (formerly The Heuga Center for Multiple Sclerosis). Tel: 800-367-3101; http://www.mscando.org. An innovative provider of lifestyle empowerment programs that empower people with MS and their support partners to transform and improve their quality of life.

Canine Partners for Life (CPL). http://www.k94life.org. Trains and places assistance dogs with individuals with mobility impairments to help increase their independence and quality of life.

Consortium of Multiple Sclerosis Centers (CMSC). http://www.mscare.org. The CMSC is made up of numerous MS centers throughout the United States and Canada. The

Consortium's mission is to disseminate information to clinicians, increase resources and opportunities for research, and advance the standard of care for multiple sclerosis. The CMSC is a multidisciplinary organization, bringing together health care professionals from many fields involved in MS patient care.

Department of Veterans Affairs (VA). Tel: 800-827-1000 for VA benefits; http://www.va.gov. Provides a wide range of benefits and services to those who have served in the armed forces, their dependents, beneficiaries of deceased veterans, and dependent children of veterans with severe disabilities.

Equal Employment Opportunity Commission (EEOC). Tel: 800-669-3362 to order publications; 800-669-4000 to speak to an investigator. http://www.eeoc.gov. Responsible for monitoring the section of the ADA on employment regulations. Copies of the regulations are available.

Inglis House. Tel: 866-2-INGLIS; http://www.inglis.org. A national information exchange network specializing in long-term care facilities for people with physical disabilities.

Multiple Sclerosis Association of America (MSAA). Tel: 800-LEARN-MS; http://www.msaa.com. A national, nonprofit organization dedicated to enhancing the quality of life of those affected by multiple sclerosis. Programs such as equipment loan, support groups, and research grants are enhanced by a wide variety of educational publications.

Multiple Sclerosis Foundation (MSF). Tel: 800-888-MSFOCUS; http://www.msfocus.org. A service-based, nonprofit organization providing a comprehensive approach to helping people with MS maintain their health and well-being. Offerings include programming and support to keep people self-sufficient and their homes safe, and educational programs to heighten public awareness and understanding about the disease.

Multiple Sclerosis International Federation. http://www.msif.org. Information about MS in foreign languages. Lists contact information for MS societies around the world.

Multiple Sclerosis Society of Canada. http://www.mssociety.ca. A national organization that funds research, promotes public education, and produces publications in both English and French. They offer MS Answers—an opportunity ask questions of MS experts, read posted answers, and access articles—on a wide variety of topics including treatment, research, and social services. Regional divisions and chapters are located throughout Canada.

National Council on Disability (NCD). http://www.ncd.gov. The Council is an independent federal agency whose role is to study and make recommendations about public policy for people with disabilities. Publishes a free newsletter.

National Family Caregivers Association (NFCA). 800-896-3650; http://www.nfcacares.org. Dedicated to improving the quality of life of America's 18,000,000 caregivers. It publishes a quarterly newsletter, a resource guide, and an information clearinghouse.

National Multiple Sclerosis Society (NMSS). 800-344-4867; http://www.nationalMSsociety.org. A nonprofit organization that supports national and international research into the prevention, cure, and treatment of MS. The Society's goals include provision of nationwide services to assist people with MS and their families, and provision of information to those with MS, their families, professionals, and the public. The programs and services of the Society promote knowledge, health, and independence while providing education and emotional support.
- Toll-free access by calling 800-344-4867.
- Web site with updated information about treatments, current research, and programs (http://www.nationalMSsociety.org).
- *Knowledge Is Power*—an eight-segment, learn-at-home program (serial mailings) for people newly diagnosed with MS and their families.
- MS Learn Online—webcasts on a wide variety of topics.

- Printed materials on a variety of topics available by calling 800-344-4867 or in the Multimedia Library section of the National MS Society Web site at http://www.nationalMSsociety.org/Library.
- Educational programs on various topics throughout the year, provided through individual chapters.
- Annual national education conference, provided through individual chapters.
- Swimming and other exercise programs sponsored or cosponsored by some chapters, or referral to existing programs in the community.
- Wellness programs in some chapters.

National Park Service, U.S. Department of the Interior. http://www.nps.gov. Provides a listing of national parks and phone numbers for obtaining up-to-date accessibility information for the individual parks.

Office on the Americans with Disabilities Act. Tel: 800-514-0301. http://www.usdoj.gov/crt/ada. Responsible for enforcing the ADA; call to order copies of its regulations.

Paralyzed Veterans of America (PVA). Tel: 800-424-8200; http://www.pva.org. A national information and advocacy agency working to restore function and quality of life for veterans with spinal cord dysfunction. Supports and funds education and research and has a national advocacy program that focuses on accessibility issues. PVA publishes brochures on many issues related to rehabilitation.

Social Security Administration (SSA). Tel: 800-772-1213; http://www.ssa.gov. To apply for social security benefits based on disability, call this office or visit your local social security branch office. The Office of Disability within the Social Security Administration publishes a free brochure entitled "Social Security Regulations: Rules for Determining Disability and Blindness." (Note: Helpful booklets for people with MS and clinicians about obtaining Social Security at the NMSS Web site at: http://www.nationalMSsociety.org/SSDI.)

Through the Looking Glass: National Research and Training Center on Families of Adults with Disabilities. http://www.lookingglass.org. A community-based, nonprofit organization that has pioneered research, training, and services for families in which a child, parent, or grandparent has a disability or medical issue.

United Spinal Association (formerly Eastern Paralyzed Veterans Association) http://www.unitedspinal.org. A private, nonprofit organization dedicated to serving the needs of its members as well as other people with disabilities. While offering a wide range of benefits to member veterans with spinal cord dysfunction (including hospital liaison, sports and recreation, wheelchair repair, adaptive architectural consultations, research and educational services, communications, and library and information services), they also provide brochures and information on a variety of subjects, free of charge to the general public.

Well Spouse Foundation. http://www.wellspouse.org. A national, nonprofit emotional support network for people married to or living with a chronically ill partner. Advocacy for home health and long-term care and a quarterly newsletter, *Mainstay*, are among the services offered.

ASSISTIVE TECHNOLOGY

Access to Recreation: Adaptive Recreation Equipment for the Physically Challenged. Tel: 800-634-4351; http://www.accesstr.com. Products include exercise equipment and assistive devices for sports, environmental access, games, crafts, and hobbies.

Adaptive Parenting: Idea Book I (Through the Looking Glass). Tel: 800-644-2666.

American Medical Alert. Tel: 800-286-2622; http://www.amacalert.com. Personal emergency response system that links a person living alone with a 24-hour emergency response center, as well as other services.

Apple Computer Disability Resources. http://www.apple.com/accessibility.

Disabled Online. http://www.disabledonline.com. Offers a wide variety of resources for people with disabilities.

IBM Accessibility Center. http://www.ibm.com/able.

Lifeline Systems, Inc. 800-543-3546; Web: http://www.lifelinesys.com. Personal emergency response system that links a person living alone with a 24-hour emergency response center, as well as other services.

Life Enhancement Technologies, LLC. Tel: 800-779-6953; http://www.2bcool.com. Manufactures a variety of cooling suits that can be used in management of heat-related symptoms in MS.

Medic Alert Foundation International. Tel: 888-633-4298; http://www.medicalert.org. A medical identification tag worn to identify a person's medical condition, medications, and any other important information that might be needed in case of an emergency. A file of the person's health data is maintained in a central database to be accessed by a physician or other emergency personnel who need to know the person's pertinent medical information.

Microsoft Accessibility Technology for Everyone. http://www.microsoft.com/enable.

National Rehabilitation Information Center (NARIC). Tel: 800-346-2742; http://www.naric.com. A library and information center on disability and rehabilitation, funded by the National Institute on Disability and Rehabilitation Research (NIDRR). NARIC operates two databases— ABLEDATA and REHABDATA. NARIC collects and disseminates the results of federally funded research projects and has a collection that includes commercially published books, journal articles, and audiovisual materials. NARIC is committed to serving both professionals and consumers who are interested in disability and rehabilitation. Information specialists can answer simple information requests and provide referrals immediately and at no cost. More complex database searches are available at nominal cost.

- ABLEDATA. Tel: 800-227-0216; http://www.abledata.com. A national database of information on assistive technology designed to enable persons with disabilities to identify and locate the devices that will assist them in their home, work, and leisure activities. Information specialists are available to answer questions during regular business hours. ABLE INFORM BBS is available 24 hours a day to customers with a computer, modem, and telecommunications software.
- REHABDATA. Tel: 800-346-2742; http://www.naric.com/research/rehab. A database containing bibliographic records with abstracts and summaries of the materials contained in the NARIC (National Rehabilitation Information Center) library of disability rehabilitation materials. Information specialists are available to conduct a database search on any rehabilitation-related topic.

Parents with Disabilities On-line. http://www.disabledparents.net. Products and solutions for making independent parenting more possible for people with disabilities.

RESNA: Rehabilitation, Engineering, and Assistive Technology Society of North America http://www.resna.org. An international association for the advancement of rehabilitation technology. Their objectives are to improve the quality of life for the disabled through the application of science and technology and to influence policy relating to the delivery of technology to disabled persons. They will respond by mail to specific questions about modifying existing equipment and designing new devices.

ENVIRONMENTAL ADAPTATIONS

A Consumer's Guide to Home Adaptation (Adaptive Environments Center). http://www. adaptenv.org. A workbook for planning adaptive home modifications such as lowering kitchen countertops and widening doorways.

American Institute of Architects (AIA). Tel: 800-242-3837; http://www.aia.org. Provides referrals to architects who are familiar with the design requirements of people with disabilities.

Financing Home Accessibility Modifications. http://www.design.ncsu.edu/cud. Identifies state and local sources of financial assistance for homeowners (or tenants) who need to make modifications in their homes.

GE Answer Center. Tel: 800-626-2005; http://www.geappliances.com. Open 24 hours a day, 6 days a week, the Center offers assistance to individuals with disabilities as well as the general public. They offer two free brochures, "Appliance Help for Those with Special Needs" and "Basic Kitchen Planning for the Physically Handicapped."

Institute for Human Centered Design. http://www.adaptiveenvironments.org. Offers workbooks for planning adaptive home modifications such as lowering kitchen countertops and widening doorways.

National Association of Home Builders (NAHB). Tel: 800-368-5242; http://www.nahb. com. Produces publications and provides training on housing and special needs. A publication entitled "Homes for a Lifetime" includes an accessibility checklist, financing options, and recommendations for working with builders and remodelers.

National Kitchen and Bath Association. Tel: 800-843-6522; http://www.nkba.org. Produces a technical manual of barrier-free planning and has directories of certified designers and planners.

TRAVEL

Accessible Journeys. Tel: 800-846-4537; http://www.disabilitytravel.com. Arranges travel for mobility-impaired travelers, and is affiliated with a network of offices in nine European countries.

Directory of Travel Agencies for the Disabled (Written by Helen Hecker, published by Twin Peaks Press). http://www.twinpeakspress.com. Lists travel agents who specialize in arranging travel plans for people with disabilities.

The Disability Bookshop. http://www.astore.amazon.com/disabilitybookshop-newtravel-20. A shop-by-mail bookstore with an extensive list of books for disabled travelers, dealing with such topics as accessibility, travel agencies, accessible van rentals, medical resources, air travel, and guides to national parks.

Information for Handicapped Travelers (available free of charge from the National Library Service for the Blind and Physically Handicapped). Tel: 800-424-8567; http://www. loc.gov/nls/. A booklet providing information about travel agents, transportation, and information centers for individuals with disabilities.

International Association for Medical Assistance to Travelers (IAMAT). http://www.iamat. org. A nonprofit organization that advises travelers about health risks and immunization requirements for all countries, and provides referrals to English-speaking, Western-trained doctors around the world.

Society for Accessible Travel and Hospitality (SATH). http://www.sath.org. A nonprofit organization that acts as a clearinghouse for accessible tourism information and is in contact with organizations in many countries to promote the development of facilities for disabled people. SATH publishes a quarterly magazine, *Access to Travel*.

Travel for the Disabled: A Handbook of Travel Resources and 500 Worldwide Access Guides.
(Written by Helen Hecker, published by Twin Peaks Press). http://www.twinpeakspress.
com. The handbook provides information for disabled travelers about accessibility.

Travel Information Service (Moss Rehabilitation Hospital). http://www.mossresourcenet.
org/travel.htm. Provides information and referrals for people with disabilities.

Travelin' Talk. http://www.travelintalk.net. An international network of people and organizations around the world who are willing to provide assistance to travelers with disabilities and share their knowledge about the areas in which they live. Travelin' Talk
publishes a newsletter by the same name and has an extensive resource directory.

Wilderness Inquiry. Tel: 800-728-0719; http://www.wildernessinquiry.org. Sponsors trips
into the wilderness for people with disabilities or chronic conditions.

VISUAL IMPAIRMENT

Canadian National Institute for the Blind (CNIB). Tel: 800-563-2642; http://www.cnib.
ca. Provides counseling and rehabilitation services for Canadians with any degree of
functional visual impairment; offers information, literature, and operates resource and
technology centers. The national office has a list of provincial and local CNIB offices.

Lighthouse International Tel: 800-829-0500; TTY: 212-821-9713; http://www.lighthouse.
org. Product catalog offers a wide variety of products for individuals with low vision.

The Library of Congress, Division for the Blind and Physically Handicapped. Tel: 888-
NLS-READ; http://www.loc.gov/nls/. The Library Service provides free talking book
equipment on loan as well as a full range of recorded books for individuals with disabilities or visual impairment. It also provides a variety of free library services through
140 cooperating libraries.

**PUBLISHING COMPANIES SPECIALIZING IN HEALTH AND
RESOURCES DISABILITY ISSUES**

Demos Health. Tel: 800-532-8663; http://www.demoshealth.com.

Grey House Publishing. Tel: 800-562-2139; http://www.greyhouse.com.

Resources for Rehabilitation. Tel: 781-368-9080; http://www.rfr.org.

Woodbine House. Tel: 800-843-7323; http://www.woodbinehouse.com.

Index

Note: Page references followed by "*f*" and "*t*" denote figures and tables, respectively.